Dynamics
of Human
Biologic Tissues

Contemporary Perspectives in Rehabilitation

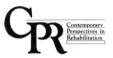

Steven L. Wolf, Ph.D., FAPTA
Editor-in-Chief

PUBLISHED VOLUMES

The Biomechanics of the Foot and Ankle
Robert Donatelli, M.A., P.T.

Pharmacology in Rehabilitation
Charles D. Ciccone, Ph.D., P.T.

Wound Healing: Alternatives in Management
Luther C. Kloth, M.S., P.T., Joseph M. McCulloch, Ph.D., P.T.
and Jeffrey A. Feedar, B.S., P.T.

Thermal Agents in Rehabilitation, 2nd Edition
Susan L. Michlovitz, M.S., P.T.

Electrotherapy in Rehabilitation
Meryl R. Gersh, M.S., P.T.

Concepts in Hand Rehabilitation
Barbara G. Stanley, B.S., P.T. and Susan M. Tribuzi, B.S., O.T.R.

Cardiopulmonary Rehabilitation: Basic Theory and Application,
2nd Edition
Frances J. Brannon, Ph.D., Julie Starr, M.S., P.T., Margaret Wiley Foley,
M.S.N., and Mary J. Geyer Black, M.S., P.T.

Dynamics of Human Biologic Tissues

Dean P. Currier, Ph.D., P.T.
Professor
Division of Physical Therapy
University of Kentucky
Lexington, Kentucky

Roger M. Nelson, Ph.D., P.T.
Professor and Chairman
Department of Physical Therapy
Thomas Jefferson University
Philadelphia, Pennsylvania

 F. A. DAVIS COMPANY • Philadelphia

Printed in the United States of America

Last digit indicates print number: 10 9 8 7 6 5 4 3 2 1

acquisitions editor: Jean-François Vilain
developmental editor: Ralph Zickgraf
production editor: Crystal S. McNichol

As new scientific information becomes available through basic and clinical research, recommended treatments and drug therapies undergo changes. The author(s) and publisher have done everything possible to make this book accurate, up to date, and in accord with accepted standards at the time of publication. The authors, editors, and publisher are not responsible for errors or omissions or for consequences from application of the book and make no warranty, expressed or implied, in regard to the contents of the book. Any practice described in this book should be applied by the reader in accordance with professional standards of care used in regard to the unique circumstances that may apply in each situation. The reader is advised always to check product information (package inserts) for changes and new information regarding dose and contraindications before administering any drug. Caution is especially urged when using new or infrequently ordered drugs.

Library of Congress Cataloging-in-Publication Data

Dynamics of human biologic tissues/edited by Dean P. Currier and
  Roger M. Nelson.
    p.   cm.—(Contemporary perspectives in rehabilitation; v. 8)
  Includes bibliographical references and index.
  ISBN 0-8036-2298-8 (hardback:alk. paper)
  1. Physical therapy. 2. Electric stimulation. 3. Human
mechanics. I. Currier, Dean P. II. Nelson, Roger M. III. Series.
  [DNLM: 1. Connective Tissue—physiology. 2. Electric Stimulation—
method. 3. Muscles—physiology. 4. Nerve Tissue—physiology.
5. Physical Therapy—methods. W1 C0769NS v. 8/WB 460 D997]
RM700.D86 1992
615.8'2—dc20
DNLM/DLC
for Library of Congress   92-10278
                                                        CIP

Foreword

That physical therapy practice is progressing from an art to a science is now beyond dispute. In August 1991, the Section on Research of the American Physical Therapy Association, with support from its parent organization, sponsored a conference/retreat in New Hampshire to evaluate and discuss muscle function. By that time this book was in the final stages of manuscript review. Several of the participants in that conference are also contributors to this text.

The organizers of the Muscle Function Conference recognized the need to reassess the scientific foundations of our treatment procedures to facilitate strength changes or control of movement. Toward this end, it was necessary to examine, from multiple perspectives, the existing body of knowledge pertinent to muscle architecture and control over its activation. This text is designed not only to provide such an examination but to explore the morphology and function of those biologic tissues that form the cornerstone of physical therapy practice. These tissues include the muscle itself as well as connective tissue surrounding muscle, the tendons forming points of muscle attachment, the articular cartilage about which muscle contracts, and the nerves that activate muscle. In this context it seemed reasonable for Dean P. Currier and Roger M. Nelson also to recruit contributions from knowledgeable physical therapist researchers on such issues as muscle fatigue, muscle responses to electrical stimulation, and the effects that such stimulation may have on muscle activation patterns or on supportive structures.

We believe that this collective work represents the most sophisticated and comprehensive presentation on muscle, tendon, and connective tissue ever written by physical therapists for students or clinicians in the health-related professions. The detailed references and analytical use of supporting information are totally compatible with the development of a scientific understanding of biologic tissue. It is only against such a background that we can hope to render explanations for how our peripheral anatomic structures respond to therapeutic interventions.

Larry J. Tillman and Gordon S. Cummings provide a comprehensive presentation of connective tissue and the degree of mutability and remodeling that these dynamic structures can achieve. With this knowledge base, the reader is better able to appreciate their discussions of the effects of shortening, immobilization, or overuse on muscle or tendon length changes and of the mechanism(s) by which thermal agents change connective tissue properties. The Tillman and Cummings chapters are logical precursors to Gary L. Soderberg's excellent review of skeletal muscle function. Soderberg offers a comprehensive picture of muscle anatomy and mechanics and the clinical consequences of immobilization or elongation. The discussion is adequately complimented by contemporary references and suggestions for how the information fits within the physical therapist's treatment approach.

Stuart A. Binder-Macleod shows why he is one of our premier thinkers and innovators as he presents a very comprehensive treatise on force-frequency responses of muscle to electrical stimulation. He demonstrates the importance of recognizing, and ultimately resolving, the relationship of stimulation rate and frequency (or, if you will, pattern) to optimal muscle responsiveness with minimal fatigue. As the role of electrical stimulation for muscle strengthening or functional participation in movement acquires greater significance in treatment regimens, the importance of force-frequency relationships will become more apparent to the student or clinical provider of electrical stimulation modalities.

Under any circumstance, electrical stimulation of muscle can yield profound changes in cytoarchitecture. David G. Greathouse and Daniel H. Matulionis offer a detailed description of muscle responses to stimulation from different generators or wave forms and the implication of such changes to restoration of function in patients with orthopedic or sports-related injuries. It is also logical to conclude that repeated electrical stimulation will induce vascular responses, some of which may be undesirable. Brian V. Reed's discussion of this issue includes a review of the effect of neuromuscular stimulation on wound healing. He also provides treatment protocols and rationales for their administration.

Fatigue is an important corollary of both volitional contractions and those induced by electrical stimulation. Carl G. Kukulka offers a detailed chapter on the interaction between muscle activity and the central and peripheral factors contributing to fatigue. The chapter by Elizabeth R. Gardner and Lucinda L. Baker will impress students and clinicians wishing for a clinical example of the use of functional electrical stimulation. These clinician/researchers have an impeccable reputation as masters at applying stimulation to spinal-cord-injured patients. Their presentation offers guidelines and training techniques that relate stimulation characteristics to optimal clinical response.

Nerve, articular cartilage, and tendon are three tissues capable of responding to electrical stimulation or other factors. Arthur J. Nitz reminds us of how the structure of peripheral nerve can be compromised through pressure and details the variables that determine how long regeneration will take. He ends his well-documented presentation with a clinical example that challenges the reader's reasoning skills. Chukuka S. Enwemeka and Neil I. Spielholz provide detailed information on how damaged tendon can be reconfigured in the healing process and the role that electrical stimulation may play in this process. Last, A. Joseph Threlkeld reviews the pathogenesis and remodeling capabilities of articular cartilage and offers original data on the effects of electrical stimulation in transforming damaged cartilage.

For students and clinicians alike, the detailed thought and references behind each contribution herald the age of a new, thought-provoking mode in which we are taught to comprehend the anatomy, pathology, and mutability of the very tissues that we wish to aid in the rehabilitation process. Our collective goal is to give you, the reader, a visual appreciation of the very tissues underlying your touch or the application of your modality of choice. Through this effort, we wish to provide a thorough, scientifically supported justification for treatment.

Steven L. Wolf, Ph.D., FAPTA
Series Editor
Contemporary Perspectives in Rehabilitation

Preface

Much of the published research in muscle, nerve, and connective tissue is fragmented and isolated, appearing in varied journals as individual articles. This volume brings together the important information and presents the concepts in a meaningful and collective manner. The purpose of this book is to present an overview of the salient normal and mutable features of muscle, nerve, and connective tissue elements as they relate to the theory and practice of physical therapy. The contributors are well known for their area of presentation, and several offer aspects of their personal research and clinical experience in the coverage of their topic. They take a unique, scholarly approach in examining the various subject areas.

Chapters 1 and 2 introduce fundamentals of the biologic and remodeling aspects of connective tissue. This survey sets the stage for Chapter 3, on the architectural and physiologic concerns that underlie patient exercise and Chapter 10, which offers new information on collagen activity in tendon regeneration by electrical stimulation. Electrical stimulation is the central theme of the remaining chapters. Chapter 4 offers a new approach to force production by muscle contractions induced by electrical stimulation. Chapters 5 and 7 provide insight into the effects of electrical stimulation on ultrastructural changes and fatigue effects on muscle, respectively. Chapter 6 synopsizes the scattered and often contradictory literature on the effect of electrical stimulation on blood flow; the chapter also presents the results of up-to-date research. Chapter 8 reviews the results of recent research on the use of functional electrical stimulation in rehabilitation of paralytic muscle. Pressure injuries and pressure effects on peripheral nerve function are discussed in Chapter 9. The final chapter introduces electromagnetic stimulation as an approach to influencing growth of injured cartilage.

All physical therapists who have studied the theory of electrical stimulation should find this information helpful in enriching their understanding of excitable and connective tissue. In particular, clinicians, clinical researchers, and academics with interest in excitable and connective tissue advances should find this book of value.

Dean P. Currier
Roger M. Nelson

Contributors

LUCINDA L. BAKER, Ph.D., P.T.

Associate Professor
Department of Biokinesiology and Physical Therapy
University of Southern California
Los Angeles, California

STUART A. BINDER-MACLEOD, Ph.D., P.T.

Assistant Professor
School of Life and Health Sciences
Program in Physical Therapy
University of Delaware
Newark, Delaware

GORDON S. CUMMINGS, M.A., P.T.

Associate Professor
Department of Physical Therapy
Georgia State University
Atlanta, Georgia

CHUKUKA S. ENWEMEKA, Ph.D., P.T., FACSM

Associate Professor
Division of Physical Therapy
Department of Orthopaedics and Rehabilitation
University of Miami School of Medicine
Coral Gables, Florida

ELIZABETH R. GARDNER, M.S., P.T.

Senior Research Therapist
Functional Neuromuscular Stimulation Department
Shriners Hospital—Philadelphia Unit
Philadelphia, Pennsylvania

DAVID G. GREATHOUSE, Ph.D., P.T.

Chief, Physical Therapist Section
Office of the Surgeon General
Falls Church, Virginia

CARL G. KUKULKA, Ph.D., P.T.

Associate Professor
Physical Therapy Graduate Program
The University of Iowa
Iowa City, Iowa

DANIEL H. MATULIONIS, Ph.D.

Associate Professor
Department of Anatomy
University of Kentucky
Lexington, Kentucky

ARTHUR J. NITZ, Ph.D., P.T.

Associate Professor of Physical Therapy
Department of Clinical Sciences
University of Kentucky
Lexington, Kentucky

BRIAN V. REED, Ph.D., P.T.

Associate Professor
Department of Physical Therapy
University of Vermont
Burlington, Vermont

GARY L. SODERBERG, Ph.D., P.T., FAPTA

Professor and Director
Physical Therapy Graduate Program
The University of Iowa
Iowa City, Iowa

NEIL I. SPIELHOLZ, Ph.D., P.T.

Associate Professor
Division of Physical Therapy
Department of Orthopaedics and Rehabilitation
University of Miami School of Medicine
Coral Gables, Florida

Formerly with the Department of Rehabilitation Medicine
New York University Medical Center
New York, New York

A. JOSEPH THRELKELD, Ph.D., P.T.

Associate Professor of Physical Therapy
Assistant Professor of Biomedical Engineering
University of Kentucky
Lexington, Kentucky

LARRY J. TILLMAN, Ph.D.

Associate Professor
Department of Physical Therapy
The University of Tennessee at Chattanooga
Chattanooga, Tennessee

Contents

Biologic Mechanisms of Connective Tissue Mutability

Larry J. Tillman, Ph.D.
Gordon S. Cummings, M.A., P.T.

Understanding the biologic and mechanical nature of tendons, ligaments, and capsules provides insights that are important to the prevention and management of injuries to these structures. This chapter describes the structural, physiologic, and histopathologic considerations of these dense, regular connective tissues. The purpose of this chapter is to review the biologic mechanisms of connective tissue mutability so that subsequent chapters addressing dense connective tissues will be better understood.

PHYSICAL PROPERTIES OF COLLAGEN

Dense, regular connective tissues consist of a complex of cells, ground substances, and fibers. The fibers include collagen, elastin, and reticulum. The mechanical behavior of these tissues is influenced by the

1. Physical properties of collagen and other fibers
2. Architectural arrangement or weave of the fibers
3. Size of collagen fibers
4. Proportion of collagen and other fibers
5. Maturity of the collagen fibers
6. Composition and hydration of the ground substance

Prior to discussing the mechanical response of collagen fibers to stress, an understanding of its basic building block, the *tropocollagen* molecule, is essential. The tropocollagen molecule is manufactured in the rough endoplasmic reticulum (ER) of connective tissue fibroblasts. In the ER organelle, amino acids are assembled in repeating sequences into long polypeptide chains. Every third residue is glycine. These chains are of uniform length. For demonstration purposes, this chain can be visualized in three dimensions, with the branches of each amino acid extending at uniform angles and distances from the axis of the chain. The branches have radicals on their terminals through which various hydrophobic, hydrophilic, and covalent interactions have the potential to attract and form chemical bonds with compatible radicals of other molecules. In the ER, three polypeptide chains become attached together in a triple helix, initially forming the *procollagen* molecule. Because of the three-dimensional shape of each chain and the relative placement of radicals that can react with each other, the chains fit together in predetermined configurations like pieces of a puzzle. Procollagen molecules are synthesized into uniform molecules with fixed dimensions of length and width. All of the atoms of the entire unit are fixed in their relation with the other atoms through a latticework of chemical bonding.

Native procollagen, therefore, is an organic crystal. The procollagen molecule is transported to the cell membrane and extruded into the interstitial space. End components of the molecule are then removed, and the slightly shortened molecule is now called *tropocollagen* (Fig. 1–1). With no changes in the internal formation of the molecule, tropocollagen remains an organic crystal. These identical tropocollagen molecules are of fixed dimensions. Attached to this crystalline molecule are small amorphous portions, thought to be the component that attaches adjacent molecules as they aggregate.

The tropocollagen crystal is the building block of collagen microfibrils. For the purpose of illustration, we can visualize the tropocollagen molecules as a set of LEGO building blocks, all of the same dimensions, and flexible so curves can be made. These blocks can only aggregate by attaching where the corresponding knobs and holes fit. The block design predetermines the types of configuration that can be built. The knobs and holes of the LEGO blocks correspond to the attachment sites on the branches of the polypeptide chains of the tropocollagen molecule. When the tropocollagen molecules are secreted into the intercellular space, they are attracted to each other and rapidly aggregate into microfibrils (Fig. 1–2). In the smallest unit of fiber

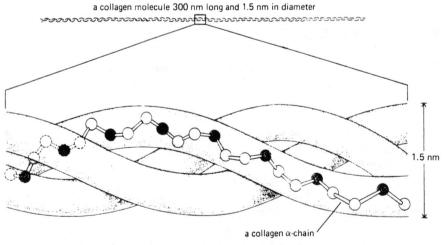

a collagen molecule 300 nm long and 1.5 nm in diameter

1.5 nm

a collagen α-chain

FIGURE 1–1. Type I collagen molecule. Tropocollagen triple helix composed of two α-1 and one α-2 (drawn) peptide chains, typically found in skin, tendon, bone, and ligaments. Every third residue in each α-chain is glycine. (From Alberts et al.,[68] p. 694, with permission.)

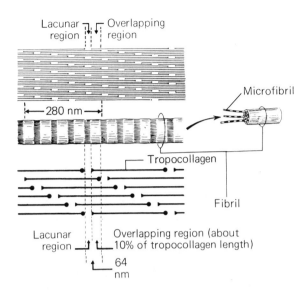

FIGURE 1–2. Formation of collagen microfibrils. Under the electron microscope, the fibrils show periodicity of dark and light bands. This 64-nm periodicity is explained by the overlapping arrangement of rodlike tropocollagen subunits, each measuring 280 nm. (From Junqueira et al.,[69] p. 97, with permission.)

organization, five tropocollagen molecules are packed together to form a highly ordered microfibril. In the microfibril, each tropocollagen molecule is staggered along its length in relation to its neighbors. The spatial relationship of the molecules in the microfibril is consistent enough, with a fixed diameter of 35 Å (3.5 nm), to be called a "crystallite."[1]

The next larger unit of organization is the subfibril (10–20 nm). Subfibrils combine

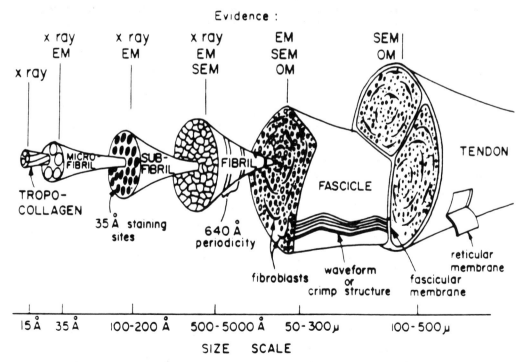

FIGURE 1–3. Hierarchial organization of tendon. (From Kastelic, J, Galeski, A, and Baer, E: The multicomposite structure of tendon. Connect Tissue Res 6:21, 1978, with permission.)

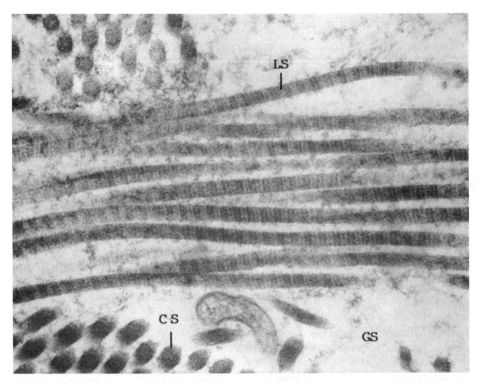

FIGURE 1–4.   Electron micrograph of human collagen fibrils in cross section (cs) and longitudinal section (ls). Each fibril consists of regularly alternating dark and light bands, which are further divided by cross sections. Amorphous ground substance (gs) completely surrounds the fibrils (magnification × 100,000). (From Junqueira et al.,[69] p. 98, with permission.)

to form fibrils, with diameters between 50 and 500 nm, that exhibit the characteristic bands seen in x-ray diffraction and electron microscopic studies (Figs. 1–3 and 1–4). These bands are thought to represent the stacking or organized packing of the tropocollagen molecules within the larger units. This stacking reflects the highly structured molecular organization throughout the hierarchy of components that form the structural fibers of tendons, capsules, and ligaments.[2]

To summarize, tropocollagen, a pure crystalline structure, is the building block of collagen. All higher levels of organization are arranged in predetermined relations and dimensions. This concept is important because the physical properties of collagen are directly governed by this ordered structure.

Polypeptide chains that aggregate to form procollagen molecules are of more than one type, each of which is capable of aggregating into different forms of collagen. One type A chain and two type B chains will produce one variety of collagen, whereas two type A chains and one type B chain will produce a second type. Currently, five classes of collagen have been identified, types I, II, III, IV, and V,[3] each of which has subclasses (Table 1–1). The larger structural, interstitial fibers of tendon and ligament contain mostly type I collagen, and in smaller quantities type II collagen.

TABLE 1–1 Main Characteristics of the Different Types of Collagen

Collagen Type	Molecular Formula	Tissue Distribution	Optical Microscopy	Ultrastructure	Site of Synthesis	Interaction with Glycosaminoglycans	Function
I	$[a1(I)]_2a2(I)$	Dermis, bone, tendon, dentin, fascias, sclera, organ capsules, fibrous cartilage.	Closely packed, thick, nonargyrophilic, strongly birefringent yellow or red fibers. Collagen fibers.	Densely packed, thick fibrils with marked variation in diameter.	Fibroblast, osteoblast, odontoblast, chondroblast.	Low level of interaction, mainly with dermatan sulfate.	Resistance to tension.
II	$[a1(II)]_3$	Hyaline and elastic cartilages.	Loose, collagenous network visible only with picro-Sirius stain and polarization microscopy.	No fibers; very thin fibrils embedded in abundant ground substance.	Chrondroblast.	High level of interaction, mainly with chondroitin sulfates.	Resistance to intermittent pressure.
III	$[a1(III)]_3$	Smooth muscle, endoneurium, arteries, uterus, liver, spleen, kidney, lung.	Loose network of thin, argyrophilic, weakly birefringent greenish fibers. Reticular fibers.	Loosely packed thin fibrils with more uniform diameters.	Smooth muscle, fibroblast, reticular cells, Schwann cells, hepatocyte.	Intermediate level of interaction, mainly with heparan sulfate.	Structural maintenance in expansible organs.
IV	$[proa1(IV)]_2proa2(IV)$	Epithelial and endothelial basal laminae and basement membranes.	Thin, amorphous, weakly birefringent membrane.	Neither fibers nor fibrils are detected.	Endothelial and epithelial cells, muscle cells, and Schwann cells.	Interacts with heparan sulfate.	Support and filtration.
V	$[a1(V)]_2a2(V)$	Placental basement membranes.	Insufficient data.	Insufficient data.	Insufficient data.	Insufficient data.	Insufficient data.

Source: From Junqueira et al.,[69] with permission.

Composition of Ground Substance

Ground substance is a mixture of water and different types of organic molecules, chiefly glycosaminoglycans (GAGs), proteoglycans, and glycoproteins. Ground substance constitutes only 1 percent of the dry weight of tendon, yet it contributes greatly to the strength of connective tissues. Seven types of GAGs, previously known as acid mucopolysaccharides, have been identified. In most tissues, GAGs are chiefly found linked to long protein or hyaluronic acid cores, as components of proteoglycans. Each type of connective tissue has characteristic GAGs present in various proportions. Also present are glycoproteins, which contain a protein portion to which carbohydrates attach. Glycoproteins, such as fibronectin and laminin, have been shown to play an important role in the interaction between adjacent connective tissue cells and in the adhesion of these cells to collagen.[4]

One of the chief characteristics of ground substance is that it is strongly hydrophilic. Hyaluronic acid, for example, takes up a hydrodynamic volume 1000 times the space occupied by the chain itself. Water constitutes 96 percent of the wet weight of normal tendon, much of it being held by the GAGs. Water held in the connective tissue is important for diffusion of molecules through the tissue, including carrying of nutrients to the connective tissue cells and export of metabolites. Water and GAGs provide space between adjacent fibers, thus reducing friction and increasing ductility of tissue.[5,6]

Glycosaminoglycans were previously thought to be an amorphous gel that lay between collagen and other structural fibers in the matrix. Recent work has indicated that in addition to forming part of the unstructured gel, GAGs form important attachments to the collagen fibers, contributing to its aggregation and strength. When collagen fibers of 200 nm length were exposed to the enzyme hyaluronidase, there was critical loss of strength and elasticity of the fiber, leading to the conclusion that hyaluronic acid may be responsible for cohesion within the fibril.[2] Myers and colleagues showed by collagen contraction studies in salt solutions that ground substance and collagen interact by chemical bonding.[7]

Whenever a connective tissue is subjected to elongation forces during formation, collagen is formed with distinct waveforms *(crimps)* in 50- to 300-μm fascicles (Fig. 1–3), which are thought to be due to attachments of GAGs to the collagen.[2,8,9] The combined effect of water and GAGs on tendon extensibility is dramatically illustrated in Figure 1–5. Wet tendon easily elongated in response to increased loading, whereas dry tendon lost all compliance. Solubility studies indicated that when a tendon is dried, a covalently linked three-dimensional network is formed, presumably between the GAGs, but no other chemical or structural changes were noted. When one considers that the GAGs constitute only 1 percent of the weight of dry tendon, it is apparent that all of the changes seen cannot be attributed only to covalent bonding. The mechanical effects of the water-gel complex on the mechanical behavior of the collagen in response to tension should be considered as well.

Progressive Changes in Bonding—Aging and Maturation

Tropocollagen molecules are initially attracted to each other by a combination of hydrophobic, hydrophilic, hydrogen, and covalent interactions. Once the tropocollagen molecules are aggregated into microfibrils, gradual and progressive changes

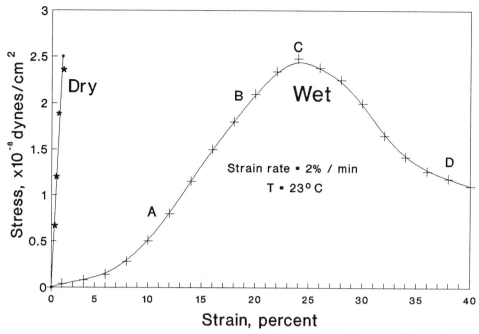

FIGURE 1–5. Stress-strain curve of wet and dehydrated rat tail tendon fibers. Note the loss of compliance in the dry tendon. (From Yannas, IV and Huang, C: Fracture of tendon collagen. J Polymer Sci 10:581, 1972. New York, John Wiley & Sons, Inc. Copyright 1972. Reprinted with permission.)

occur in the intermolecular and intramolecular bonding. These changes include the conversion of unstable hydrogen bonding to stable covalent bonding, as well as the formation of new attachments provided by the molecules of the ground substance and reticular fibers that interact with the collagen. These interactions result in increased chemical and mechanical stability of the structure.

The biologic age of collagen has been determined by tests of swelling, fatigue, solubility, and thermal denaturation. The process of increasing stability of collagen is referred to, rather inconsistently, as both aging and maturation. Maturation generally refers to changes seen in an animal between birth and sexual maturity; aging refers to changes in an animal after sexual maturity is reached. Figure 1–6 shows how rat tail tendon becomes progressively more rigid and strong due to these changes from youth through maturity. As an animal matures from 1.7 to 37 months, increased stress is required to produce a similar amount of elongation.

The same process of progressive stabilization of bonding occurs in the fibers of newly synthesized connective tissue in adult animals. The length of the crimp increases with age in rats, and newly formed scar tissue forms with a similar crimp length in the tails of rats.[2] Figure 1–7 demonstrates the progressive increase in strength of newly formed scar tissue in adult rats. The increase in strength seen in this figure could be due to any combination of three factors: alignment of more collagen fibers along stress lines, increased size of those fibers, and increased strength of the bonding. Solubility and chemical analysis studies clearly show that increasing density and stability of bonding is present as one of the factors.[11] This process is also found in artificially reconstituted collagen ribbons, demonstrating that it is in large measure a

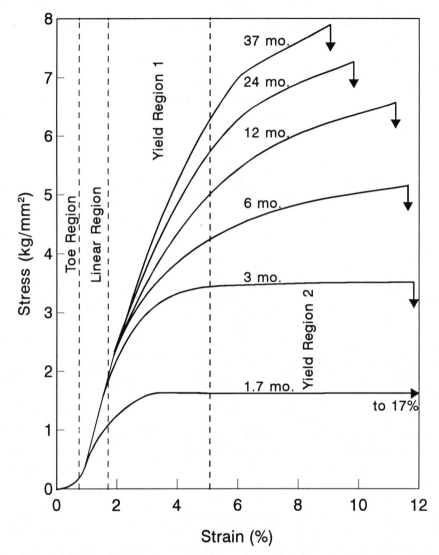

FIGURE 1–6.   Stress-strain behavior as a function of age. (From Betsch, DF and Baer, E: Structure and mechanical properties of rat tail tendon. Biorheology 17. Copyright 1980, Pergamon Press, Inc.)

physical-chemical property of the bonding and not secondary to the aging of the animal.[12]

     Stress as a physical stimulus is a significant factor in the formation and maintenance of collagen in dense connective tissue. Woo and associates[13] showed that increasing stress levels caused an increase in collagen in tendon and ligaments and that deprivation of stress caused weakening of the connective tissue. Enwemeka[14] showed that 4 weeks of immobilization of rabbit soleus tendon, in the absence of trauma, caused marked disorganization of collagen fibers in the tendon.

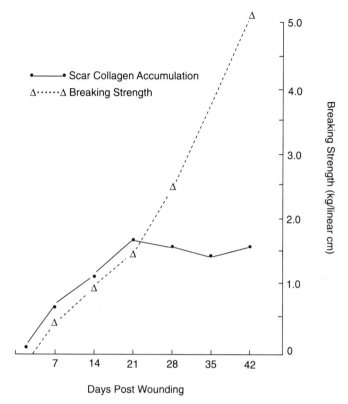

FIGURE 1–7. Comparison of scar collagen accumulation *(solid line)* and breaking strength *(dotted line)* of wounds. (From Madden, JW and Peacock, EE: Studies on the biology of collagen during wound healing: III. Dynamics metabolism of scar collagen and remodeling of dermal wounds. Ann Surg 174:511–520, 1971, with permission.)

Response of Collagen to Mechanical Elongation

A common method to study the mechanical behavior of tendon is to elongate the tendon to rupture, while measuring increases in length and tension during stretch. The values of change in length and tension can be plotted to produce a *stress/strain curve*. *Stress* refers to the amount of tension or load per unit cross-sectional area that is placed on a specimen. *Strain* refers to the proportional elongation that occurs. An idealized stress/strain curve characteristic for tendon is shown in Figure 1–8 and does not vary much between vertebrates.

There are five distinct regions of the stress/strain curve:

Toe region: There is very little increase in stress with elongation. This region represents 1.2 to 1.5 percent strain, and occurs during loading for 1 hour staying within the physiologic limit of the tissue.

Linear region: The stiffness of the tendon is basically consistent, and stress rapidly increases with increased elongation. Microfailure begins very early in this region.

Progressive failure region: Failure involves disruption of sufficient material to decrease the slope of the curve. The tendon, however, appears to the naked eye to be intact and normal.

Major failure region: The slope flattens dramatically. The tendon remains intact, but narrowing of the tendon at points of shear and rupture are visible.

Complete rupture region: The gross tendon breaks.

Comparisons between different stress/strain studies are very difficult, because

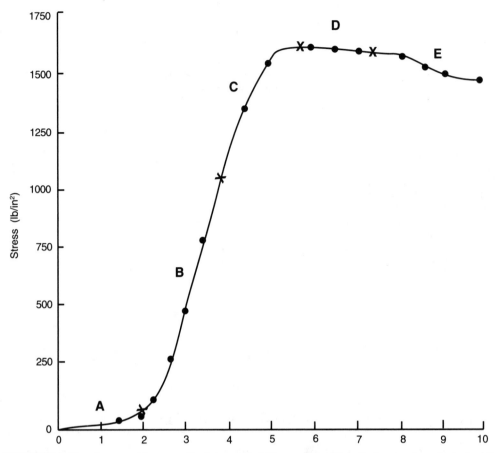

FIGURE 1–8.   Stress-strain curve for human Achilles tendon. Five distinct regions include (A) toe region, (B) linear region, (C) progressive failure region, (D) major failure region, and (E) complete rupture region. (Adapted from Ellis,[20] p. 7.)

the results vary significantly with changes in the experimental design. Values for the stress and strain in Figure 1–8 are presented in Table 1–2.

Recovery

If a stress/strain procedure is followed, but the stress is removed before partial rupture (*yield*) occurs, the tendon will return to its original length after a rest period during which there is no load. The return of the tendon to its original length is called *recovery*. Figure 1–9 illustrates the recovery of tendon following the removal of both cyclical and sustained stress. Recovery followed a cyclical load that produced 1.5 percent strain, and a sustained load that produced 2.6 percent strain. Rigby and associates[18] showed that the stress/strain curve could be repeated in tests of rat tail tendon as long as the strain was kept below 4 percent, and a 10-minute rest period was allowed between each subsequent application. They tested at strain rates between 1 and 20 percent per minute.

When stress/strain studies are initiated on totally unstressed tendon, the results

TABLE 1-2 Summaries of Stress/Strain Values

Author's Name	Tissue Type	Strain Rate	0 Point	Toe	Linear	Yield	Rupture Strain	Rupture Load
Kastelic*	Rat tail tendon	8%	Tendon first pulled	0–1.2%	1.2–1.6%	1.6–4.5%	10.9%	
Diamant*	Rat tail tendon	8%	Tightest point keeping native band structure	0–1.2%	1.2–1.6%	1.6–4.5%	10.9%	
Nathana*	Rat tail tendon	160%	Tendon first detected				12–14%	4–6.3 kg/mm²
Chapvil*	Rat tail tendon	8–16% 2–8%						600–1200 g/min 180–600 g/min
Betsch	Rat tail tendon			2%				
Dunn	Human psoas tendon	10%		5%				
Lehman	Rat tail tendon	6.7%						413 g/12 cm 178 g/6 cm
Nordin†	Human tendon			2%	2–6%	6–8%	8%	
Nordin‡	Human ant. cruciate ligament			1%	1–6%		8%	
Van Brocklin	Human toe extensor		Slack tendon	1.5% est				0.17 and 0.9 mdyne/cm²/min
Yamada	Human FHL§		(Unknown experimental design)				9.4%	6.7 kg/mm²
	Human EHL¶						9.9%	6.4 kg/mm²
	Human FPL**						9.6%	6.4 kg/mm²
	Human EPL††						9.9%	6.2 kg/mm²
	Human tendo Cal.						9.9%	5.3 kg/mm²

*Betsch citings, †citing Abraham, ‡citing Noyes, §Flexor hallicus longus, ¶Flexor hallicus longus, **Flexor pollicis longus, ††Extensor pollicis longus.
Source: Modified from Ellis.[20]

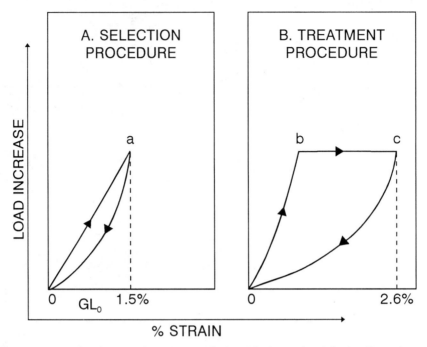

FIGURE 1–9. Graphs illustrate the recovery of (A) cyclical stretch—Selection Procedure and (B) sustained stretch—Treatment Procedure. (Adapted from Warren, et al.,[17] p. 466.)

are inconsistent. This problem can be eliminated by conditioning the tendon with gentle stretching prior to testing. Rigby and associates[18] found that the conditioning stretch resulted in a length increase of 0.4 to 0.8 percent, which did not recover when the stress was removed.[18] Hooley and associates[8] reported this increase to be 0.5 percent.

The word *recovery*, unfortunately, seems to imply that no permanent damage or permanent elongation has occurred. Recovery is in fact used to describe the regaining of different functions, for example, recovery of melting temperatures.[1,17,19,21] *Recovery of one function does not imply recovery of the other functions.* Rigby and associates[18] concluded that recovery had occurred because the tendon returned to the conditioned starting length, and the stress/strain curve was reproduced on each subsequent test. However, this recovery does not rule out the presence of some microfailure, inasmuch as the tendon showed full recovery even when safe limits were exceeded. Other studies[16,17] have confirmed that recovery of length does occur even after microfailure has begun.

Rate of Stretch

Van Brocklin and Ellis[25] showed that the stress/strain curve changed dramatically when the rate of stretch was changed. Human toe extensor tendons were subjected to cyclical ramp loading at two different rates. The slow rate loaded the tendons were subjected at 0.170 megadyne/cm^2 per second and unloaded at 0.223 megadyne/cm^2 per second. The fast rate loaded and unloaded at 9.2 megadynes/cm^2 per second (Fig. 1–10). The duration of the stretch was approximately 100 seconds for the slow rate

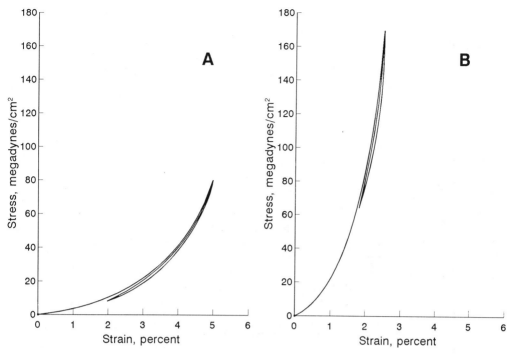

FIGURE 1–10. Stress-strain data from the extensor digitorum muscle tendon; (A) slow rate and (B) fast rate. (Adapted from Van Brocklin and Ellis,[25] p. 371.)

and 20 seconds for the fast rate.[25] Figure 1–11 shows changes in the viscoelasticity or "stiffness" of tendon that occur with different levels of applied stress. This example illustrates the difficulty of comparing the results of different authors who have used different experimental procedures.

Creep

An ideal spring shows resistance to elongation that does not depend on the speed of stretch, and maintains the same tension no matter how long the spring is held at a given length. Collagen does not act as an ideal spring in either regard. When a tendon is subjected to constant loading or to uninterrupted cyclical loading, the tendon gradually lengthens. This slow elongation in response to constant or repeated stress is called *creep*. Two methods are commonly used to study this phenomenon: load-deformation studies and stress-relaxation studies.

In the load-deformation test, a constant load is applied and the specimen is allowed to elongate (Fig. 1–12A). In stress-relaxation procedures, a specimen is stretched to a given length, which is then held constant. As the specimen creeps in response to the initial load, the tension drops (Fig. 1–12B). This creep elongation is described as plastic or viscous behavior of dense connective tissue.

Sanjeevi and co-workers[13] compared the stress-relaxation curves of different lengths of collagen fibers removed from rat tail tendon after treatment to remove surface proteins. The lengths of the fibers were 1, 2, 5, and 10 cm. Tests were performed at 25°C. Specimens were stressed to 4 percent, and tension development and relaxation

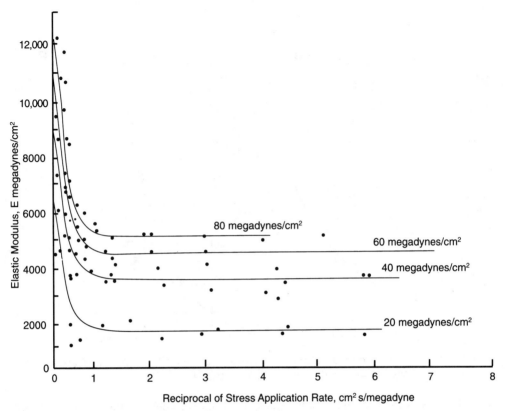

FIGURE 1–11.   Elastic modules as a function of the reciprocal of stress applications at several levels of stress for the extensor digitorum muscle tendon. (Adapted from Van Brocklin and Ellis,[25] p. 372.)

were recorded.[13] Their results showed how creep values also varied significantly between specimens of different length (Table 1–3).

Rigby[1] clearly differentiated between creep due to recoverable changes in tendon and that from disruption of the structure. He studied the stress-relaxation of rat tail tendon strained to 1 percent and to 10 percent at room temperature, with relaxation allowed to continue for increasing periods from 5 min to 30 hours. Subsequent to the stress-relaxation procedure, Rigby studied the melting temperatures of the treated samples to determine whether the stress-relaxation treatment had caused damage to the tendon (see section "Effects of Temperature"). All samples strained to 10 percent showed reduced melting temperatures, indicating disruption of the structure of the tendon. Samples strained to 1 percent showed minimal damage.[1]

Rigby then studied recovery by allowing tendons to rest without strain for up to 12 hours and found that samples strained to 1 percent showed full recovery to normal thermal transition temperature, but no samples strained to 10 percent showed recovery (Fig. 1–13).[1] He suggested that the molecular distortion occurring with a 1 percent strain is sufficiently minimal to allow reestablishment of the affected bonding, given appropriate time without stress for recovery. In an earlier work, Rigby and associates[18] showed that recovery from stress/strain at 1 percent, measured by reproducibility of the stress/strain curve, only occurred if the duration of loading was less than 60 minutes. This test indicated that damage occurred if a 1 percent strain was maintained

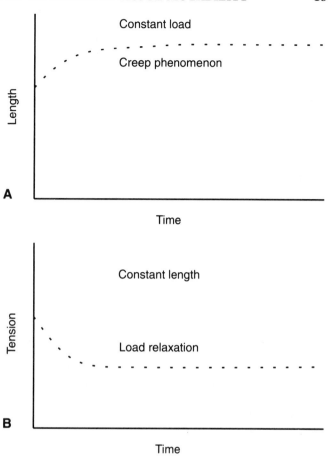

FIGURE 1–12. *(A)*. The creep phenomenon takes place when a tendon is subjected to a constant low load over an extended time period. Creeping of the soft tissues is greatest during the first 6 to 8 hours of loading but may continue at a low rate for months. *(B)*. A corresponding load relaxation of the soft tissues takes place with time. (From M. Nordin and V. Frankel: Basic Biomechanics of the Musculoskeletal System, 2nd edition. Philadelphia, Lea & Febiger, 1989. Reproduced with permission.)

for over 1 hour. They also showed that even short-term strain at 3 percent or greater caused irreversible damage to tendon.

Rigby's studies[1,18] shed important light on the nature of the "stability" of bonding in mature, dense connective tissue. Stability has previously been interpreted to mean not only stronger bonding but also fixed bonding. These studies suggest that the stability of bonding in connective tissue is much more dynamic than previously thought, because mature connective tissue can be partially disrupted and still reform. This observation promises to have important implications for understanding creep, recovery, damage from repetitive stress, and the effects of stress on connective tissue.

Rigby[1] found that up to 12 hours were needed for full recovery from long periods of stress-relaxation, and after only 10 minutes following single cyclical strain. Hooley and colleagues[9] found that following load elongation of rat tail tendon for up to 33

TABLE 1–3 Stress-Relaxation (kg/mm²)

Tissue	Initial	25 Sec	150 Sec	400 Sec
			Loads	
1 cm	6.8	6.0	5.66	5.60
10 cm	6.5	4.91	4.61	4.55

Source: Data from Woo, S L-Y, et al.[13]

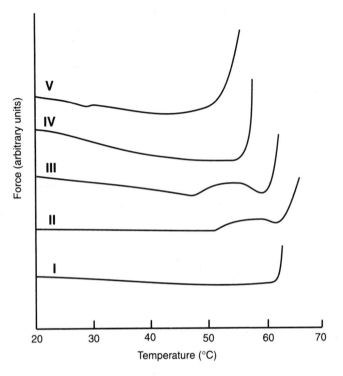

FIGURE 1–13. Isometric tension-temperature curves for rat tail tendon in 0.9% saline, obtained after various strain histories. (I) unstretched, (II) 1% strain for 22 hours, (III–V) 10% strain for 4, 17, and 69 hours, respectively. (Adapted from Ellis,[20] p. 31.)

hours, up to 2 hours were required for recovery to original length. Lehman and co-workers[14] concluded that stress-relaxation within these physiologic limits, and at 25°C, does not result in any permanent lengthening. Because Lehman and co-workers allowed only a 10-minute recovery time, this finding supports their conclusion that *all creep found in physiologic limits and at 25°C is only transient.*[14]

In summary, the phenomenon of creep occurs at two levels in tendon, starting with an elongation that shows recovery, and going on to damage and permanent elongation or progression to rupture. If the term "recovery" implies that no damage is done, then various tests of recovery can be listed in order, from least sensitive to most sensitive:

1. Recovery of original postconditioned length
2. Reproducibility of stress/strain curves
3. Recovery of thermal transition temperatures

By these tests it appears that *the physiologic limit of strain for tendon below 37°C is between 1 and 3 percent.* These studies are on long, compact tendons. Values are higher for less dense tendons, such as in the iliopsoas, which may have a less compact collagen fascicular architecture.

Effects of Temperature

When an unconstrained tendon is gradually heated, it will undergo an abrupt and irreversible shrinkage at the critical temperature of 59°C to 60°C. This point of change is often called the "melting temperature," because the shrinkage is assumed to reflect the breaking of chemical bonds that maintain the structure of the fiber at some level of organization (Fig. 1–14).

Temperatures between 37°C and 40°C can affect the viscoelastic properties of tendon. When a tendon is held under tension in stress-relaxation and load-deformation studies, the amount of relaxation is nearly temperature independent until 37°C. Above 37°C, as the temperature is increased, the stress-relaxation increases. Figure 1–15 demonstrates the stress-relaxation procedure. The initial tension minus the final tension, $F_0 - F_t$, is the stress-relaxation. Figure 1–16 shows the stress-relaxation found at different temperatures when tendons were held at a 3 percent strain, achieved at a rate of 9 percent per minute. Thermal transition occurred between 37°C and 40°C.[1]

Rigby[1] found that thermal transition in the stress/strain studies was reversible below critical values of temperature, strain, and time. At strains between 1 and 4 percent, cooling the tendon caused a return to original levels of stress (recovery), for temperatures up to 37°C. When stress-relaxation occurred at 40°C, however, the change was irreversible. The change was also irreversible if strain was greater than 4 percent.[1]

Thermal transition also dramatically affects the rupture strain of tendon. Rigby[1]

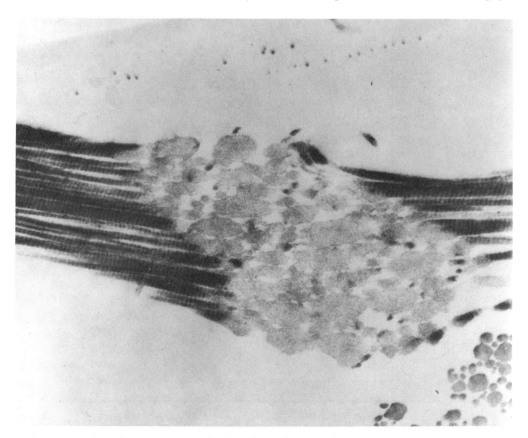

FIGURE 1–14. Electron micrograph of tendon collagen at the major transition (Ts). Melting is shown by the amorphous areas which coexist with unmelted crystalline areas (×63,000). (From Nordschow,[19] p. 370, with permission.)

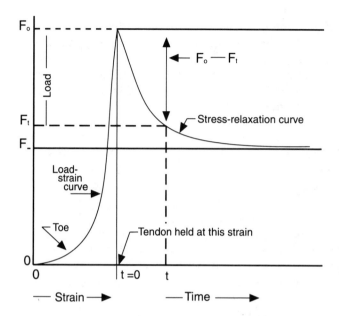

FIGURE 1–15. Schematic diagram of the curve obtained in a typical load-strain, stress relaxation experiment. The tendon is stretched at a predetermined rate to the desired strain, thus producing the load-strain curve shown at the left. The tendon is then maintained at this particular strain and measurements on the stress are continued, resulting in the stress-relaxation curve shown at the right. F-infinity (F_∞) would represent the stress when time approached infinity, e.g., the limited stress. (Reproduction from the *Journal of General Physiology*, 1959, vol. 43, pp. 265–283, by copyright permission of the Rockefeller University Press.)

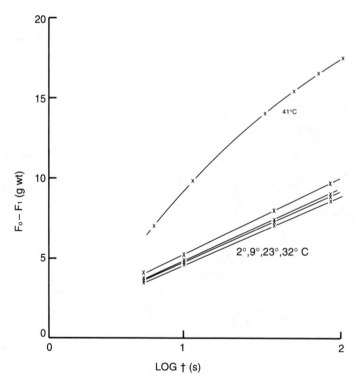

FIGURE 1–16. Stress relaxation curves (decrease, $F_o - F_t$, in load plotted as a function of the logarithm of time) for rat tail tendon at 3% strain at several temperatures. (Reproduction from the *Journal of General Physiology*, 1959, vol. 43, pp. 265–283, by copyright permission of the Rockefeller University Press.)

found that tendon at 40°C had a rupture strain of only 3 to 4 percent, whereas below 37°C specimens could be repeatedly strained to 4 percent with no change in their stress/strain curves. As indicated earlier, tendons at lower temperatures have rupture strains in the range of 8 to 14 percent.

Warren and associates[17] performed a series of experiments on rat tail tendon showing the effect of thermal transition temperatures on rate of creep, and on rupture load and rupture strain. Their rate of strain was 6.7 percent per minute. To standardize load to the dimensions of each tendon, they stressed each tendon with the load needed to produce a 1.5 percent strain with the tendon at 27°C. The tendon was then subjected to a stress-relaxation treatment at that predetermined load until a 2.6 percent strain was achieved. Table 1–4 summarizes their findings.[17]

The first column in Table 1–4 reflects an increase of the creep rate with increasing temperature as reflected by the decreasing time needed to achieve a 2.6 percent strain, thus supporting the findings of Ellis.[20] The reduced rupture loads and strains, measured after return of the tendon to 25°C, show damage in all cases. This observation suggests that the 30-g load or the 2.6 percent strain used in this series exceeded the working load of tendon within the temperature range and strain rate studied. When tendon had cooled to 25°C and was tested for damage, the first yield point was 2 percent, compared with normal values of 8 to 12 percent. After the 2.6 percent strain was achieved, however, the length was maintained for 2 minutes, during which time the temperature was reduced to 25°C. This precooling of prestrained tendon may inhibit the reestablishment of structural bonds, thus increasing the weakness shown when the rupture tests were performed just 10 minutes after release of tension.

The time needed for full recovery after strain under different conditions of time and temperature is unclear. Whatever the critical factors for a rupture load, the results in Table 1–4 demonstrate increased fragility of the tendon when stressed at or above thermal transition temperatures. In a previous study, the rupture load of tendon at 45°C was only about one fourth of the value found when the tendon was tested at 25°C.[14] In another study, the maximum physiologic load for tendon at 45°C was only about one third of the "safe load" for tendon at 25°C.[17]

The effect of time on reversibility of stress-relaxation on tendon heated to 40°C was not reported in detail by Rigby.[1] He did report, however, that recovery occurred following 4 percent strain for stress-relaxation periods of up to 60 minutes. When stress-relaxation exceeded 60 minutes, recovery did not occur. Although Rigby found load-deformation and stress-relaxation behavior nearly temperature independent below

Table 1–4 Effect of Temperature on Rupture Load and Rupture Strain[17]

Condition	Temperature			
	39°C	41°C	43°C	45°C
Achievement of 2.6% strain (min)—heated	9.3	4.78	2.86	1.48
Rupture load (% normal)—cooled	31.9	39	73	89.6
Rupture strain (% elongation)—cooled	3.3	3.1	7.0	11.45
Rupture strain (% normal)	21.1	19.9	45.5	63.4

Source: Data from Warren, et al.[17]

37°C, he also found slight differences in the final values of stress in the fully relaxed tendons. The tendon length varied slightly at different temperatures.[1]

Increasing temperatures affect not only the total stress-relaxation, but the rate of creep.[17,20] In Ellis's[20] report, the tendon was subjected to creep for 200 seconds at 20°C and then heated to 35°C. On heating, there was an immediate increase in the amount and rate of stress-relaxation (Fig. 1–17). Clearly, the tendon becomes more ductile when heated, creeping more rapidly. This observation is consistent with the breaking strain of tendon reducing dramatically at 40°C. Paradoxically, Warren and associates[21] showed that stress applied at the upper limit of thermal transition temperatures results in less damage, but only within strict limits of stress. They applied a "working load" of one-fourth the rupture load of tendon at 25°C in stress-relaxation tests until 2.65 percent strain had occurred. One set of tendons was loaded at 25°C, and the temperature was then increased. For the other tendons, the temperature was first raised, and then the load was applied. Two temperatures were used: 39°C and 45°C. After 2.6 percent strain was achieved, the load was removed, the temperature reduced to 25°C, and the residual strain measured after 10 minutes. To detect damage, they tested the rupture load after measuring residual strain. Although there was no difference in the residual strain between groups, there was a dramatic difference in

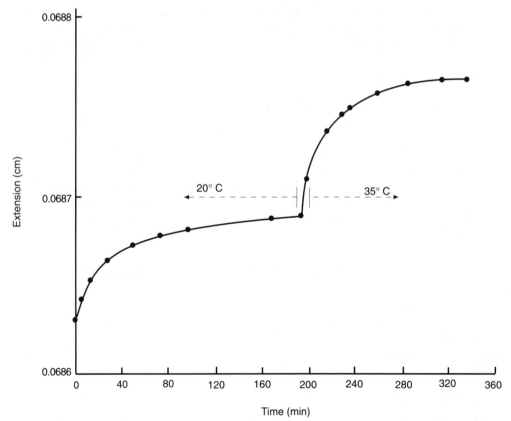

FIGURE 1–17.   Extension as a function of time for a collagen specimen permitted to creep at 20°C and then heated to 35°C. (Adapted from Ellis,[20] p. 27.)

TABLE 1–5 Rupture Tests

Condition	Rupture Load (% normal)		Rupture Strain (% normal)	
	39°C	45°C	39°C	45°C
Loaded at 25°C, then heated to temperature shown above	31	74	22	59
Loaded after heating	67	113	50	97

Source: Data from Warren, et al.[21]

damage sustained during the procedures.[21] Results of Warren and associates' rupture tests for damage are shown in Table 1–5.

Damage is prevented when the tendon is heated to 45°C prior to loading, but not when preheated to 39°C (which is still within the thermal transition temperature range). In further experiments Warren and associates[21] showed that one-half and one-fourth working loads resulted in damage reflected by rupture loads of about 78 percent and rupture strains between 64 and 78 percent. The average time of stress-relaxation to 2.64 percent was 7.6 minutes for loads of "½ safe load" and 29.7 minutes for "¼ safe load." Because these experiments were conducted at lower loads, and other conditions were the same, it is assumed that the damage was caused by increased time of stress-relaxation. This finding implies that *stress applied at 45°C can result in reduced damage, but only for short periods of time and at strains of 2.6 percent or less.*

Creep occurs in heated tendon not only with constant loading but also with repeated cyclical stretching with no rest period between each successive stretch. Figure 1–18 shows shows how the tendon gradually elongates with repeated cyclical stretching. Within the first few percentages of elongation, the curve is reproducible and damage does not occur. If treatment continues, however, the elongation gradually changes from transient recoverable strain to strain caused by yield and rupture.

FIGURE 1–18. Load-elongation records for a tendon subjected to cyclic loading at 1 cycle per minute; *(A)* before plasticlike elongation was initiated, *(B)* after plasticlike elongation had proceeded for some time. Tests at 32.4°C. (Reproduction from the *Journal of General Physiology,* 1959, vol. 43, pp. 265–283, by copyright permission of the Rockefeller University Press.)

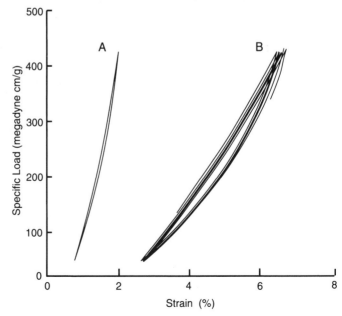

Lehman and co-workers[16] found that there is no difference in the creep elongation of tendon subject to cyclical stretching versus stress-relaxation when tendon was stressed to the maximum physiologic limit for 10 minutes. There was no significant difference between methods at both 27°C and 45°C.[16]

Biomechanical and Ultrastructural Correlations

The studies just reviewed have clear significance for the clinical management of dense connective tissues. The first principle derived from this review is that *collagen fibers in dense connective tissue are highly ordered structures that cannot be permanently lengthened without denaturing the fibers and greatly weakening them.*

Several authors have reported correlations between the stress/strain curves and changes in the ultrastructure of tendon. Hooley and Cohen[8] assumed that the toe region of the stress/strain curve corresponded to the flattening of the crimp waves, whereas the linear region reflected stretching of the straightened fibers. In a later study[9] they demonstrated that the activation energy of viscoelastic deformation is different in the toe and linear regions, confirming that the mechanisms of elongation are different.

Light and electron microscopic observations have confirmed the correspondence of the toe region of elongation to flattening of the crimp pattern.[18] The toe region of the stress/strain curve also represents the physiologic limits (safe limits) of elongation in natural tendon, in the estimation of several authors.[18,24,27] The most direct correlation of this relationship was reported by Viidik,[27] who found that the stress needed to flatten the crimp was equal to the force produced by a maximum tetanic contraction of the corresponding muscle. This observation may shed light on injuries in so-called "overuse syndromes" or repetitive stress injuries, in which a joint is held in its close-packed position after fatigue of the muscles controlling the joint. In this situation, the safe levels of loading between muscles and tendons may be exceeded by the application of outside force.

When strain exceeds 3 or 4 percent, the crimp form is permanently lost. This ultrastructural change indicates damage. Denaturing of collagen fibers with lost crimp is reflected by reduced thermal transition temperatures and reduced rupture strains and loads.[1,12,20,27,28]

Once the tendon reaches the linear region of the stress/strain curve, strain occurs due to stretching of the straightened fibers.[2,8,12,18] Many studies have examined discrete collagen fibers teased from tendon. In these fibers, a clear transition occurs between loss of crimp and strain in the straightened fiber, and this can be correlated to values on the stress/strain curve. In an intact tendon, however, all fibers do not lie in perfect parallel,[29] and the constituent subfibers are not equally straightened. In intact tendons and other structures, therefore, the constituent fibers are stressed somewhat sequentially, and the fibers first straightened should also first yield or rupture. In such whole tendons, direct correlation of stress/strain curves to ultrastructural changes cannot be made.[2]

As mentioned in the review of the ultrastructure of collagen, tropocollagen is a crystalline molecule with small amorphous components at the ends of the chain. Apparently the crystalline portion of the molecule is the most rigid and stable. After straightening the crimp waveform, the next unit at which strain occurs appears to be the amorphous components through which adjacent tropocollagen crystals attach.

This proposed mechanism is supported by x-ray diffraction studies performed after straightening of the crimp[27] and after elongation.[17,24,30]

According to Rigby,[1] application of mechanical force brings about structural changes equivalent to those produced by heat or chemical denaturation. To detect and identify the ultrastructural level of damage resulting from mechanical strain, the thermal transition temperatures of tendons after being subjected to stress-relaxation were compared to strains of 1 and 10 percent for up to 15 hours at room temperature. Tendons strained to 1 percent showed recovery to normal thermal transition temperatures if allowed to recover without strain for up to 3 hours. Rigby suggested that recovery results from the strain occurring between tropocollagen molecules and with minimal displacement. This minimal displacement of molecules allows reestablishment of the bonds during the recovery period and is reflected in the appearance of lower melting temperatures of the unstabilized, isolated tropocollagen equal to that in the tendon strained to 10 percent. Rigby explained that the difference between the native material that melts at 60°C and the conditioned material that melts at lower values depends on the number of specific structural units that are broken. These units are taken to be the "end structures" that project from the tropocollagen molecule and are responsible for polymerization and fibrogenesis.[1]

When a collagen fiber is stretched, we can postulate that these small disordered regions, being mechanically weaker than the tropocollagen molecules and crystallites (groups of tropocollagen molecules), will be disrupted first. If sufficient numbers of these regions are disrupted, crystal melting takes place. If fewer regions are disrupted, intermediate melting temperatures will be obtained. If the extension is maintained for long periods of time, damage in these regions will accumulate until individual or small groups of tropocollagen molecules are isolated and allowed to melt. The pattern of melting temperatures indicates melting of attachments between the tropocollagen molecules. Rigby[1] presented evidence that mechanical strain results in breaking bonds at the same levels as occurred with thermal transition temperatures and some forms of chemical denaturation.

Rigby and colleagues[18] advanced an additional argument in favor of straining the tendon in the linear region, where stress rapidly increases with elongation. The length of the tropocollagen molecule is a function of the latticework of the molecular attachments of its polypeptide chains. When melting occurs in an unstrained tendon, the latticework structure is destroyed and the subunits collapse on themselves because of their mutual attraction. This condition accounts for the shrinkage that occurs with melting. If strain results in extension within the tropocollagen molecules with destruction of its bonds, the molecule will collapse and recovery will proceed to lengths less than the original length of the material. In stress/strain experiments in which elongation was measured at the point at which crimp wave pattern were straightened, Rigby found no tendency for the tendon to contract below its initial length, indicating that the tropocollagen molecule itself is not disrupted in strain and that slippage occurs at higher levels of bonding.[18]

These studies demonstrate several principles. First, *bonding between tropocollagen molecules is sufficiently dynamic to allow reformation and recovery of the original ultrastructural architecture, so long as the fiber is not mechanically distended too far* or heated to temperatures that allow collapse of the crystal. The tropocollagen molecule collapses, however, at the melting temperature, and the fiber is irreversibly denatured. Mechanical extension sufficient to cause permanent elongation results in disruption of the ultrastructure and denaturing of the fiber. These factors may be important to consider in cases of "overuse" syndrome.

Slippage at higher levels of organization has also been identified. Yannas and Huang[10] studied rupture of 200-μm fibers that were teased from tail tendons of 3-month-old rats. They removed the reticular membrane in acid solution and studied fracture patterns with electron microscopy. Fracture occurred primarily in 10-μm fibers that had slipped in relation to each other. Much smaller fibers with diameters clustered around 1 μm also slipped.[10] Whether the same pattern would be found in untreated tendon fibers is not clear.

Second, *increasing the temperature of dense connective tissues to 40°C or higher dramatically increases the chance that permanent damage will be done by stretching the tissue.* This is reflected by the approximate three-fourths reduction in rupture strain and stress that is found in tendon heated to these thermal transition temperatures. *Reduction in rupture strain occurs unless the temperature can be carefully controlled to 45°C, the strain to 2 percent or less, and the time of maintained stretch to less than 60 minutes.* In a clinical situation, only the last parameter can be controlled with confidence.

PHYSIOLOGIC AND HISTOPATHOLOGIC CONSIDERATIONS

Scar Tissue Formation

Given the evidence that the structural integrity of dense connective tissue results from collagen fibers that are very rigid and stable, the question arises, How are contractures treated to allow greater freedom of motion? In cases of contractures involving tissue that can be surgically removed without causing disability, it can be argued that the restricting components are being stretched and denatured. In an ideal treatment of Dupuytren's contracture, for example, the restricting connective tissue is stretched and denatured while leaving the original tissues of the palmar fascia intact. In this case the traditional explanation of "stretching out" the contracture is supported by the known characteristics of collagen.[31] In a case of advanced adhesive capsulitis, on the other hand, the capsule itself has shortened so that it limits motion. In this example, "stretching out" the capsule results in the destruction of a tissue that is essential to joint function. The fact that motion can be restored in such cases without loss of joint stability indicates that lengthening of the tissue as a whole occurs without collagen denaturation. These changes are the result of biologic processes that cause tissue restructuring.

The next section reviews the biology of connective tissue mutability, which must be understood by the clinician who wishes to prevent or treat contractures of dense connective tissues. Included in the biology of connective tissue mutability are the mechanisms of change at both the cellular level and the resultant structural level.

Cellular Control Mechanisms in Scar Tissue Healing and in Dense Connective Tissue Fibroplasia

Understanding connective tissue mutability requires knowledge of both the sequence of cellular and biologic events and the stimulus-response mechanisms controlling each step of the process. The complexity of the puzzle results in part from the many different factors that have been identified as possible stimuli for the initiation of remodeling. Likewise, different cells have been identified as taking part in remodeling different tissues. Consequently, an understanding of connective tissue mutability has emerged very slowly and is incomplete. Considerable light has been shed on the process by Hunt, Banda, and Silver.[32] They have identified a sequence of events common to most forms of dense connective tissue mutability associated with inflammation. These mechanisms apply to the formation of scar tissue after an acute injury, or to the remodeling of dense connective tissue in response to chronic irritation.

Their experiments consisted of placing, into a rabbit ear, a chamber containing windows through which cells could be observed migrating into the wound space. Cells migrated from the wound edges into the space in a specific sequence. *Macrophages* were on the leading edge of the tissue, followed by newborn *fibroblasts*, then replicating fibroblasts clustered around capillary endothelial buds, and finally functioning blood vessels and mature fibroblasts.[32] Forrest[33] reported that *myofibroblasts* appear 24 to 48 hours after leukocytes, and 48 to 72 hours before the deposition of collagen fibers. Similar sequences have been reported by others.[34-36] Collagen could be identified immunologically among young fibroblasts, and morphologically among mature ones. The leading edge of the scar tissue was chiefly cellular, with collagen fibers appearing in the older part of the tissue. Four weeks after implanting the rabbit ear chamber, the tissue filled with scar tissue and healed. At this point, the active cell population disappeared, vascularization diminished, and healing merged into reorganization as collagen synthesis and lysis decelerated.

In that experiment, Hunt and associates[32] were able to determine the sequence of cellular migration and activity. The leukocyte population changed from 75 percent granulocytes in the first week to 86 percent macrophages by the third week. When the wound space closed, the macrophages disappeared and tissue proliferation stopped. Two questions remained. First, do leukocytes and fibroblasts respond independently to chemical stimulants or do the leukocytes control the fibroblast activity? Second, because macrophages can be found in small numbers in normal tissue, must they be activated by an inflammatory environment before they will produce the chemicals that initiate fibroplasia?[32]

Hunt and associates[32] performed a series of experiments to investigate conditions under which microphages or polymorphonuclear leukocytes stimulated a fibrotic reaction. They compared the reaction of connective tissue to the introduction of macrophages and polymorphonuclear leukocytes from both normal tissue and inflamed tissue. Macrophages from normal tissue were obtained from the peritoneal space of rabbits. Macrophages and polymorphonuclear leukocytes from inflamed tissue were obtained from an experimentally produced, inflamed tissue space under the rabbits' skin. Each of these cell populations was injected into the cornea of the rabbit from which they were obtained. There was no response to the injection of polymorphonuclear leukocytes from either source or to macrophages from normal tissue. Macrophages from the inflamed tissue, however, quickly caused angiogenesis and fibroplasia, resulting in a severalfold increase in collagen synthesis.[32]

This reaction suggests that "activated" macrophages stimulate fibroplasia in normal dense connective tissue. Rennard and co-workers[37] arrived at the same conclusion in studies on mechanisms of pulmonary fibrosis. They identified activated macrophages as an attractant for fibroblast proliferation and collagen production. They concluded that *the development of fibrosis is almost always preceded by an accumulation of inflammatory cells within a tissue.* Although the involved inflammatory cells and the biomechanical mediators probably differ among diseases, the general phenomenon of fibroblast recruitment and replication is likely to be a common pathogenic mechanism.

In a separate experiment, Hunt and associates[32] compared the reaction of scar tissue as it grew toward two different materials placed in the center of the wound space chamber. One material was biocompatible silicone and the other was silica, which acted as a foreign body. This model is important for understanding both acute, post-traumatic fibrosis and chronic inflammation, in that reactions continued to be observed well after the end of healing. When the scar tissue grew up against the silica plug, a high rate of cellular activity persisted at the interface. Macrophages remained in high numbers, and fibroblasts remained active. Withdrawal of the silica plug resulted in an immediate healing reaction, and the wound space filled quickly.[32]

In contrast, when the scar tissue grew up against the silicone plug, cellular activity diminished as in normal healing. At this point the silicone plug was removed, leaving a space in the center of the scar tissue. There was no cellular reaction for up to 2 months, and complete healing took months longer. This result indicates that activated macrophages are necessary to initiate activity of the connective tissue cells. Hunt and associates[32] confirmed this by showing that activated macrophages added to the plug space caused vasodilation within 12 hours, angiogenesis by 3 days, and healing by 14 days. This very important observation is the basis for a fundamental theory for the management of fibrotic adhesions, such as adhesive capsulitis, which is discussed in the section ''Clinical Implications'' (Chapter 2).

Farkas and associates[38] reported a similar reaction in connective tissue sheaths that grew around implanted silicone rods in chickens. They noted that the inner layer of the resulting connective tissue tunnels consisted of tissue macrophages that persisted indefinitely, perhaps induced by inflammatory reaction in the adjacent scarring volar soft tissue. On removing the silicone rods, they found that the inner surfaces of the connective tissue tunnels adhered to each other after 14 days and that the space was obliterated by 21 days. Similar reactions occurred in tunnels in place for 1, 2, and 4 months. Observations by several investigators suggest that similar interactions between activated macrophages and fibroblasts occur in chronically inflamed, anatomically normal, dense connective tissue structures.[36–38]

Chemical Control Agents

By what mechanisms do the activated macrophages stimulate fibroplasia? For some time it has been thought that chemical mediators are involved. Hunt's group[32] investigated this question by studying reactions to extracellular fluid from the wound sites and from cultures of activated macrophages. Both reactions elicited a 20-fold increase in replication of fibroblasts and endothelial cells of normal dense connective tissue. The protein that caused this reaction was not isolated or identified. Tsukamoto and co-workers[36] identified the exact protein that stimulated fibroblast migration into a wound area. They showed that activated macrophages produced unattached, soluble fibronectin. Fibronectin is both a chemoattractant for fibroblasts and a stimulant for their proliferation and fibroblastic activity. This finding was a surprise because it was originally thought that fibronectin was produced only by fibroblasts and myofibroblasts. There is a difference, however, in either the exact form of fibronectin or in the cellular response to it. Although the activated macrophages produce fibronectin, they do not appear to have significant amounts attached to their cell surfaces, nor do they form an intercellular maxtrix containing fibronectin as do connective tissue cells in culture. The function of the soluble fibronectin produced by the activated macrophages therefore appears to be merely an attractant and stimulant of connective tissue cells. Alitalo and colleagues[39] have reported that blood monocytes also produce fibronectin.

Other interstitial environmental factors identified as stimuli to initiate or maintain inflammation are local P_{O_2}, P_{CO_2}, pH, and lactate levels. Increased fibroplasia is commonly associated with areas of diffusion deficits. These relationships have been demonstrated by Hunt and associates.[32] The wound chamber method allowed them to place micropipettes across the wound space and to measure P_{O_2}, P_{CO_2}, pH, and lactate levels at each point from the periphery to the center of the growing scar.

During the period when the wound space is filling, marked gradients are found. The P_{O_2} gradient runs from 80 mm Hg at the periphery to 5 mm Hg in the area of replicating macrophages. The P_{CO_2} gradient was from 70 mm Hg in the center of the wound to 40 mm Hg at the periphery. In the center, pH was as low as 5 and lactate levels were high. Once the wound space closed and fibrosis ceased, the P_{CO_2} and P_{O_2} gradients disappeared, and pH and lactate levels returned to normal values. These observations do not reveal whether the P_{O_2} and P_{CO_2} gradients were simply the result of cellular activity or were themselves stimulants to that activity.

In a series of experiments, Hunt's group showed that low P_{O_2} is the chemoactivator for angiogenesis, in a sequence mediated by macrophages.[32] When a small hole was drilled through one of the windows at the growing margin of the scar, allowing oxygen to enter, angiogenesis stopped within 24 hours. Injecting medium from macrophages cultured in low P_{O_2} into the cornea of the rabbit eye stimulated angiogenesis, whereas medium from macrophages cultured at normal P_{O_2} did not. Not only were the gradients identified chemoattractants for macrophages but the macrophages were in turn a controlling stimulus for initiation and cessation of angiogenesis and fibroplasia. Once healing was completed, angiogenesis resulted in adequate oxygen diffusion and cellular activity diminished, as seen in the silicone plug experiments. In the contrasting silica plug experiment, it is probable that the high metabolic activity of the macrophages maintained gradients in that area, which became part of the vicious cycle resulting in persistent chronic inflammation and fibroplasia.

Low P_{O_2} has been implicated as a stimulant for continuous fibrosis in other forms of chronic inflammation. Kischer and Speer[40] studied the microvascular changes in Dupuytren's contracture because others had reported the paradoxical finding of hypervascularization of the tissue combined with a low P_{O_2}.[40] Light and electron microscopic studies consistently revealed occlusion of the lumen of microvessels by excessive layering of the basal laminae and endothelial cells. These changes were only found in the nodules of contracted tissues and accounted for diffusion deficits existing simultaneously with the hypervascularization. Forrest[33] reviewed literature related to wound healing and found that the wound space was hypoxic and acidotic. Collapsed microvessels have also been reported in hypertrophic and keloid scar tissue, both of which exhibit continuous fibroplasia.[41-43]

Important as it is to understand the sequence of events elucidated by Hunt and associates,[32] it is also significant that this is not the only pathway to fibroplasia. Besides activated macrophages, other agents have been identified as attractants for fibroblasts. Among these are serum complement,[36] platelets,[37] disrupted tissue components,[37] monocytes,[37] and various lymphocytes.[32,36,37] As the relative place of each of these agents is identified, implications for treatment may emerge.

For additional information on the chemical cycles found in inflammation, the reader is referred to Wilkerson's[44] review of chemical reactions in acute and chronic inflammation. Both acute and chronic inflammation are initiated and controlled by a chain of reactions so numerous, and forming so many parallel pathways, that they are referred to as "cascades." Fibroplasia can be initiated by vascular sources, mast cells, white cells, platelets, and by injured interstitial tissues and cells. The only common denominator is that *either acute trauma or repetitive chronic irritants always initiate an inflammatory reaction, which subsequently results in fibroplasia.* The exact sequence of the chain of events is still unclear.

Cellular and Extracellular Components in Remodeling Scar Tissue

Scar tissue is a specialized dense connective tissue that is important to clinicians. Scar tissue changes in composition from the newly formed to the final quiescent stage of the mature scar. The clinician must have a clear understanding of what scar is at each stage and how it behaves, either naturally or in response to treatment.

The understanding of tissue mutability has caused a profound change in our understanding of tissue structure. We used to think that once a tissue had formed in an adult animal, it was as fixed and unchangeable as statuary marble. We now realize that the form of a structure is a result of constant activity and renewal in the tissue, the shape being more analogous to a water fountain, which is sustained only by the constant flow of water. This is particularly true of scar tissue, which changes totally in content, activity, and physical characteristics as it evolves from the initial scar through the final stages of mature scar.

SCAR TISSUE COMPOSITION AND ACTIVITY:
2 TO 4 DAYS AFTER WOUNDING

Immediately following a tissue wound, the space fills with blood products, which quickly form a clot. This space is immediately invaded by leukocytes and macrophages, which reach peak concentrations by the end of 48 hours. Following the Po_2 gradient, activated macrophages migrate toward the center of the wound, where the lowest oxygen levels are found furthest from the wound edges. Nearby fibroblasts are stimulated to replicate, and the replicating myofibroblasts follow the macrophages into the wound space.[32] This process is quite rapid. Levenson and co-workers[45] found large concentrations of mature and young fibroblasts, as well as epithelial cells, leukocytes, and mast cells, in 5-day-old scar in rats. Madden, DeVore, and Arem[46] stated that, as a rule, fibroblasts are active in scar within a few days. Based on evidence of new collagen production, some investigators state that a period of 48 hours is needed before fibroblasts become active in collagen production.[11,34] Forrest[33] reported fibroblast appearance 24 to 48 hours after leukocytes appeared, and 48 to 72 hours before the deposition of collagen fibers.

One reason collagen has not been seen in morphologic studies until after 2 days is because the type of collagen produced appears to change during this period. Collagen deposited during the first 2 days is type III (reticular fibers), which has not been generally recognized as collagen by earlier morphologic tests, such as argyrophilic staining. This early deposition of reticular fibers probably acts as a scaffold on which type I collagen is laid to form larger collagen fibers. Injuries, various diseases, and different stages of development govern the types of collagen found in any given tissue. The dynamic, biologic changes are only now being recognized and may have significant clinical implications for the study of physical characteristics of tissue and in clinical management.[33,47–49]

Capillary budding is stimulated by macrophages, as reported by Hunt and associate,[32] and begins within hours of wounding. Some capillary buds canalize and carry blood while others resolve. Madden, Devore, and Arem,[46] and Hunt and associates[32] reported capillary budding after fibroblast migration, although exact times were not reported.

The establishment of a significant population of fibroblasts requires 2 to 3 days, and the peak of collagen production and deposition only occurs after this period. Collagen is identifiable only by immunofluorescent methods, among the replicating fibroblasts at the edge of a wound. Morphologically identifiable collagen deposition occurs among the more mature fibroblasts near blood capillaries. The earliest identification of collagen formation was reported in wound scar 2 days after injury by Madden and Smith,[34] using saline extraction, and by Madden and Peacock,[11] using radioactive isotope labeling. Levenson and co-workers[45] identified small collagen fibers by staining in 5-day-old scar tissue. They also reported droplets of degenerated collagen showing synthesis and degeneration were present in this early stage.[45] This observation was supported by Madden and Smith.[34] Madden, DeVore, and Arem[46] reported the development of collagen fibers occurring rapidly from day 5 onward. The general agreement appears to be that structural collagen fibers are present no earlier than the fifth day. From that time on, type I fibers form rapidly.

During the first few days of wound healing, therefore, scar tissue has no significant extracellular matrix of collagen fibers to provide strength and stability. At this stage, the scar tissues are held together predominantly by intercellular attachments and the formation of a fibroblast-reticulin network. The tissue is therefore fragile. Levenson and colleagues[45] reported on the fragility of scar at 5 days and noted that the wound margins were loosely held and easily disrupted during preparation of tissue for slides. In recent years, details of these intercellular attachments have been reported. Baur and Parks[4] reported that myofibroblasts comprise 100 pecent of the fibroblast population at the height of fibroplasia, and that these cells can both migrate and attach to each other and to collagen fibers in the matrix. Adjacent cells attach at gap junctional complexes that form between the cell membranes. Intercellular actin bundles reinforce the cell membranes at the point of attachment and apparently provide attachments necessary for contraction within the cells. The contractions are then transmitted through a series of adjacent cells, thus providing a basis for scar tissue contraction. For the therapist who is physically stressing scar to bring about remodeling, it is important to visualize the highly cellular, fragile structure of new scar. Use of stress to "stretch" scar tissue at this stage will cause elongation of the scar by one of only two mechanisms: disruption of cell membranes and cell death, in response to high or sudden loads, or cell migration, in response to gentle and prolonged loads.

FIBROPLASIA: THE GROWTH PHASE OF SCAR FROM 5 TO 21 DAYS

In rat skin wound studies of the biology of scar tissue, Madden and Peacock[11] showed that scar tissue rapidly increased in bulk for 21 days, a phenomenon known as fibroplasia. A period of 3 to 4 weeks of fibroplasia was confirmed by other authors using various experimental models and animals.[32,45,51] As the scar tissue enters the fibroplasia stage, it changes composition. From the first appearance of collagen fibers around day 4 or 5, until day 21, the quantity of collagen present increases, paralleling the increase in the scar tissue bulk.[11] The parallel between the size of the scar and the quantity of collagen implies that the percentage of collagen remains relatively constant through this period. The rate of collagen deposition peaks at 14 days.[50] There is simultaneous collagen degradation during this period, resulting in a tremendous amount of collagen remodeling, with lysis of some fibers, aggregation of new fibers, and increases in the size of other fibers. During this highly active stage of collagen synthesis and degradation, architectural changes occur in the fiber attachments, alignment, spacing, and placement.[51] The fibers are first small, closely packed, and randomly aligned.[11,33,34,45,46,52] These small fibers begin to form larger bundles of fibers, alignment becomes more parallel, and spaces begin to appear between them. Levenson and co-workers[45] reported the first formation of loose fascicles at 14 days and interlacing fascicles with spaces by the 21st day.

The cell population changes by the gradual disappearance of inflammatory cells. From day 5 onward, fibroblasts become the predominant cell, replacing the leukocytes.[45] In 5-day-old scar tissue, numerous fibroblasts, endothelial cells, undifferentiated adventitial cells, monocytes, and lymphocytes are still found. There are fewer eosinophils, polymorphonuclear leukocytes, and—in the margins of the wound—mast cells. By day 14 Levenson[45] found only fibroblasts to be present. Macrophages form the majority of residual cells from early on and persist at this stage.[32] By the end of the second week, inflammatory cell participation has ceased and cellular modulation has peaked. This leaves a fairly homogeneous population of fibroblasts and myofibroblasts, which are active in response to the activated macrophages.

There is some confusion about the nature of the connective tissue–producing cells. Older literature exclusively used the term *fibroblasts*. Since the recognition of myofibroblasts as an entity has gradually entered the literature, these new cells have been mentioned with increasing frequency, and comparisons between authors are no longer possible. In 1983, Baur and Parks[4] reported that myofibroblasts constituted the major percentage of the cells observed at the peak of fibroplasia. The difference between fibroblasts and myofibroblasts is clinically significant, because the latter are known to cause scar tissue shrinkage, whereas fibroblasts cause only remodeling without active shrinking.[53] The appearance of myofibroblasts corresponds with the onset of the contraction phase, which begins on about day 5, and diminution of their population marks the end of the contraction phase and the start of the maturation phase.[4,37,53–55] Based on descriptions of scar changes by Peacock and Van Winkle,[55] the contraction phase is roughly equal to the fibroplasia stage, from about day 5 to day 21. In some cases this process continues indefinitely (see "Scar Tissue Contraction and Shrinkage," Chapter 2).

THE CONSOLIDATION PHASE: DAY 21 TO DAY 60

Assuming normal healing, the scar stops increasing in size at about 21 days.[11] Scar tissue shrinkage diminishes quite rapidly and myofibroblasts disappear, leaving a predominance of fibroblasts. During the consolidation phase, the tissue gradually changes from a predominantly cellular tissue to a less cellular fibrous tissue, with collagen constituting the bulk of fibers embedded in the proteoglycan/glycosaminoglycan matrix. At day 21 the cell population in thin skin-incision scars is only slightly greater than in the adjacent skin.[45] Well-organized cells and fibers are found in 4-week-old scar around silicone implants. Four weeks seems to be the minimum time required for the organization of the tissue.[50] With the reduction of cellular numbers, the vascularity slowly diminishes, equaling that in adjacent skin by day 42.[45] Despite the diminishing cell population, marked changes in the shape of the scar continue during this period due to the high activity of fibroblasts. The collagen turnover rate remains elevated, resulting in architectural restructuring of the collagen network. This turnover rate is reflected in gradually increasing strength and suppleness of the scar.[45,46]

MATURATION PHASE: DAY 60 TO DAY 360

After day 60 the activity of the connective tissue cells gradually diminishes. Collagen turnover remains high to around day 120 and then gradually tapers off. Eighty-five percent of original collagen in a skin graft is replaced with new collagen by about day 150.[54] All of these changes are time dependent. Between 180 and 360 days, few cells are seen and the tissue has become tendonlike.[38,45] The collagen fibers are compact and large, and the scar has only a few scattered cells imbedded in it; fully mature scar is only 3 percent cellular, and blood vessels are sparse. Thus scar tissue changes from a predominantly cellular tissue in the first few days to an almost totally collagenous connective tissue by the end of maturity.

The changes occurring in scar are very gradual in the consolidation and maturation stages. The age of scar tissue is impossible to identify by histologic appearance between day 42 and day 360, individual scar changes being greater than age-related ones during these last two phases.[45,46]

Scar Tissue Contraction and Shrinkage

For an eloquent review of the history of scar tissue shrinkage investigations, the reader is referred to Peacock and Van Winkle.[55] Once scar tissue has formed, at about 5 days, it begins to shrink. This shrinking is an active process in which the scar develops significant centripetal forces, pulling the wound edges together. This shrinkage appears to result from the actual contraction of the myofibroblasts, which are found in large numbers in the tissue during this 5- to 21-day period. The myofibroblasts anchor to each other and to fibrillar structures in the extracellular matrix, so that the contraction of each cell is transmitted to the tissue as a whole. This contraction is limited by the amount each cell contracts, and by the compaction of the extracellular fibers and ground substance.[4] Scar tissue shrinkage is progressive, however, resulting in a significant reduction in size of the scar over time.

Progessive contraction can be explained by envisioning the continuous contraction of myofibroblasts with simultaneous collagen turnover. As the tissue is pulled together, preexisting collagen fibers are absorbed allowing further compression of the bulk of the tissue. New collagen fibers are laid down, fixing the smaller dimensions. The myofibroblasts attach to the new fibers and pull them. The process continues in this lockstep, ratchet-type progression.[42]

Untreated, newly formed scar will normally contract for about 3 weeks. In some cases, persistence of myofibroblast shrinkage continues for longer periods, in response to various poorly understood circumstances. This prolonged shrinkage seems to happen in cases of very large scars, such as those occurring after burns to extensive surface areas. These large scars become very tight and tense, which impedes circulatory supply in the area. The findings of Hunt and colleagues[32] suggest that the persistence of contraction for long periods in these cases is due to poor diffusion, with continuous gradients of O_2, Co_2, and pH acting as chronic irritants and prolonging the active phase of contraction.[32]

Effects of Stress and Motion on Scar Remodeling

Mechanical tension and compression affect scar tissue remodeling at almost all levels of organization. Apparently the spatial orientation of connective cells within a tissue is affected by stress. Fibroblasts orient in the direction of tension, and even their mitotic bundles align parallel to tension lines.[56] Daughter cells separate along the same lines. The long axis of cells lies predominantly parallel to the direction of wound contraction.[4] Flint[57] noted that in the portion of calf tendon that passed around a bony pulley, cells on the compressed side were more rounded that those on the outer portion of the tendon. Collagen under compressive loading tends to stain differently from collagen under tension in the same tissue.[57] This difference in staining suggests different distributions of electrical charge on the collagen fibers in the two circumstances.

The metabolic activity of connective tissue cells is also affected by mechanical forces. Magonne and colleagues[58] cultured chondrocytes from the leg bones of chicks in tube-shaped culture vessels. After 14 days, the culture formed a solid block of tissue that could be removed and maintain its structural integrity under cyclical strains of up to 5.5 percent. They subjected the tissue culture cylinders to cyclical strain for 24 hours and reported an increase in chondrocyte activity. This chondrocyte activation included proteoglycan production, as reflected by a 1.4-fold increased uptake of $^{35}SO_4$, a 1.7-fold increase in ^{14}C-glucosamine, and a 2.4-fold increase of ^{3}H-thymidine incorporation into DNA in the stressed cultures. On the other hand, collagen synthesis did not increase during the same time period as reflected by unchanged uptake of ^{3}H-glycine uptake. Magonne and co-workers[58] cited unpublished studies, however, that showed cyclical straining in excess of 24 hours resulted in an increase in collagen synthesis, with simultaneous changes in the collagen organization in the stressed tissue.

Slack and co-workers[59] cultured whole chick embryo tendons, which were placed under a cyclical load for 48 to 72 hours. The tendons showed a 50 percent increase in DNA synthesis and a 200 percent increase in protein synthesis when loaded. Glycosaminoglycan synthesis in response to tension depended on the exact age of the embryo when the tendon was harvested. Overall synthesis increased in the tendons of 17-day-old chicks, whereas in tendons from 18-day-old chicks, total synthesis did not change; there was, however, a change in the relative amounts of different GAGs.

Collagen fibers are laid down in response to stress lines of mechanical loads. This formation of collagen fibers has been attributed to various mechanisms, all of which involve transduction of physical forces into electrochemical events at the molecular level. Direct current potentials flowing from piezoelectric crystals, such as collagen fibers, were previously thought to direct the aggregation of new collagen fibers in an automatic, physical aggregation of the highly electrostatic tropocollagen molecules. This is an attractive theory for tissue containing preexisting collagen fibers, but it does not explain the orientation of collagen fibers in newly forming tissue. A mechanism of initial collagen alignment has been proposed based on cellular control. Baur and Parks[4] found that the long axis of cells lies along lines of force in scar, and that the fibronectin-anchoring strands of myofibroblasts lay predominantly parallel to the direction of wound contraction. They presented evidence that the myofibroblast strands were a scaffold upon which collagen fiber aggregation occurred. This model can explain how cellular orientation can lead to orientation of collagen fibers in the early development of dense connective tissues.

Farkas and co-workers[38] implanted silicone rods in chicken feet to stimulate development of connective tissue tunnels around the rods. The silicone rods were subsequently removed, and tendon transplants were passed through the tunnels. The dorsal aspect of the tunnels under tension became thicker, denser, and more tendonlike, whereas the plantar portion, which was compressed, became thinner. This observation supports the view that physiologic loads of tension cause increased aggregation of collagen, whereas compression has the opposite effect. Unfortunately, the correlation between collagen deposition and the presence of tension or compression in a tissue is not a simple one. Factors such as the amount of force and the duration of application also have varying effects on collagen deposition.

Interactions between stress lines and scar tissue hypertrophy have been investigated clinically and histologically.[60] When split skin grafts are oriented to the direction of the predominant collagen fibers of the grafted area, hypertrophic scarring is prevented. Conversely, multiple Z-plasties of hypertrophic scar cause that scar to progressively thin and soften. This thinning and softening is a paradoxical finding, because an incision in the scar will normally produce increased scarring. However, if the Z-plasty is performed to relieve lines of tension within the scar, thinning and softening result. Biopsies show that this reaction is associated with changes in the orientation of collagen fibers. The new orientation is along physiologic crease lines as early as 14 days following Z-plasty. The relative proportion of GAGs also returns to normal following Z-plasty.

In contrast, when recent or late scar is subjected to intermittent tension over a joint, there is an immediate production of collagen fibers of abnormal size, structure, and staining characteristics, with a random alignment of fibers, resulting in a thick and hardened scar. Based upon these observations, control of the amount and direction of stress are primary considerations in either the prevention or the treatment of hypertrophic scar. Brody and associates[61] have pointed out that hypertrophic scar occurred exclusively in areas where there was intermittent compression of the developing scar. Scar that was subjected to tension (e.g., the extensor surface of the elbow) formed normally, whereas that on the flexor surface was likely to become hypertrophic. This observation is in agreement with Longacre's correlation of the presence of alternating tension in different directions, with the refinement of noting that the compression component of the alternating movements is corrected with the hypertrophy.[60] When one considers the elbow, the protective response of a patient is to hold the joint in flexion, resulting in compressive forces in the antecubital area. Brody and associates'[61] observations of hypertrophic scar in areas around the breast where constant compression exists support this hypothesis. A systematic analysis of the relative durations of compression and tension and the appearance of hypertrophic scar, however, is lacking in the literature.

Tissues that are compressed tend to fold upon one another. This folding, rather than simply the presence of compression, may be the critical factor that promotes interfibrillar adhesions. This model, presented by Brody and associates,[61] is supported by the fact that therapeutic compression of burn scars, in which the scar is compressed in a flattened configuration by splints or bandages, results in gradual thinning and elongation of the scar rather than hypertrophy.[40,41]

Tension has been shown to control both the direction of collagen fiber alignment and the tendency to form large bundles. Arem and Madden[56] subjected blocks of subcutaneous scar in rats to constant tension for 6 hours per day for 4 weeks.[56] The collagen fibers within the scar became oriented parallel to the line of tension. Forrester and co-workers compared strength and collagen architecture of skin incision scars that were closed by suture with those closed by tape.[52] Suture-closed wounds were compressed by the sutures, whereas tape-closed wounds were subjected to moderate tension during normal activity. The suture-closed scar initially showed disorganized, closely packed collagen fibers with little sign of aggregation of fibrils to make larger fibers (Fig. 1–19A). The fibers became progressively densely packed with time, and at 100 days postinjury formed irregular masses of collagen with little evidence of fibril structure. In contrast, tape-closed wounds at 10 days postinjury displayed fiber organization with many fibers lying along tension lines across the wound (Fig. 1–19B). Aggregation of fibers into large bundles lying along tension lines was also seen at 10 days. At 100 days, better fiber definition was seen, with more interfibrillar spaces.

Goldstein and Barmada[62] reported greater organization of collagen fibers in the margins of repaired medial collateral ligaments of rabbits that had been mobilized after repair, compared with those cast. The structure of tendon is dependent upon the functional loading of the tissues. According to Magonne and associates,[58] any alteration in the degree or type of physiologic loading is followed by changes in cellular metabolism, matrix morphology, and functional capacity. This statement is quite revolutionary, because it implies a great deal more mutability of mature, dense connective tissue than had been previously appreciated. It was supported, however, by Enwemeka,[14] who cast immobilized ankles of rabbits with the tendon of the soleus muscle slack. At 4 weeks, Enwemeka found that the collagen fibers were disorganized, with shorter fiber bundles randomly aligned. Active fibroblasts were also found in greater numbers. The structural organization of the tendon connective tissue returned to normal 4 weeks after the ankle joints were recast so that slight tension was applied to the soleus tendon.

Kirscher and Speer[40] noted in the contracted tissues of Dupuytren's contracture that the microvessels were oriented parallel to the long axis of the contracture bands. We can see, therefore, that *cells, GAGs, and collagen type and architecture are all affected by the direction and magnitude of physical stress applied to a tissue.*[40] These factors appear to be operational during the development of a new scar, an old healed scar, and in normal dense connective tissues.

Effects of Stress on Strength of Collagen in Scar Tissue

Many factors cause scar tissue to gain strength with time. Several factors were identified in Madden and Peacock's[11] studies on the dynamic metabolism of scar collagen in sutured rat skin wounds. During the first 3 weeks after wounding, scar

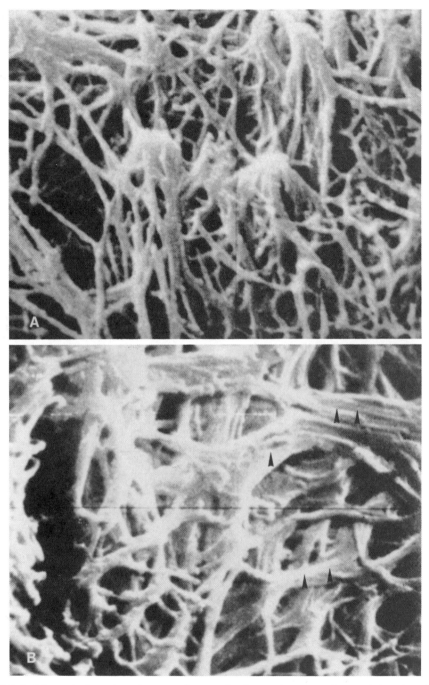

FIGURE 1–19. *(A)* Scanning electron micrograph of a 10-day sutured wound showing the randomly oriented collagen fibrils. They show little tendency to aggregate. Cross-banding is not apparent (×7500). *(B)* Scanning electron micrograph of a representative portion of a 10-day tape-closed wound. The fibrils are aggregating to form small bundles oriented across the wound. Compare with the suture-closed wound shown in *(A)* at the same magnification (×7500). (Adapted from Forrester et al.,[52] pp. 733, 734.)

increased in strength in direct proportion to the increasing bulk of collagen deposited in the scar.

Figure 1–20 shows a high deposition of collagen during the first 3 weeks and a high rate of collagen turnover in scar during the next 3 weeks. The turnover provides a second mechanism for increase in strength of scar. Consider a newly forming scar after an incision. If we take into consideration that removal of sutures after a few days allows tension to be present across a wound scar, we can assume that the collagen fibers reorient across the wound and that larger fiber bundles form, as shown by Forrester and co-workers.[52]

Figure 1–20 illustrates the difference between the predicted volume of scar, based upon the deposition rate of newly formed collagen, and the actual volume of scar that forms. The actual volume of scar is less than that predicted, due to the remodeling process in which old collagen is degraded and absorbed. These changes provide an

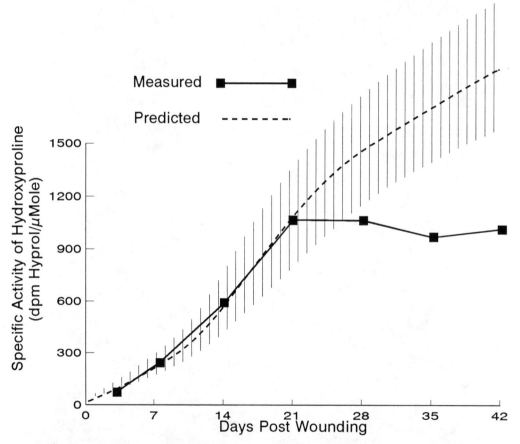

FIGURE 1–20. Comparison of scar collagen accumulation predicted from rate measurements and actual values. The predicted volume of scar based on the rate of deposition of new collagen is shown by the hatched lines; the solid line shows the actual volume of scar formed. The amount of collagen that has been degraded and absorbed in the remodeling process is indicated by the gap between these two lines. On day 42, remodeling has removed a volume of collagen equal to the entire volume of collagen remaining in the scar. (From Madden, JW and Peacock, EE: Studies on the biology of collagen during wound healing: III. Dynamics metabolism of scar collagen and remodeling of dermal wounds. Ann Surg 174:511–520, 1971, with permission.)

architectural explanation for the increasing strength of the scar, without a concurrent increase in volume. This argument is supported by Madden and Peacock's[51] finding that strength increased only as long as new collagen fibers were being deposited. Also, collagen bonding became more prevalent and more stable with maturation of newly formed collagen fibers, providing a chemical explanation for scar strength increase.

In summary, evidence supports *three explanations for increasing the strength of scar: (1) increasing scar collagen volume; (2) increasing chemical bond stability; and (3) selective aggregation of collagen fibers along stress lines.*

The effect of stress on strength of new scar is a function of the intensity and duration of stress applied. If excessive stress is applied to newly formed and weak tissue, the scar is pulled apart and weakened. As previously mentioned, Goldstein and Barmada[62] compared the strength of repaired medial collateral ligaments of rabbits that were either allowed free activity with the joint unsupported, or were casted for varying periods. Three weeks after repair, the ligaments of the animals that were allowed free activity had a breaking load of 2.7 kg, compared to 6.1 kg for those that were casted for the same period of time. The possibility that unrestricted activity had subjected the scar to excessive strain and damaged the fragile tissue was supported by histologic studies. The scar from the unconstrained animals showed less evidence of healing, less fibroplasia, and evidence of persistent inflammation. At the same time, collagen fibers at the periphery were more organized. The immobilized scar was more cellular, with a thick fibroblastic reaction that was immature and poorly organized. One is tempted to conclude that the two scars represent the two extremes of poor methods of management: prolonged immobilization leading to poorly organized tissue, and excessive early motion leading to disruption of the scar.

In their study of sutured versus tape-closed skin incision scars, Forrester and colleagues[52] noted that in the deeper layers of the scar at the level of the subcutaneous muscle, the scar was elongated by the muscle pull in the tape-closed wounds.[52] In this case, the restricted levels of stress resulted in a breaking strength that was much greater for the tape-closed wounds. At 150 days, the tape-closed wounds had recovered 90 percent of the strength of the unwounded skin, while the suture-closed scar had recovered only 70 percent. Remarkably, the difference in management for only the first 7 days (until sutures and tape were removed) had a long-lasting effect on the strength of the scar. Forrester and colleagues' study illustrated the benefits of restricted levels of stress and identified differences in collagen architecture, in response to stress, as the biologic explanation for the increased strength.[52]

Changes in Shape of Scar by Remodeling

Hunt and associates'[32] study indicates that the hole left in the center of the scar in the wound space chamber can fill by two different mechanisms. In the presence of chronic irritants, the hole fills rapidly due to fibroplasia. In contrast, when the tissue around the hole has normal metabolic gradients, it requires 2 months for the space to begin to fill, and complete filling requires several more months. Nonetheless, it does gradually fill. This gradual filling is probably accomplished by normal scar tissue remodeling, which proceeds faster than the collagen turnover rate of the adjacent skin for 4 months after wounding. After this, collagen continues to turn over at rates equivalent to that of the skin, for up to a year.[46] This gradual change in shape of scar by remodeling is probably similar to the gradual filling of a pierced ear hole, which occurs when one stops wearing earrings.

With two exceptions, the change in shape of scar is not well documented in the literature. Articles have been published on the flattening and lengthening of burn scars in response to therapeutic compression.[63] The change in shape results from remodeling and is well documented by histologic and scanning electron microscopic studies[52,56,64] of the collagen architecture at different stages (Fig. 1–21). When newly formed scar is subjected to noncyclical strain, the scar gradually changes shape, becoming long and attenuated. Madden[64a] attributed this change in shape entirely to the remodeling of collagen. As shown in Figure 1–22, however, the scar does not simply grow longer but assumes the hourglass shape of any malleable structure that is stretched. One is tempted to conjecture that cell migration flows along lines of stress into the hourglass shape. This hypothetical cellular orientation could then be

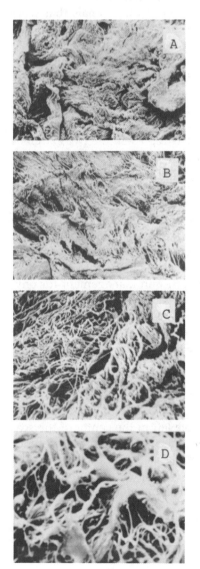

FIGURE 1–21.   Scanning electron micrographs showing remodeling of collagen in burn scars. *(A)* Biopsy of scar of patient before pressure showing increased, compact collagen. *(B)* After 3 to 4 weeks, compact collagen beginning to loosen. *(C)* After 6 weeks of pressure and splinting, the collagen is less compact, and individual fibers are now visible. *(D)* After 3 months' pressure and splinting, fibroblasts are seen in a loose collagen network (magnification ×6000). (From Larson et al.,[64] p. 13.)

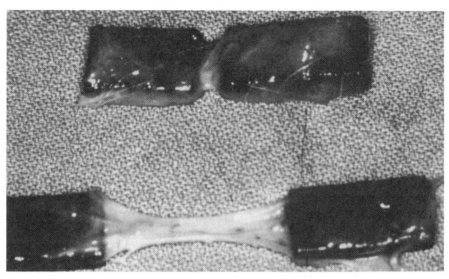

FIGURE 1–22. The effect of stress on healing wounds. Rat study with sponges. The scar was stressed 6 hours per day × 4 weeks. When a newly formed scar is subjected to stress, the scar grows longer and attenuates in the center. (From Arem and Madden,[56] p. 97.)

translated by the fibronectin-collagen scaffold mechanism into organized matrix, resulting not only in increased length but also in attentuation of the central portion of the scar.

Change in shape of scar by remodeling is a slow and gradual process. In the absence of stress stimulus, scar takes months to fill in a small space.[32] In postoperative scars in fingers, scar elongates in response to tension, allowing an average gain in range of motion of three degrees a week.[46] Conversely, gradual shortening and increasing density of scar occurs by remodeling, as has been reported in many types of scar in which myofibroblasts are found.

Time Factors Governing Ability of Scar to Change Shape

Because changes in the shape of scar occur only by remodeling, it follows that two conditions must be met for these changes to occur. First, *there must be a sufficient population of active connective tissue cells to remodel the tissue.* Second, *there must be a relationship between the ability of scar to respond to stress and the relative density, stability, and size of collagen fibers that compose its fibrillar matrix.* As scar matures, it reaches a stage in which the collagen fiber architecture and the size and stability of its fibers result in a tissue that responds to stress so slowly and to such a limited degree that conservative management is often unsuccessful.

In the case of normal scar tissue, it is possible, within limits, to identify the time scar will remodel in response to applied strain. Madden, Devore, and Arem[46] compared the response to noncyclical strain of 4-week-old scar and 14-week-old scar. In each case, the scar was subjected to strain for 6 hours a day for 4 weeks. The 4-week-old scar elongated significantly, whereas the 14-week-old scar remained unaffected.

The population of fibroblasts in scar diminishes significantly between 6 and 8 weeks after wounding. Collagen turnover remains elevated for a longer period. Collagen turnover, as reflected by saline solubility studies, is highest between 3 and 9 weeks, dropping significantly in the ninth week.[52] Radioisotope studies show elevated collagen turnover for up to 16 weeks.[46] However, the elevated turnover rate does not result in remodeling of scar stressed at 14 weeks. This may be a function of either the reduced population of connective tissue cells, or the development of a sufficiently strong collagen fiber architecture to resist the applied strain. Whatever the mechanisms might be, Madden, DeVore, and Arem's study suggests that normal scar no longer responds to therapeutic application of tension after 14 weeks.[46]

In many situations, scar tissue remains active indefinitely, and time factors do not appear to be useful in predicting whether the scar will respond to treatment. Persistently active scars have been reported in the plaque of Peyronie's disease, in fibrosed intrinsic muscles of the hand, in the transverse band in carpal tunnel syndrome, in fibrous tissue around breast implants, and in extensive burn scars.[53] Persistent, high gradients of metabolites acting as chronic irritants are common to all of these diagnoses. One of the predominant factors causing continuous activity may be the tension produced by the myofibroblasts. High turnover rates and scar hypertrophy occur almost indefinitely in these circumstances.[41,60] Hypertrophic burn scars continue to actively harden and shorten for years.[60] In these cases, the scar tissue may also continue to respond to therapeutic application of stress as long as it remains active.

Biologic Behavior of Ligaments and Capsules

In the mature vertebrate, normal ligaments and capsules are comprised chiefly of densely packed collagen fibers with a sparse population of connective tissue cells. The cells are predominantly fibrocytes, indicating low activity levels in producing connective tissue components. Vascularity varies with the exact structure but is always sparse.[65] This histologic picture suggests that the tissue is stable, offering little chance for tissue changes in strength, length, or extensibility. Whether remodeling occurs in dense connective tissues of normal adults, and how inflammatory states affect that remodeling, is the focus of this section.

Noting some basic differences in the arrangement of collagen fibers between tendons, capsules, and ligaments is useful. In tendons collagen bundles are closely packed and roughly parallel. In capsules there is a very loose weave of interlaced collagen fibers with less parallel alignment. Extensibility of the capsule depends upon the individual fibers remaining free to slide over one another.[24,65,66] The architecture of ligaments lies between that of capsules and tendons. Normal function of ligaments is dependent upon freedom of the constituent collagen bundles.

Loss of range of motion in a joint may be due to two distinct types of change in the capsules or ligaments. First, loss of mobility between adjacent fibers may limit extensibility of the tissue, despite the persistence of fibers of normal length. Interfibrillar mobility may be limited by several means: by attachment of new collagen fibers; by increased friction due to increased attachment of proteoglycans to the fibers; or by loss of water and unattached proteoglycans, which some consider to have a significant lubricating function. Second, the fibers may be shortened by remodeling. For detailed descriptions of these two distinct hypothetical mechanisms the reader is referred to Akeson and associates,[5] Bornstein and Sage,[48] Frank and colleagues,[65] Brand,[66] and Le Lous and co-workers.[67]

SUMMARY

The mechanical behavior of dense connective tissue including tendons, ligaments, and capsules, is influenced by the physical properties of collagen. The building block of collagen microfibrils is the tropocollagen molecule. Tropocollagen is a crystalline structure, with highly ordered units of chemically bonded atoms. This physical arrangement of atoms accounts in part for the stability and strength of the dense connective tissue. Ground substance, consisting of glycosaminoglycans, proteoglycans, and glycoproteins, also contributes to the stability and strength of dense connective tissue.

Stress as a physical stimulus plays a significant role in the formation and maintenance of collagen in dense connective tissue. An increase in stress increases collagen production and organization, whereas a decrease in stress causes a decrease and disorganization of collagen fibers in tendon, thereby producing a weakened connective tissue. Stress/strain curves are used to study the mechanical behavior of tendons and ligaments. *Recovery* is the return of a tendon to its original length following the removal of stress prior to rupture. *Creep* is the slow elongation of a tendon in response to constant or repeated stress, and is transient when seen within physiologic limits of strain, between 1 percent and 3 percent, and below 37°C. Temperatures between 37°C and 40°C affect the viscoelastic properties of tendon; as the temperature increases, creep increases. Increasing the temperature above 40°C increases the chance that permanent damage will be done to the dense connective tissue. However, stress applied at 45°C can actually result in reduced damage if strains of 2.6 percent or less are applied for short periods (less than 1 hour). Initially, temporary straightening of collagen fibers involves stretching out the "crimp form" at the level of the collagen fascicle. However, once a tendon reaches the linear region of the stress/strain curve, the collagen can be permanently lengthened only by denaturing and weakening the fibers, which occurs when the tissue is subjected to excessive strain and temperature.

There is a sequence of cellular and biologic events that take place during dense connective tissue repair. The development of fibrosis is usually preceded by an accumulation of inflammatory cells within a tissue. Activated macrophages stimulate the migration of fibroblasts into the area, resulting in an increase in collagen synthesis. An understanding of both acute, post-traumatic fibrosis and chronic inflammation is necessary for the successful clinical management of fibrotic adhesions.

The clinician must have a clear understanding of what scar tissue consists of during each stage of development, and how it responds to treatment. Scar tissue changes in composition from the newly formed to the final quiescent stage of the mature scar.

Day 2–4. Scar tissue composition: A clot forms in the wound. Connective tissue cells infiltrate the area, with macrophages attracting fibroblasts. In this initial stage of scarring, the tissue is very fragile and easily disrupted due to the predominance of weak and unstable type III collagen. Adhesion is by cellular attachments, and stretching of the scar causes tearing of the cells.

Day 5–21. Fibroplasia and contraction: This stage is very cellular. The scar increases in bulk due to fibroplasia, with an increase in the quantity of collagen fibers. This is a highly active stage of collagen synthesis and degradation. Treatment to increase range of motion and function of a joint can be very effective during this stage due to the collagen remodeling process.

Day 21–60. Consolidation: The scar contains well-organized collagen. The tissue gradually changes from predominantly cellular to fibrous, with a large amount of collagen fibers. There is a gradual increase in strength of the scar due to an increase in stable covalent bonding. During this time there will be a continuous decrease in the ability of the scar to respond to treatment.

Day 60–360. Maturation: Type I collagen fibers are compact and large. The fully mature scar is only 3 percent cellular and almost totally collagenous. Response to treatment is poor, and hypertrophic and keloid scar tissue will worsen when stretched in multiple directions.

Tension controls both the direction of collagen fiber alignment and the formation of collagen into large bundles. The cells, glycosaminoglycans, and collagen architecture are affected by the direction and magnitude of physical stress applied to a tissue. Scar strength is a function of the intensity and duration of stress applied. Scar strength increases with the increase of collagen volume, stable chemical bonding, and aggregation of collagen fibers along lines of stress. The change in shape of scar tissue by remodeling is a slow and gradual process. If remodeling is to occur, there must be a sufficient population of active connective tissue cells to remodel the tissue. In addition, the scar must be malleable enough for therapeutic stress to stimulate remodeling.

REFERENCES

1. Rigby, BJ: The effect of mechanical extension upon the thermal stability of collagen. Biochim Biophys Acta 79:634–636, 1964.
2. Betsch, DF and Baer, E: Structure and mechanical properties of rat tail tendon. Biorheology 17:83–94, 1980.
3. Gay, S, Gay, RE, and Miller, EJ: The collagens of the joint. Arthritis Rheum 23:937–941, 1980.
4. Baur, PS and Parks, DH: The myofibroblast anchoring strand: The fibronectin connection in wound healing and the possible loci of collagen fibril assembly. J Trauma 23:853–862, 1983.
5. Akeson, WH, Amiel, D, and Woo, S L-Y: Immobility effects on synovial joints: The pathomechanics of joint contractures. Biorheology 17:95–110, 1980.
6. Amiel, D, Akeson, WH, Harwood, FL, et al: Stress deprivation effect on metabolic turnover of the medial collateral ligament collagen. Clin Orthop 172:265–270, 1983.
7. Meyers, ER, Mow, VC, Roth, V, et al: Transactions of 27th annual meeting. Orthopaedic Research Society 6:21, 1981.
8. Hooley, CJ and Cohen, RE: A model for the creep behavior of tendon. International Journal of Biological Macromolecules 1:123–132, 1979, and personal communication, 1981.
9. Hooley, CJ, McCrum, NG, and Cohen, RE: The viscoelastic deformation of tendon. J Biomech 13:521–528, 1980.
10. Yannas, IV and Huang, C: Fracture of tendon collagen. Journal of Polymer Science 10:577–584, 1972.
11. Madden, JW and Peacock, EE: Studies on the biology of collagen during wound healing: III. Dynamic metabolism of scar collagen and remodeling of dermal wounds. Ann Surg 174:511–520, 1971.
12. Viidik, A, Danielsen, CC, and Oxlund, H: On fundamental and phenomenological models, structure and mechanical properties of collagen, elastin and glycosaminoglycan complexes. Biorheology 19:437–451, 1982.
13. Woo, S L-Y, Matthews, JV, Akeson, WH, et al: Connective tissue response to immobility. Arthritis Rheum 18:257–264, 1975.
14. Enwemeka, CS: Ultrastructural changes induced by cast immobilization in the isolated soleus tendon. APTA Annual Conference Abstract R-123, Anaheim, CA, June 24–28, 1990, p 65.
15. Sanjeevi, R, Somanathan, N, and Ramaswamy, D: Viscoelastic model for collagen fibers. J Biomech 15:181–183, 1982.
16. Lehman, JF, Masock, AJ, Warren, CG, et al: Effect of therapeutic temperatures on tendon extensibility. Arch Phys Med Rehabil 50:481–487, 1970.
17. Warren, CG, Lehman, JF, and Koblanski, JN: Elongation of rat tail tendon: Effect of load and temperature. Arch Phys Med Rehabil 52:465–484, 1971.
18. Rigby, BJ, Hirai, N, and Spikes, JD: The mechanical behavior of rat tail tendon. J Gen Physiol 43:265–283, 1959.

19. Nordschow, CD: Aspects of aging in human collagen: An exploratory thermoelastic study. Exp Molec Pathol 5:350–373, 1966.
20. Ellis, DG: Temperature effects on the dynamic and transient mechanical behavior of tendon. Technical report No. 11. Orthotics Research Project, Dept PM&R, Medical School. Univ of Michigan, Ann Arbor, MI, May, 1970.
21. Warren, CG, Lehman, JF, and Koblanski, JN: Heat and stretch procedures: An evaluation using rat tail tendon. Arch Phys Med Rehabil 57:122–126, 1976.
22. Dunn, MG and Silver, FH: Viscoelastic behavior of human connective tissues: Relative contribution of viscous and elastic components. Connect Tissue Res 12:59–70, 1983.
23. Dunn, MG, Silver, FH, and Swann, DA: Mechanical analysis of hypertrophic scar tissue: Structural basis for apparent increased rigidity. J Invest Dermatol 84:9–13, 1985.
24. Fung, YC: Biomechanics: Mechanical properties of Living Tissues. Springer-Verlag, New York, 1981, p 433.
25. Van Brocklin, JD and Ellis, DG: A study of the mechanical behavior of toe extensor tendons under applied stress. Arch Phys Med Rehabil 46:369–370, 1965.
26. Frankei, VH and Nordin, M: Basic biomechanics of the skeletal system. Lea & Febiger, Philadelphia, 1980, pp 87–110.
27. Viidik, A: Interdependence between structure and function in collagenous tissues. In Viidik, A, and Vuust, J (eds). Biology of Collagen. Academic Press, London, 1980, pp 257–280.
28. Diamant, J, Keller, A, Baer, E, et al: Collagen: Ultrastructure and its relation to mechanical properties as a function of aging. Proc Soc London [Biol] 180:293–315, 1972.
29. LaBan, MM: Collagen tissue: Implications or its response to stress in vitro. Arch Phys Med Rehabil 43:461–466, 1962.
30. Jones, CW: Physical changes in isolated human collagen subjected to clinical dosages of ultrasound. Master's thesis, Department of Biology, Midwestern State University, Wichita Falls, TX May, 1976.
31. Neviasier, JS: Adhesive capsulitis of the shoulder: A study of pathologic findings in periarthritis of the shoulder. J Bone Joint Surg (B) 27:211–222, 1945.
32. Hunt, TK, Banda, MJ, and Silver, IA: Cell interactions in post-traumatic fibrosis. Clin Symp 114:128–149, 1985.
33. Forrest, L: Current concepts in soft connective tissue wound healing. Br J Surg 70:133:146, 1983.
34. Madden, JW and Smith, HC: The rate of collagen synthesis and deposition in dehisced and resutured wounds. Surg Gynecol Obstet 136:487–493, 1970.
35. Neuman, Z, Ben-Hur, N, and Tritsch, IE: Induction of tendon sheath formation by the implantation of silicon tubes in rabbits. Br J Plast Surg: 313–316, 1965.
36. Tsukamoto, Y., Helsel, WE, and Wahl, SM: Macrophage production of fibronectin, a chemoattractant for fibroblasts. J Immunol 127:673–678, 1981.
37. Rennard, SI, Bitterman, PB, and Crystal, RG: Current concepts of the pathogenesis of fibrosis: Lessons from pulmonary fibrosis. Myofibroblasts and the biology of connective tissue. Alan R Liss, New York, 1984, pp 359–377.
38. Farkas, LG, McCain, WG, Sweeny, P, et al: An experimental study of the changes following silastic rod preparation of new tendon sheath and subsequent tendon grafting. Br J Surg 55:1149–1158, 1973.
39. Alitalo, K and Vaheri, A: Pericellular matrix in malignant transformations. Adv Cancer Res 37:111–158, 1982.
40. Kirscher, CW and Speer, DP: Microvascular changes in Dupuytren's contracture. J Hand Surg 9A:58–62, 1984.
41. Caffee, HH: External compression for the prevention of scar capsule contracture: A preliminary report. Ann Plast Surg 8:453–457, 1988.
42. Baur, PS, Larson, DL, and Stacey, TR: The observation of myofibroblasts in hypertrophic scars. Surg Gynecol Obstet 141:22–26, 1975.
43. Peacock, EE: Wound Repair, ed 3. WB Saunders, Philadelphia, 1984.
44. Wilkerson, GB: Inflammation in connective tissue: Etiology and management. Athletic Training 20:298–301, 1985.
45. Levenson, SM, Greever, EF, Crowly, LV, et al: The healing of rat skin wounds. Ann Surg 161:293–308, 1965.
46. Madden, JW, DeVore, G, and Arem, AJ: A rational postoperative management program for metacarpophalangeal joint implant arthroplasty. J Hand Surg 2:358–366, 1977.
47. Anderson, JC: Glycoproteins of the connective tissue matrix. International Review of Connective Tissue Research 7:251–322, 1976.
48. Bornstein, P and Sage, H: Structurally distinct collagen types. Ann Rev Biochem 49:957–1003, 1980.
49. Frank, C, Woo, S L-Y, Amiel, D, et al: Medial collateral ligament healing: A multidisciplinary assessment in rabbits. Am J Sports Med 11:379–389, 1983.
50. Hernandez-Jaurequi, P, Esperabsa-Garcia, C, and Gonzales-Angulo, A: Morphology of the connective tissue grown in response to implanted silicone rubber: A light and electron microscope study. Surg 75:631–637, 1974.

51. Madden, JW and Peacock, EE: Studies on the biology of collagen during wound healing. I. Rate of collagen synthesis and deposition in cutaneous wounds of the rat. Surg 64:288–294, 1968.
52. Forrester, JC, Zederfeldt, BH, Hayes, TYL, et al: Tape closed and sutured wounds: A comparison by tensiometry and scanning electron microscopy. Br J Surg 57:729:737, 1970.
53. Rudolph, R: Contraction and the control of contraction. World J surg 4:279–287, 1980.
54. Bryant, WM: Wound Healing. Clinical Symp 29(3), 1977.
55. Peacock, EE and Van Winkle, W: Wound Repair, ed 2. WB Saunders, Philadelphia, 1976.
56. Arem, AJ and Madden, JW: Effects of stress on healing wounds: I. Intermittent noncyclical tension. J Surg Res 20:93–102, 1976.
57. Flint, MH: The basis of the histological demonstration of tension in collagen. In Longacre, JJ (ed): The Ultrastructure of Collagen. Charles C Thomas, Springfield, IL, 1976, pp 60–66.
58. Magonne, T, DeWitt, MT, Handeley, CJ, et al: In vitro response of chondrocytes to mechanical loading: The effect of short term mechanical tension. Connect Tissue Res 12:98–109, 1984.
59. Slack, C, Flint, MH, and Thompson, BM: The effect of tensional load on isolated embryonic chick tendons in organ culture. Connect Tissue Res 12:229–274, 1984.
60. Longacre, JJ (ed): The Ultrastructure of Collagen. Springfield, IL, Charles C Thomas, 1976.
61. Brody, GS, Peng, STJ, and Landel RE: The etiology of hypertrophic scar contracture: Another view. Plast Reconstr Surg 67:673–684, 1977.
62. Goldstein, WM and Barmada, R: Early mobilization of rabbit medial collateral ligament repairs: Biologic and histologic study. Arch Phys Med Rehabil 65:239–242, 1984.
63. Kirscher, CW and Shetlar, MR: Microvasculature in hypertrophic scars and the effects of pressure. J Trauma 19:757–764, 1979.
64. Larson, DL, Abston, S, and Dobrkovsky, M, et al: The prevention and correlation of burn scar contracture and hypertrophy. Shriners Burns Institute, U of Texas, Med Br, Galveston, TX, 1973.
64a. Madden, JW: Personal communication, April, 1989.
65. Frank C, Amiel, D, Woo, A L-Y, Akeson, W: Normal ligament properties and ligament healing. Clin Orthop Rel Res 196:15–25, 1985.
66. Brand, P: Clinical Mechanics of the Hand. CV Mosby Co, St. Louis, MO, 1985.
67. Le Lous, M, Ailain, J-C, Cohen-Solal, L, et al: Hydrothermal isometric tension curves from different connective tissues, role of collagen genetic types and noncollagenous components. Connect Tissue Res 11:199–206, 1983.
68. Alberts, B, Bray, D, Lewis, J, et al: Molecular Biology of the Cell. Garland, New York, 1983, p 694.
69. Jungueira, LC, Carneiro, J, and Long, JA: Basic Histology, ed 6. Los Altos, CA, Lange Medical Publications, 1989, pp 92–104.

CHAPTER 2

Remodeling of Dense Connective Tissue in Normal Adult Tissues

Gordon S. Cummings, M.A., P.T.
Larry J. Tillman, Ph.D.

Dense connective tissue is composed of cells (fibroblasts, macrophages, mast cells); fibers (collagen, elastin); and ground substance (glycosaminoglycans, proteoglycans, glycoproteins). Collagen fibers provide strength and maintain the form of tendon, ligaments, bone, and skin. The strength and shape of these structures can be changed by remodeling of the dense connective tissue (DCT), which occurs at different rates in the different tissues. This chapter reviews the effects of remodeling on tissue strength and joint motion. The conditions that stimulate these changes are identified, and the therapeutic implications of these findings for prevention of injury and for treatment are discussed.

COLLAGEN AND GLYCOSAMINOGLYCANS (GAGs) TURNOVER RATES IN NORMAL, NONIMMOBILIZED TISSUE

The turnover rates of collagen and ground substance are significant because these rates determine the speed at which connective tissue changes in strength and excursion. Collagen and ground substance turnover enables DCT to reform in response to differing conditions of stress, excursion, or immobilization. The process of restructuring is called *remodeling*. For example, DCT remodeling is rapid during growth periods, allowing joint capsules and other structures to increase in size and strength. DCT also changes in response to new activity levels, such as beginning a new sport or working in a new job with different load demands. From a clinical perspective one

45

might ask two questions: First, is the process of remodeling that is causing strength changes the same as the remodeling causing changes in tissue excursion? Second, is the rate of turnover fast enough to cause clinically significant limitations of movement within time periods for which joints are normally immobilized?

The static histologic appearance of DCT is deceptive, inasmuch as this tissue is continuously remodeled at various rates. Neuberger and Slack[1] found constant collagen turnover in bone, skin, and tendon of young and adult rats. Madden and Peacock[2] also found collagen turnover in skin of adult rats. The turnover rate in all tissues slows as the animal matures, although it remains fairly high in bone but lower in skin and tendon. Svobada and colleagues[3] reported that the relative turnover rate of collagen is progressively higher in order for rat skin, gingiva, and molar periodontal ligaments. They also found a trend for fibril diameter to be in inverse relation to the rate of turnover of GAGs and collagen. Plaas and Sandy[4] made an additional observation, explaining one factor in the reduced rate of remodeling in adults. They found a progressive decrease in the percent of synthesized proteoglycans that became link-stabilized in the matrix of cultures of chondrocytes from donor dogs of increasing age. The important principle emerging from these studies is that remodeling of the DCT continues at all ages. The above studies suggest that in the mature animal, remodeling proceeds at rates that are characteristic of the tissue, age, and species of the animal. However, as will become apparent from the following discussion, rates of remodeling are dramatically accelerated by changes in the stress experience of the tissues or by the presence of inflammation. Understanding these changes helps to explain how injuries occur and how loss or increase in tissue excursion is regulated.

Strength Changes in Dense Connective Tissue

Noyes and associates[5] measured the strength and compliance of the anterior cruciate ligaments of monkeys in response to differing degrees of activity. They used newly captured, late adolescent, and adult rhesus monkeys. After 8 weeks of immobilization in full body casts, the strength of the anterior cruciate ligaments was 61 percent of normal, as measured by the load at rupture. Breaking strain, the percent increase in length at rupture, was unaffected. There was a 40 percent increase in compliance of the ligaments, reflecting significant changes in the extracellular matrix, probably including collagen remodeling. Resumption of activity resulted in a reversal of the changes in the ligaments. When the monkeys were allowed 20 weeks of unrestricted activity in 1.8 × 2.3-m cages following the immobilization, the breaking strength returned to 86 percent of normal values, and compliance returned to normal. Thus Noyes and associates showed that remodeling significantly affects the strength of normal ligaments, in response to changes in the stress and excursion to which they are subjected.

The study by Noyes and associates[5] does not explain why 20 weeks of activity failed to result in full recovery of breaking strength. Because Noyes and associates are often cited to support rehabilitation for more than 5 months, an explanation of why 20 weeks was not sufficient for full recovery is important. Their finding, in fact, may be a misleading result of the research design. Their results may have occurred because stress on the ligaments from activity in the cages is much less than in the wild, where monkeys commonly leap distances of 10 m. Recently captured monkeys were used in the study, and these stress levels may be reflected in the values of the normals. If Noyes' and associates normal values were tested at the beginning of the experiment, they were not true controls for the effect of cast immobilization. The cage confinement during the 20 weeks of activity caused a marked reduction of stress, and may account for the lack of recovery to the previous level of breaking strength. To test this effect, Noyes and associates[5] studied failure load and compliance of the anterior cruciate ligaments of 58 monkeys that had been confined in cages for 10 to 218 weeks. They found a linear correlation between duration of confinement and changes in stress/strain behavior of the anterior cruciate ligaments. For each week of captivity, there was an average loss of 0.17 kg breaking load and a loss of 0.056 cm/kg force in energy absorbed. The linear correlation confirms that the strength of DCT is remodeled to match the stress levels the animals experience. Further research, therefore, is necessary to confirm how many weeks of rehabilitation are necessary to restore normal cruciate strength.

Findings by Noyes and associates[5] of DCT changes in ligament are mirrored in Maggone's studies of tendon. Maggone and co-workers[6] concluded that the structure of tendon "is dependent on the continued maintenance of functional loading of the tissues and that any alteration in the degree or type of physiological loading is followed by changes in cellular metabolism, matrix morphology and functional capacity." Enwemeka's[7] recent observations of stress-modulated organization changes in the collagen fibers of the soleus tendon support this important principle. Enwemeka immobilized the hind limb of nontraumatized rabbits so that the soleus tendon was slack and deprived of stress. Electron microscopy showed that within 4 weeks the soleus tendon collagen became grossly disorganized. The tissue became so fragile that specimens were difficult to fix for study. When the hind limb was recast with the soleus under tension, the tissue reorganized within 4 weeks. The architectural changes in the collagen fibers observed by Enwemeka present one clear mechanism explaining the changes in strength of DCT in response to varying load experience.

CLINICAL IMPLICATIONS: STRENGTHENING DENSE CONNECTIVE TISSUE

Information from the above studies explains why DCT injuries can be prevented by gradual increases in activity levels for individuals training for a sport, industrial work, or military maneuver. Time must be given for the DCT to remodel in proportion with the increased demands of the new situation. Conversely, a gradual loss of strength during periods of inactivity can be expected. The clinician must appreciate that DCT weakening is especially critical during the rehabilitation of individuals who have marked disuse atrophy secondary to paralysis or long-term bed rest. Tabary and co-workers[8] found that the cat soleus that had been immobilized for 4 weeks ruptured at only 20 percent of normal, passive strength. Programs designed to increase the strength of an individual must increase the strength of the DCT as well as that of the muscle. Muscle contraction strength may increase faster than strength of DCT, thereby increasing the chance of injury. Future surveys of the types of injuries that occur under different programs may help to identify the various rates of change in the different tissues. It is hoped that future research will identify protocols specific to remodeling DCT or muscle.

Remodeling eventually protects tissue by increasing its strength, but, paradoxically, the process itself often involves a period of increased susceptibility to injury. The remodeling process involves not only disposition of new collagen, but also degradation of preexisting tissue. In programs that involve intensive training or work, it is important to consider that degradation often results in temporary weakening of a tissue. Overuse injuries, including stress fractures and tendon ruptures, have been prevented in military training by planned reduction of exertion during peak periods of DCT remodeling during a training program.[9,10] Similar reductions in the incidence of overuse injuries among industrial workers might also be possible but await future research.

Atrophy Versus Contracture of Dense Connective Tissue

There may be two distinct processes of remodeling of DCT. One process results in atrophy of ligaments and tendons; the other results in limited motion or joint stiffness. Ligament and tendon atrophy can occur without shortening or fibrotic adhesions in the tissue as no contractures were reported in the monkeys that had been confined in cages.[5] In the group of monkeys that were immobilized in plaster casts, however, contractures of the joints developed at the end of the 8 weeks of immobilization. These contractures would certainly have involved adaptive shortening of muscle, with an unknown contribution from changes in the DCT. Three of 11 monkeys, however, had residual contractures of the elbows and hips at the end of the 20 weeks of free activity. The persistence of contractures in these three cases suggests the presence of DCT contractures. Studies by Noyes and associates[5] show that different conditions stimulate different types of remodeling. When the monkeys were caged, which reduced the stress to the tissues but allowed full joint motion, strength was reduced but not joint excursion. By contrast, cast immobilization, which reduced both stress and excursion of the joints, resulted in loss of both strength and excursion of the DCT.

The morphologic observations by Enwemeka[7] suggest two types of changes occurring in the DCT of the cast immobilized monkeys. As previously mentioned, the gross disorganization of unstressed collagen bundles after 4 weeks of immobilization accounts for the weakness and fragility of the observed tissues. Disorganization may represent the initial reaction in the tissue. Given additional time, a second stage of remodeling possibly sets in, resulting in consolidation of the randomly aligned fibers into a shorter structure, resulting in contracture. The hypothesis of second-stage consolidation is supported by the following citations.

Studies by Videman[11] and Finsterbush and colleagues[12] make two important contributions to understanding the remodeling characteristics of DCT in response to stress deprivation. First, they showed with immobilization studies of rabbits that *the types of changes discussed above can be generalized to all of the DCT structures at the joint, including the articular cartilage, capsule, synovium, and ligaments.* Second, their histologic studies confirm that *there is a time-dependent transition between initial disorganization of the tissue and subsequent reorganization with restricted motion.* In response to cast immobilization, cellular responses occur within days, followed after 2 weeks by progressive disorganization of the collagen. Contracture of the DCT was found at 4 weeks in a few animals, and in all animals after 6 weeks. Reynolds[13] also found limited excursion in the DCT of the ankles of rats that had been cast immobilized for 6 weeks, but not at 4 weeks.[13] Interarticular adhesions were found by Finsterbush and co-workers[11] after 8 weeks.

There is some difficulty in interpreting the histologic changes reported above.

Does the observation of tissue changes correlate well with clinically significant contractures, which require intensive care? Partial answers are supplied in parallel studies by Langenskiold and co-workers.[14] When animals that had been immobilized for up to 6 weeks were freed, motion was regained within 3 weeks, thus indicating that the changes seen histologically had not reached significant stability. However, after 7 weeks of immobilization there was an abrupt transition in the histologic changes, reflected by the fact that the animals no longer regained full motion of the joints even after 7 weeks of free activity. Changes are similar to those found in contractures, of uninjured capsules which require intensive rehabilitation only after 7 weeks of immobilization.

CLINICAL IMPLICATIONS: THE EFFECTS OF IMMOBILIZATION ON VARIOUS TISSUE TYPES

The relation between duration of immobilization and type of tissue response is clinically relevant. There is general agreement that rates of change are slower in humans than in small animals, justifying an estimate that immobilization of noninflamed human joints does not cause DCT contractures in less than 6 or 7 weeks. Beyond this time, DCT contractures become more common. Such time factors may help in setting clinical priorities and goals. For example, passive range of motion exercises for someone with a flaccid paralysis and normal joints can be deferred for several weeks without fear of DCT contractures. On the other hand, as will be shown later, this decision might lead to severe DCT contractures in a patient with accelerated rates of remodeling due to trauma.

As can be expected from the tissue-specific turnover rates, different structures remodel at different rates. Tardieu and associates[15] reported shortening of stress-deprived tendon and noted that remodeling occurred at different rates in different portions of the tendon. They surgically shortened the bones of rats and found that the musculotendinous unit shortened in response. They compared the amount of shortening of the exposed tendon, the tendon that was buried in the muscle belly, and the muscle fibers and found that up to 75 percent of the shortening of the total unit was the result of shortening of the tendon, as opposed to the muscle fibers. The predominant changes in tendon length occurred at the musculotendinous junction in the buried portion of the tendon. Apparently the turnover rate of collagen is much higher at the musculotendinous junction than in the exposed tendon.

Shortening of tendon is another cause of joint contracture. The mismatch between rates of lengthening of muscle and tendon can also cause problems during lengthening. In some cases, the tendon grows more rapidly than the muscle, resulting in excessively long tendons, with short muscle bellies and poor function.

One factor that seems to determine whether shortening occurs during remodeling is whether the tissue is placed in a shortened or stress-deprived position during immobilization. This factor was elegantly illustrated in Enwemeka's[7] study and is also supported by a study using human subjects. Flowers and Pheasant[16] investigated the effect of 6 weeks of plaster cast immobilization on the fingers of uninjured subjects. After removal of the casts, all fingers were initially limited in motion and were stiff, but full range of motion was restored by passive exercise within several minutes. Since motion was restored so easily, the stiffness could not have been due to change in the collagen architecture or length. The absence of DCT contractures in these subjects is probably a function of the position of immobilization. Flowers and Pheasant casted the fingers in extension, where the extensor hood can be expected to slide proximally without folding, the volar and lateral tissues are elongated, and only the dorsal portion of the rather vestigial capsule is folded. Remodeling occurred in response to immobilization and may have caused atrophy of the major ligaments. The transient stiffness may have been due to a reduced rate of proteoglycan synthesis and impaired rate of aggregation of proteoglycans, such as reported by Palmoski and Brandt[17] after 6 weeks of cast immobilization of the knees of dogs. However, all the major ligaments were in a lengthened position during immobilization, so no shortening occurred.

The lack of contractures found in Flowers and Pheasant's[16] study suggests that in other cases too, DCT contractures can be minimized or prevented by choosing immobilization positions that place significant structures in their lengthened position. Careful attention to the details of the DCT anatomy should suggest optimal positions for many joints.

The *degree of rigidity* of immobilization is another factor that may affect the tendency of DCT remodeling to result in shortening. Miura[18] reported limitation of extension of the proximal interphalangeal joint as a result of a band of DCT in the volar fat pads of children and teenagers, whose interphalangeal joints had been held in flexion for periods of 6 months to several years. There was no history of pain, and active motion occurred within the limitations of the fibrous band. In these cases, despite very prolonged periods of restricted motion, the joint capsules and volar plate did not remodel to the shortened positions in which the finger was held. Full range of motion was restored in most cases by sectioning the DCT band, without need to cut the volar plate or collateral ligaments. Thus active motion, even though restricted in range, may be sufficient to prevent shortening of DCT.

Physical therapists have traditionally used quadriceps femoris muscle setting exercises for patients in long leg casts to prevent muscle atrophy. The above studies[7,14,16,18] suggest that the use of isometric exercises for all immobilized muscle groups may significantly reduce atrophy of both muscle and DCT, and may also minimize DCT contracture formation. Clinical experience tends to support the use of this stratagem at the knee. Furthermore, our clinical impression is that isometric exercises of the long finger and wrist muscles minimize DCT contractures of uninjured wrist capsules in a person with a forearm cast.

Summary: Changes in Mature, Nontraumatized DCT

All DCT remodels to match changes in stress and motion. With changes only in activity level, these changes are continuous and gradual. The remodeling can be responsible for overuse injuries when appropriate pacing is not introduced into the training regimen. Changes in extensibility and length occur independently of changes in compliance and breaking strength. When nontraumatized tissue is immobilized in a shortened position, changes in architecture result in persistent contractures of joints only after approximately 7 weeks.

IMMOBILIZATION OF INTACT DENSE CONNECTIVE TISSUES IN A TRAUMATIZED LIMB

The rate and extent of changes in DCT are accelerated by a history of trauma. The condition of trauma, therefore, has a strong influence on the types of problems seen clinically. For this reason, data on post-traumatic problems are addressed as a separate unit. Most experimental evidence on the nature of DCT changes comes from experiments involving trauma to the immobilized limb or tissue. In the most common protocol, the limb was immobilized by placing a pin through the bones adjacent to the joint. There was no direct surgical trauma to the periarticular tissues studied. However, as Hunt and associates[19] showed, serofibrinous exudate from the incision sites is sufficient to stimulate rapid fibroblast proliferation and remodeling in the articular tissues. Therefore, all such studies are classified as post-traumatic. In other procedures reviewed below, various surgical manipulations were performed directly on the involved tissues. The common condition of the following studies is that they all involve post-traumatic immobilization.

Remodeling

Remodeling is a biologic process, and the rate of remodeling is presumed to be a function of the density and activity level of fibroblasts. The greater the density of cells and the higher their activity level, the faster the remodeling. Knowing how these factors compare between immobilized normal tissue and tissue that has been traumatized prior to immobilization might explain how these conditions affect the tissues. Unfortunately, there are too few data to make quantitative comparisons between the amount of fibroblast proliferation in post-traumatic and nontraumatic immobilized tissues.

Increases in density and activity of fibroblasts after nontraumatic immobilization have been reported by Enwemeka,[7] Finsterbush and colleagues,[12] and Langenskiold and co-workers.[14] Tipton and associates[20] measured the space between fibroblasts in tendon and found that this was reduced when the tendon had been immobilized.[20] The reduced distance may have been due to reduction in the size of the collagen fiber bundle, as they concluded, or there may have been an increased density of cells in the tissue. Although no quantitative data were reported in any of these studies, a trend is evident.

There is even more sparce data on the increases in cell density or activity level after trauma. However, the descriptions of healing tissue imply a much greater increase in number and activity level of fibroblasts after injury than after immobilization without injury. In new scar tissue, the cell population is estimated to be about 30 percent of the tissue volume. These changes are represented by Figures 2–1 and 2–2 (see also Fig. 10–4). How much change occurs in tissues that are bathed in serofibrinous exudate but not directly traumatized is unknown.

Increased cellular density was reported in studies of animal medial collateral ligaments that were cut and repaired. The joints were immobilized for 2 weeks, after which separate groups were subjected to 6 weeks of continued immobilization, or to free activity, or to treadmill exercise. At the end of the eighth week, cellularity was highest in the continuously immobilized ligaments.[7,20,21] The increased cellularity may reflect an interaction to which both the initial trauma and the immobilization contributed.

The observation of cellular density alone is a limited predictor of rates of remodeling, because the level of cellular activity has been shown to vary significantly. Plaas and Sandy[4] showed that in explants of articular cartilage, proteoglycan synthesis was six times greater in tissue from 6-week-old dogs than in tissue from 50-week-old dogs,

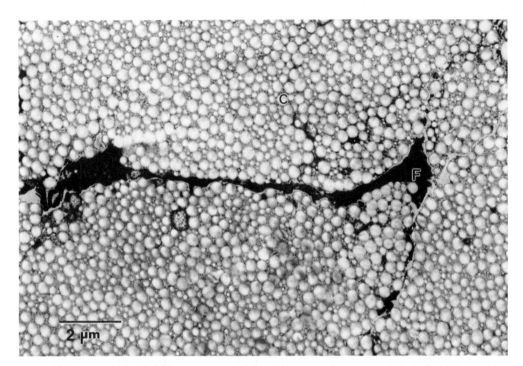

FIGURE 2–1. Normal adult rabbit Achilles tendon showing a cross section of collagen fibers. The compact, homogenous arrangement of large and small fibers (C) and the compact fibroblast (F) are shown (magnification × 11,650). (Courtesy of CS Enwemeka, P.T., Ph.D., University of Miami, FL.)

despite similarity in the histologic appearance of the tissues. The cell density in the explants of immature cartilage was only twice that of mature cartilage. These data suggest that chondrocytes in immature tissue are significantly more active than are chondrocytes in mature tissue. The difference in chondrocyte activity occurs despite the similar morphologic appearance of the tissue at different ages. Videman[11] and Finsterbush and colleagues[12] found increased metabolic rates of fibroblasts in response to immobilization of the nontraumatized limb. Hunt and associates[19] also found both increased numbers and increased metabolic activity of these cells in response to trauma. Whether the effects of trauma and immobilization are additive is not clear. Such an effect would account for the faster changes seen in post-traumatic immobilization. Clarification of the roles of cell density and metabolic activity under nontraumatic and post-traumatic immobilization may have important clinical implications.

Another factor determining the type of remodeling occurring in DCT is the *type* of cell present. Rudolph[22] suggested the necessity of making a distinction between contractures caused by active contraction by myofibroblasts and those caused by collagen remodeling in response to passive positioning. Her electron microscopic studies of DCT in pin-immobilized rabbit knees failed to demonstrate the presence of myofibroblasts. Her finding demonstrated that contractures can form in the capsules and ligaments after a few weeks of post-traumatic immobilization without the contractile mechanism provided by myofibroblasts.

Myofibroblasts on the other hand, have been found in the DCT of many contractures that are difficult to manage clinically. These conditions include Dupuytren's

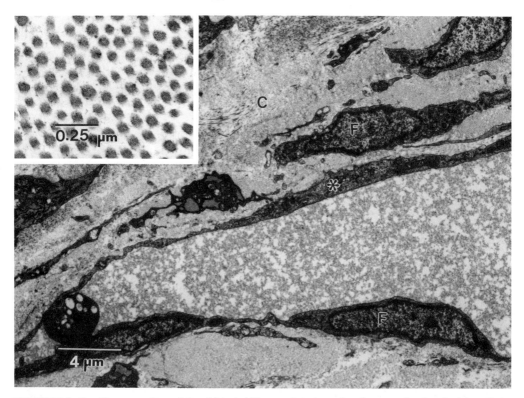

FIGURE 2–2. Regenerating adult rabbit Achilles tendon (sample taken proximal to incision site) that was surgically transected, sutured, and allowed to heal while immobilized by a cast for 21 days. The nuclei of numerous fibroblasts (F) reflect active synthesis associated with healing and fibrillogenesis. The asterisk indicates an elongated cytoplasmic process of a fibroblast ($\times 5660$). The insert is a high-magnification profile of collagen fibers of that tendon. Note the less well defined perimeter of the individual fibrils and the loose arrangement. This profile was magnified $\times 60,600$ to yield fiber sizes that are related to those of the normal intact tendon shown in Figure 2–1, in which magnification was only $\times 11,650$. (Courtesy of CS Enwemeka, P.T., Ph.D., University of Miami, FL.)

disease, Peyronie's disease, fibrosis of the lung, hypertrophic scar, keloid scar, and contractures of DCT around silicone implants. The clinical characteristics of these conditions suggest that the presence of myofibroblasts causes an exaggeration of the types of contractures found following remodeling in the absence of myofibroblasts. Nevasier[23] studied patients with frozen shoulders and found capsular shortening and adhesions between capsular folds. These are typical of the changes found in connective tissue remodeling, except that in those cases remodeling should stop well before actual tissue tension occurs. Nevasier found that the capsule had shortened so severely that marked tension was present. An incision in the capsule was pulled open by the tension and could not be subsequently approximated. Such tension results from the persistent, active contraction of myofibroblasts. *Progressive contraction and self-perpetuating contracture are clinical signs that myofibroblasts are present.*

CLINICAL IMPLICATIONS: POST-TRAUMATIC REMODELING IN DENSE CONNECTIVE TISSUE

Progressive, self-perpetuating contractures are important for the clinician to recognize. The initial treatment objective must be to reduce the population density and activity level of myofibroblasts. In thick and massive scars, such as large burn scars, compression bandages apparently reduce the myofibroblast contraction state and fibroblast activity by causing partial ischemia of the tissue.[24] In problems such as frozen shoulder or lateral epicondylitis, one clinical approach is to eliminate the chronic irritants that are the stimulus for continued myofibroblast presence. Only after myofibroblast activity and density have been reduced is direct treatment to denature or remodel the restricting tissue appropriate.

Changes in Glycosaminoglycans in Post-traumatic Immobilization

Akeson and co-workers[25] reported a 41 percent reduction in hyaluronic acid and a 30 percent reduction in chondroitin-sulfate four and six in the periarticular connective tissue of rabbits after 9 weeks of pin immobilization. Because degradation of GAGs was not accelerated, as shown by labeled tritium, they assumed that the loss reflected a reduced rate of synthesis. These findings were similar to those found in nontraumatized, immobilized limbs reported by others.[11,12] In contrast, Gamble and colleagues[26] reported that in rabbits pin-immobilized for 8 weeks, lactic dehydrogenase and malic dehydrogenase decreased, while lysosomal hydrolase increased. Gross and microscopic changes in the ligaments were seen as early as 2 weeks after immobilization. Thus, doubt remains about the mechanisms that cause reduced GAG concentrations in DCT after post-traumatic immobilization. The following study, however, shows that reduced GAG concentrations play important permissive or causative roles in the development of DCT contractures.

Amiel and associates[27] tested the effect of injected hyaluronic acid on both GAG content and contracture of periarticular tissues in pin-immobilized rabbits. When hyaluronic acid was injected weekly or biweekly, there was a 90 percent reduction in the loss of GAGs, and a 50 percent reduction in joint stiffness after 9 weeks of immobilization. The injected hyaluronic acid may stimulate GAG production by the tissue. It is possible, however, that the hyaluronic acid is absorbed into the tissue and acts as a core to which GAGs attach to form proteoglycans. The latter mechanism is suggested by the following two reports.

Plaas and Sandy[4] used pulse-chase radiolabeling of proteoglycans from cultured rabbit chondrocytes in an investigation of age-related GAG concentration levels, in 6- to 50-week-old rabbits. There was no correlation between age of donor and rates of proteoglycan synthesis. There was, on the other hand, an inverse relation between age of donor and the amount of proteoglycan incorporation. This inverse relation reflected the low production of link protein by the more mature cells. Low production was identified because addition of link protein to these cultures resulted in incorporation of proteoglycans into the matrix. Buckwalter and co-workers[28] showed that introduction of link protein to fetal bovine chondrocyte cultures resulted in proteoglycan aggregates which were five times longer and contained three times as many monomers per aggregate than without link protein. This proteoglycan aggregation indicated that the introduction of link protein affected not only attachments of GAGs, but enhanced development of longer hyaluronic acid cores in the aggregates. These studies suggest the possibility that hyaluronic acid injection, as performed by Amiel and associates,[27] may provide a ready-made, full-length core, thus providing more ready aggregation of GAGs and increasing the percentages of synthesized GAGs that become link-stabilized in the matrix.

CLINICAL IMPLICATIONS: PREVENTING DENSE CONNECTIVE TISSUE CONTRACTURES

Changes in the concentration and balance of GAGs have been shown to play an important role in the development of DCT contractures. Modalities of treatment that stimulate GAG production or aggregation in DCT may prove to be powerful tools for the prevention of DCT contractures. Diathermy has been shown to increase GAG levels; this modality and others should be subjected to clinical trials to determine their efficacy for prevention and treatment of contractures.

Water Content of Dense Connective Tissue in Post-traumatic Immobilization

Akeson and colleagues[29] found a 4 to 6 percent reduction in water content of periarticular tissues after 9 weeks of post-traumatic immobilization. This modest reduction in water content is not fully explained by the loss of GAGs in the tissue, because a 30 to 40 percent reduction in GAGs should cause a very much greater loss of water. The reported loss of GAGs may not have taken into account the presence of non–link-stabilized GAGs in tissue, the presence of which would hold more water in the tissue.

Collagen Changes in Dense Connective Tissue in Post-traumatic Immobilization

A series of studies published by Akeson and co-workers[29] showed that DCT contractures are chiefly the result of remodeling. The authors found a significant increase in the reducible, intermolecular cross-links of collagen in the periarticular connective tissue of rabbits, after 9 weeks of pin immobilization. This finding indicates the presence of increased percentages of newly formed collagen, as well as an increased rate of collagen turnover in post-traumatic immobilization, as confirmed by radiolabeled studies.[29,30] In the medial collateral ligaments of young rabbits, after 9 weeks of pin immobilization, there was a 14 percent decrease in old collagen, reflecting a turnover rate double that of the controls. Total collagen was not statistically different at 9 weeks, indicating that collagen synthesis and degradation remained roughly in balance at this time. After 12 weeks of pin immobilization, there was a shift in the balance between synthesis and degradation, resulting in a 28 percent loss of old collagen and a net increase of 1 percent of new collagen. As suggested by these percentages, there is a reduction in the total collagen present after 12 weeks.

In a study by Amiel and co-workers,[30] old collagen was found to be preferentially lost. This finding suggests a theoretical model to explain the development of contractures and weakness in DCT. The old fibers that are of functional length, alignment, and strength are selectively lost, while new fibers form attachments and anchor the tissue in the folded position. Subsequently the folded fibers are degraded. In addition, the lack of stress can be expected to result in random alignment of the newly formed collagen fibers, which thus contribute little strength to the tissue. This random alignment tethers adjacent, preexisting fibers, limiting their extensibility with a loose basket-weave architecture. This basic process is similar to that proposed by Brody and associates[31] to explain changes in scar. There is no reason to suspect that the quality of changes is different in the nontraumatically immobilized tissue. Unfortunately, similar studies of turnover rates of nontraumatically immobilized tissues are not available for comparison under the two conditions.

One histochemical method commonly used to identify the quantity of new collagen fibers is to test the amount of salt-soluble collagen in the tissue, newly formed collagen being highly soluble. However, this test has been shown to have significant limitations. Amiel and co-workers[30] compared salt solubility values with radiolabeling of collagen in the periarticular tissues of pin-immobilized young rabbits. They found no difference in the salt solubility of the collagen, suggesting that no collagen synthesis was present, although collagen synthesis *was* found by radiolabeling. The salt solubility method may be inappropriate in this case because of the relatively high rate of turnover in growing, young rabbits. Alternatively, cross linking to stability levels above salt solubility may occur more rapidly than has been previously thought. Regardless of the mechanism, results and conclusions from studies that use this method must be interpreted carefully. The validity and sensitivity of this test for new collagen in adults has not been reported.

CLINICAL IMPLICATIONS: TREATING ADHESIONS

The studies of Akeson and colleagues[25,29] have contributed greatly to our ability to picture the changes that occur in DCT during the formation of contractures. One clinical implication for treating these contractures is that "the adhesion" is the structure itself. When we talk, for example, of "breaking the adhesions" in an advanced frozen shoulder, we are really talking about tearing the capsule. In many such cases, it is better to preserve the structure and to regain motion by stimulating a reversal of the changes, using therapeutic remodeling. The new, short, randomly aligned collagen fibers that limit tissue excursion must be absorbed. At the same time, the collagen must be replaced by new fibers of correct alignment and size, thus rebuilding tissues of functional length, flexibility, and strength. The amount, duration, and direction of stress applied in treatment need be only sufficient to stimulate and guide this remodeling process. As will be discussed later, these forces are significantly less than those traditionally applied, when the reigning concept was to "stretch out" the contracture. These low levels of force are preferable because they cause optimal rates of improvement, while protecting the weakened tissue from the trauma of excessive force.

Effects of Post-traumatic Immobilization on Stiffness and Strength in Intact Tissue

The implications of the aforementioned histochemical studies for DCT contracture are confirmed by studies that directly correlate those changes to changes in joint motion or DCT strength. Woo and associates[32] measured torque and hysteresis during passive movement of osseoligamentous preparations of rabbit knees, after 9 weeks of pin immobilization. Changes in resistance to passive motion were due to remodeling in both periarticular and intra-articular DCT. Torque in the osseoligamentous preparation of immobilized limbs was four times greater than in the control preparations; hysteresis was increased 10 times. Resistance was increased equally during both flexion and extension, indicating that the connective tissue changes were generalized. The immobilization procedure was the same in this and the previously cited experiment, suggesting that the increased stiffness was largely a result of remodeling.

Lavigne and Watkins[33] studied contracture development over time intervals that are closer to clinical experiences. They measured DCT contractures in monkey knees that were pinned and casted for 0, 4, 8, 16, 32, and 64 days. Osseoligamentous stress/strain experiments were performed for each period of immobilization. No measurable differences occurred before 16 days. At day 16, there was a slight increase in torque at the ends of motion. At 32 days, joint excursion was reduced to 30 degrees, with marked increases in torque at the ends of motion, and increased torque throughout range. Extensibility of the collateral ligaments of the knees gradually decreased with increasing periods of immobilization. Inasmuch as Lavigne and Watkins's longest immobilization period corresponds with the 9-week period used by Woo and colleagues,[32] these two studies show the progression of changes during post-traumatic immobilization. The changes were delayed in onset and were gradual and progressive, supporting the hypothesis that they were the result of gradual remodeling of the connective tissue. Limited joint motion occurred 19 days earlier in traumatized than in nontraumatized tissue, illustrating the accelerated rates of change after trauma.

Frank and associates[34,35] found that after 9 weeks of pin immobilization of rabbit knees, the medial collateral ligament had only 50 percent of the normal breaking strength, and increased compliance. These changes suggested changes in collagen structure and architecture similar to those changes in remodeling of nontraumatized DCT. Akeson (personal communication, September 1981) found similar changes in the DCT whether pin immobilization or cast immobilization was used. There is, therefore, evidence of similar changes in proteoglycans, water, and collagen in both post-traumatic immobilization and immobilization of normal tissue. Many of the same physical and biologic mechanisms appear to be operational in both circumstances. The fact that the changes are found more consistently and extensively in post-traumatic immobilization supports the view that trauma accelerates the rate of these changes. *These studies demonstrate that both trauma and immobilization lead to atrophy and contractures of DCT, because of remodeling. The speed and severity of contracture development are faster in the limb that suffers both trauma and immobilization.*

Effects of Stress and Motion on the Nature of Healing in Dense Connective Tissue

The above studies show how stress and motion affect DCT mutability and offer exciting insight into mechanisms of tissue change and treatment. The following studies are perhaps even more stimulating to the clinician. They show that treatments not only cause changes in length and strength of DCT, but actually change the type of tissue that develops. Traditionally, repaired lacerated tendons have been immobilized for several weeks, because healing of tendon was thought to occur exclusively by invasion of the incision space by scar tissue from the surrounding area. Recent studies have shown, however, that healthy, vascularized tendon can heal by intrinsic tendinous tissue.[36-38] Healing of cut tendon has been observed even in lacerated tendons maintained in culture.[36] One major factor that determines the type of healing is the presence or absence of physiologic levels of stress during healing.

Gelberman and co-workers[37] showed that healing occurs by dramatically different mechanisms, depending on the postoperative management. They compared mechanisms of healing of repaired flexor tendons in dogs. Half of the dogs were immobilized and half were moved passively through limited excursions 50 times, once a day, starting immediately postoperatively. In the immobilized tendons, healing occurred by scar tissue invasion. The scar did not penetrate the deeper recesses of the incision by day 10, but did thereafter. The ends of the cut tendon did not change significantly in appearance through day 42. Healing by scar resulted in a union that was initially weak, and which remained relatively weak for several months. Each union was associated with a scar tissue adhesion, because the scar grew in from the periphery. By contrast, in the mobilized tendon, the sheath developed well-oriented, circumferentially aligned fibroblasts and collagen fibers by day 10. Scar tissue adhesions were usually absent. On day 21, the surface of the tendon was smooth and was comprised of uniform patterns of cells with interdigitating cytoplasmic extensions. Cells extended peripherally along the surface of the tendon, and collagen fibers lay in normal longitudinal orientation between the cells. The deeper recesses of the incision were subsequently filled by ingrowth from the epitendineum between days 21 and 42. By day 42, longitudinal orientation of the collagen fibers and cells from the epitendineum was seen in the deepest region of the healing area. These unions were superior in early and late strength and were not associated with scar tissue adhesions.

The difference between the types of healing is explained, in part, by differences in the rates of collagen synthesis and degradation that were found in the tendon ends. Surprisingly, the cellular activity within the tendon gap on day 21 was much greater in the immobilized tendon than in the mobilized tendon. There was a difference, however, in the balance between synthesis and degradation of collagen in the two situations. In the immobilized tendon, even at 42 days, collagen degradation remained increased and synthesis was modest. In the mobilized tendon, by contrast, active collagen synthesis was seen on days 21 and 42. The mobilized tendon developed new tendon tissue, which closed the incision. In the immobilized tendon, cut surfaces did not unite by tendinous tissue, but were "glued" together by scar tissue.[37] The persistent high level of degradation probably softened the tendon ends, increasing the chance of a suture pulling loose during the third week.

In vitro studies of tendon suggest that changes in DCT are intrinsic to the tissue and are not dependent on hormonal or neural mediators.[38,39] Chick embryo tendons and their response to cyclical tension in culture were studied by Slack and associates.[39] Tendons subjected to cyclical tension showed increased production of protein and increased deoxyribonucleic acid (DNA) production. After 2 days, changes were noted in the staining characteristics, indicating an acceleration of the maturation process of the collagen. These results showed the effect of stress, not only on cellular activity, but also on the physical-chemical process of collagen maturation. Either factor could account for the better healing of DCT when stressed after injury. This in vitro study suggests that intrinsic changes in the tendon, such as available charge distributions on the surrounding collagen fibers, are responsible for the changes.

The presence or absence of motion has also been shown to make a dramatic difference in the type of repair in other tissues. Salter and co-workers[40] demonstrated that when holes were drilled in the articular cartilage of rabbits, healing occurred by scar tissue when the joint was immobilized, and by considerable ingrowth of surrounding cartilage when the joint was continuously moved after the injury. The cartilage that was moved had greater quantities of collagen and GAGs, less cellularity, and fewer scar tissue adhesions.

Repaired medial collateral ligaments demonstrate greater collagen production in exercised joints, than immobilized joints. Repairs were larger and total collagen content greater 8 weeks after injury.[21] Goldstein[41] noted that when medial collateral ligaments in rabbits were tested for breaking strength, 6 weeks after repair, the rupture site was always at the tenoperiosteal junction, rather than at the repair site. This observation suggests that remodeling after repair involves not only the repair site but also the entire ligament. When ligaments were allowed to heal by scar tissue ingrowth, remodeling of the scar eventually resulted in tissue that appeared histologically similar to ligament. Differences, however, persisted. Even 40 weeks after injury, scar-healed ligaments contained different types and proportions of collagen and GAGs. The highly organized collagen architecture of ligament was never reproduced within the scar, and there were differences in the periodicity of the crimp in the collagen fibers.[34,41]

CLINICAL IMPLICATIONS: STRESS AND MOTION

The relevance of stress and motion to DCT healing will be readily apparent to the clinician. The studies noted above show dramatically that better formed healing occurs more frequently when the tissue is stimulated by physiologic levels of stress during the healing process. Stress stimulates a more functional alignment of collagen fibers, maximizes healing by development of the correct type of DCT, and minimizes scar tissue adhesions. The clinician should note that only a few repetitions of movement were necessary to stimulate the processes resulting in these dramatic differences. However, more research is needed to identify the threshold number of repetitions that are necessary. For example, Woo and associates[43] and Gelberman and co-workers[44,45] used 50 repetitions per day, yet in earlier clinical studies Madden and associates[42] achieved positive results with as few as 15 repetitions per day. Future clinical or basic research should identify the most efficient and cost-effective numbers of repetitions for different types of injuries. The amount of force and the timing of stress are also important to success. These factors are discussed in the next section.

Effects of Stress on Strength and Architecture in Dense Connective Tissue Healing

The morphologic observations cited above show that the introduction of stress early after injury will result in stronger unions of tendon and ligament, and fewer scar tissue adhesions. On the other hand, totally unrestricted activity during the healing stages is detrimental. Stress exceeding the safe working loads of the healing tissue may result in reduced breaking strength of the ultimate union, actual failure, or increased scar tissue volume.

To match levels of stress to the strength of healing of tendons, it is necessary to remember that sutured tendon heals much more slowly than does a wound in the skin. In one study, when dogs were allowed unrestricted activity following 3 weeks of immobilization, five of six tendon repairs ruptured.[43] The surviving repair was strong, but the predominance of failure clearly precludes adoption of this management. The weakness of the tendon union after 21 days of immobilization is explained by the morphologic findings cited above: softening of the tendon ends and only partial-thickness repair by poorly attached scar tissue. At 21 days following suture, the breaking strength of repaired tendons that have been immobilized is at best only equal to that of freshly sutured tendons. The studies suggest that tendon mobilization should either be initiated immediately, or after 42 days, but not at the 21-day period.

Unrestricted activity immediately after repair of ligaments also results in inferior healing. Goldstein and Barmada[41] compared the effects of 6 weeks of continuous immobilization with those of 6 weeks of unrestricted activity on the healing of lacerated medial collateral ligaments of rabbits. They found persistent signs of inflammation in the scar and less healing in the ligaments of rabbits that were allowed unrestricted activity. The comparative breaking strengths of ligaments were as follows: for controls 8.97 kg, for continuously immobilized subjects 6.45 kg, for those allowed unrestricted activity 5.6 kg. Scars in the continuously immobilized ligaments were more cellular, poorly organized, but larger than those in rabbits allowed unrestricted activity. Goldstein and Barmada attributed the greater strength of these scars to the larger scar size.

Note that the breaking strength of both groups of Goldstein and Barmada's repaired ligaments was greater than the 50 percent residual breaking strength reported by Amiel and colleagues[30] after 9 weeks of pin immobilization, with no surgical trauma of the periarticular tissues. Comparison of these breaking strengths will remind the clinician of the severely weakened state of DCT that can result from disuse atrophy alone.

Superior healing occurs when activity level is reduced to physiologic limits, however. Two studies showed that protected mobilization introduced immediately after repair resulted in stronger unions than did delayed mobilization or prolonged immobilization.[35,37] Repaired tendons were subjected to either immobilization, protected mobilization, or combinations of the two. The shortest time period for initiating any treatment was 0 days, and the maximum duration of treatment was 105 days. The weakest breaking strength, 6 percent of control tendons, was found immediately after suture and also after 21 days or 42 days of immobilization. The highest breaking strength, 48 percent of controls, was found when protected mobilization was begun immediately after suture and continued for 84 days. Tendons that were first immobilized and subsequently mobilized had intermediate breaking strengths, the highest being 34 percent of controls, after 84 days of immobilization followed by 21 days of protected mobilization.

Introduction of immediate, protected mobilization promotes healing of DCT by intrinsic tissues. Compared with the outcome of delayed activity, such healing results in the strongest unions, in faster healing, and in reduced scar tissue adhesions.

Introduction of protected motion also appears to enhance healing of DCT that has not been sutured. When ankle strains were managed with airsplints and protected ambulation, the duration of inflammation decreased and function returned more rapidly, compared with management by immobilization in casts.[46,47] Reduced periods of inflammation, decreased DCT atrophy, and increased range of motion have also been reported when traumatized joints were managed using constant passive motion (CPM) machines.[33,48–51] These findings are consistent with the basic science studies showing the devastating effects of remodeling in DCTs immobilized in the presence of inflammatory exudates.

Unfortunately, and quite surprisingly, there is no persuasive documentation to support most of the protocols for CPM. Most characteristics of treatment protocol have yet to be systematically evaluated, including how soon after injury CPM should be instituted, what rate of motion should be used for different purposes, what arcs of motion should be used, when should they be changed, how many repetitions a day are optimal, and what are the optimal durations of rehabilitation with CPM.

The disappointing lack of systematic investigation of CPM seems due to two factors. First, there has been no apparent attempt to differentially diagnose types of contractures that are to be treated or prevented. Second, arising from this lack of precision, there is confusion in treatment goals. CPM gained clinical acceptance based on studies of articular cartilage healing, and yet it has been adopted without modification for the postoperative management of total joint replacements, treatment of adhesive capsulitis, tendon repairs, and other post-traumatic conditions. In these cases, goals include promotion of healing of DCT by intrinsic tissue, prevention of muscle shortening, and prevention of scar tissue adhesions. Scar tissue adhesions may be prevented by a few daily repetitions of a few millimeters of motion, whereas articular cartilage regeneration requires constant motion. Future studies are needed to demonstrate how variations in protocol are related to specific tissue effects.

CLINICAL MANAGEMENT OF CHANGES IN DENSE CONNECTIVE TISSUE

Before reviewing management of contractures resulting from changes in DCT, it is worth pointing out that scar tissue adhesions and periarticular tissue remodeling represent only two of the five classes of contracture. Soft tissue contractures may also result from adaptive shortening of muscle, pseudomyostatic contracture of muscle, and persistent joint subluxation. Different programs of management are indicated for each diagnosis, and optimal rates of improvement also vary with the type of contracture. The material reviewed in this section reflects only information regarding changes in DCT. Contractures form in muscle much more rapidly than in DCT; therefore, any contracture involving changes in the DCTs will be associated with adaptive shortening of muscle. Techniques designed to stimulate lengthening of muscle should be incorporated in the management of nearly all patients with DCT contractures.

The optimal management of each type of contracture is difficult to document because many stiff joints contain a mixture of contracture types. For example, after post-traumatic immobilization, one can anticipate that there will be scar tissue adhesions, shortening of DCT (fibrotic adhesions), and shortening of the musculotendinous units. However, it is not possible to determine the precise contribution of each to the limitation, even in the relatively known injuries in the experimental animal model. Resistance to passive motion was compared between the intact limbs and osseoligamentous preparations of rabbits that had been pin-immobilized for 9 weeks.[32] The torque measured during forced passive motions was 10 times normal in the intact limbs, but only four times normal in the osseoligamentous preparation. This result suggests that the pin-track scar and muscle shortening contributed greater resistance to passive motion than did the remodeling of the periarticular connective tissues.

However, it is not possible to determine the relative contributions of the pin-track scar and the musculotendinous shortening, or the exact portions of the periarticular tissues that had shortened. Because of diagnostic uncertainties, the following clinical rules for the management of DCT contractures should only be taken as general guidelines.

Physical Responses of Dense Connective Tissue to Therapeutic Stress

The physical response of DCT to different therapeutic modalities is discussed first; subsequently, these observations will be applied to treatment programs for different types of contractures. This separation is important because clinicians generally fail to differentiate physical from biologic effects, which may lead to a great deal of confusion. For example, a given treatment may cause a purely transient physical increase in tissue length. Recovery of the tissue to the original length by the next visit might lead the therapist to abandon the treatment as being ineffective, and yet that treatment may be the precise stimulus necessary to stimulate a permanent increase in length by the biologic process of remodeling! The therapist who is aware of this fact will wait a sufficient time for the biologic process to occur before changing treatment. Optimal management of DCT requires clinicians to clearly understand and to differentiate physical from biologic events in contracture management.

The data reviewed suggest the following physical responses of DCT to stretching:

1. Collagen fiber elongation of 1 to 1.5 percent for less than 1 hour causes no permanent deformation.
2. Elongation of as little as 1.5 to 2 percent that is maintained for more than 1 hour will cause transient melting of the tropocollagen bonds. If recovery is prevented by maintaining the tissue only slightly less stretched, or by initial stretch periods in excess of an hour, denaturing and thus permanent elongation will result.
3. Following elongation of up to 2 percent, recovery may occur by reestablishment of the bonding. This requires between 1 and 24 hours, depending on the amount of melting. Stretching intended to denature the tissue must therefore be followed by sustained or intermittent stretching during the subsequent 24 hours.
4. At normal temperatures, elongation of 3 to 8 percent will cause lengthening by tearing of portions of the tissue but preserving its gross continuity. As strain increases, increasing weakening of the tissue occurs. Because this amount of lengthening is well above physiologic limits, inflammation usually results.
5. Permanent stretching of DCT occurs by two processes: tearing of the gross structure, or disruption of the intermolecular bonds between the tropocollagen units. Both of these processes result in denaturing of the collagen and weakening of the tissue.

The first decision a clinician must make in planning the treatment of a contracture is whether to stimulate remodeling of the tissue or to destroy the tissue by denaturing or rupturing the collagen. After this decision has been made, the rules of the physical properties of DCT can be used to establish the treatment regimen.

Destruction of Nonessential Restricting Tissues

In some clinical situations, joint motion is restricted by the presence of DCT adhesions, which can be sacrificed with no loss of joint stability or function. In the earlier stages of Dupuytren's contracture, for example, the palmar fascia becomes thickened and adherent, but the flexor muscle tendons and capsular structures are not involved. At this stage, the adhesive and thickened palmar fascia can be sacrificed without significant loss of function in the hand. In other cases, the restricting tissue can, without detriment, be weakened by treatment, so long as the gross integrity of the tissue is preserved. For example, stretching and denaturing the collagen of early burn scars is probably an acceptable treatment goal, so long as the scar is not broken open. This denaturing of the collagen is acceptable because during the first 8 months of scarring, up to 85 percent of the collagen is replaced by the normal remodeling process, and functional connective tissue will result despite the collagen denaturation in the early phases of treatment.

The treatment goal in this class of contracture is to stretch and denature the collagen of the restricting tissue, preferably without causing an inflammatory reaction. However, when blood vessels and cells in the connective tissue are damaged, an inflammatory reaction is inevitable. These factors demand a balance between amount of force used and frequency of treatment. Care must also be taken to prevent damage to surrounding functional tissue.

In these cases, little recovery of length will occur between treatments because the treatment is aimed at denaturing or rupturing the collagen fibers. Therefore, an increase in tissue excursion is to be expected not only immediately after treatment, but also on the following visit.

Short-term Stretching

Short-term stretching, as occurs in manual therapy or a few minutes of traction, is commonly used to stress contractures. In theory, a short-term strain of 4 to 6 percent can be used to permanently increase the length of the tissue by denaturing the collagen and by fracturing some of the collagen bundles. However, this degree of strain can be expected to cause damage to cells and vessels in the tissue, causing a significant inflammatory reaction. There is no evidence that such strenuous treatments are warranted. Strenuous treatments are particularly contraindicated for patients with conditions that make them more susceptible to inflammatory reactions (such as rheumatoid arthritis, autonomic dysreflexias, and hemophilia), and in tissues that are already chronically or acutely inflamed.

Strains of 1.5 to 2 percent will also destroy collagen, if maintained for an hour or longer, and this level of strain can be expected to cause much less cellular and vascular trauma than higher strains. Sustained stress for more than 1 hour, however, is contraindicated, because such high strains occlude the circulation and lead to ischemic trauma and unnecessary inflammation. Careful monitoring for inflammatory reactions should be sufficient to recognize and avoid such excessive treatment. It has been possible to reverse early Dupuytren's contracture in several patients using this approach, when more conservative approaches were not successful. This approach, therefore, is a viable option, despite the difficulties. However, further clinical and applied research is needed to verify the benefits of this approach.

The biologic and physical characteristics of DCT suggest the need to modify the amount of force used during each succeeding session. For example, when sufficient strain is used to enter the linear region of the stress/strain curve, the *initial treatment will probably cause weakening of the tissue. Subsequent treatments at the same level of stress will probably result in a traumatic inflammatory reaction.* When the DCT is weakened by denaturing collagen, subsequent stretching may traumatize cells and vessels that survived the first treatment. Logic suggests that treatment be modified to allow for remodeling of cellular and vascular components in the area. These considerations suggest that sessions of maximal strain should be staggered with sessions of less strain. An alternative approach would be to schedule sessions less frequently. Clinical research is needed to determine optimal protocols for treatment frequency and progression when sacrifice of the tissue is desired.

Restoring Function through Remodeling of Essential Structures

In the majority of cases, restricted motion results from adhesions or remodeling of such essential structures as ligaments, joint capsule, and the musculotendinous portion of tendons. As discussed earlier, the goal of therapeutic stress, in these cases, is to restore motion by stimulating a reversal of the remodeling process. Denaturing the collagen, which weakens the tissue, must be prevented. For example, in repairs of cruciate ligaments with DCT grafts, excessive stretching during early rehabilitation has been blamed for eventual failure, because the ligament continues to lengthen after the normal range of motion has been reached, so that the joint consequently becomes unstable.[52] Data from the literature suggest that the excessive strain in early treatment denatures the collagen, thereby weakening the structure, which gradually fails. When essential structures are involved, the goals of treatment must include both increasing the range of motion and promoting healthy and functional tissues in the final result.

Based on our review,[53–59,61–65,67] treatment that causes stress-relaxation of the collagen is the safest method. Stress-relaxation occurs if a constant, fixed load is applied to the tissue, which then elongates by creep. The force applied in this treatment is not increased as increasing resistance is generated by the tissue. The studies suggest that elongation should be limited to the very beginning of the linear region of strain, that is, from 1.5 to 2 percent.

Clinical reports have confirmed that there are less frequent traumatic, iatrogenic injuries when stress-relaxation forms of treatment are used. Although they have not generally been described as "stress-relaxation" therapies, they have been employed for many years. These treatments include techniques such as traction, splinting, and casting.[53–64] Because these modalities are normally applied for longer than 1 hour, strains of 1.5 to 2 percent are sufficient to stimulate remodeling and even a minimal amount of denaturing. Because these levels of strain are only at the end of the toe region of strain, very low levels of force are sufficient to produce them.

Load Limits in Prolonged Positioning

In the clinical situation, we cannot identify the exact percent strain of a given tissue in most circumstances. Knowing the physical characteristics of collagen helps explain why the use of low levels of force works in these methods. However, determining the amount of force to use in the clinic is usually made according to less quantitative, clinical criteria. Guidelines reviewed here are for splints worn for a minimum of 12 hours per day, or casts worn for 1 to 2 weeks.

For finger contractures, 250 g of extension force used while the finger is placed in a plaster cast is the maximum force that can be applied without a significant incidence of skin ulceration, or inflammatory reaction occurring in the deeper tissues.[53,54] This force is sufficient to stimulate remodeling.

For most joints, more subjective criteria have been found adequate. Hepburn[58] has shown the efficacy of using very low forces applied by a dynamic splint. His protocol called for stress that was not perceived as a "stretching" force by the patient until the splint had been worn for 1 hour or more. The subject should remain comfortable for up to 12 hours of positioning, with only a feeling of stiffness or mild ache for a short time after removal of the appliance. Hepburn's experience is supported by that of others. They report positioning the limb at the maximum position, with the patient remaining essentially comfortable for the duration of the splinting.[55,56,58–60,62–65] In using splints for knee contractures in a variety of patients, Savill[59] reported splinting the limb in the position of maximum extension, so that "slight manual pressure" caused the heel to lift a short distance out of the splint. When the cast was removed at 5-day intervals, increased extension was found beyond the angle of immobilization. In all of these protocols, the magnitude of the stretching force was well below what either the therapist or the patient would consider "a significant stretch." Yet, as discussed later, these levels of force have been shown superior to traditional strenuous stretching. In the above reports, the strain in the collagen fibers was in all probability no more than 0.5 percent. The chief mechanism of response is certainly remodeling of the tissue.

The use of excessive force, or too long a duration of stress, is easily identified by the ensuing inflammatory reaction. The more difficult problem is to identify when one is using too little force, or too short a period of stress. One way to identify sufficient treatment dosage is to compare the rate of gain in motion to that reported by others for the same condition. If the reported rate is equaled or exceeded, it is reasonable to assume that sufficient force is being exerted on the correct target tissues.

Unfortunately, the possible rates of gain in length for DCT contractures is unclear, because of the lack of differential diagnosis in most publications. In a few papers, however, DCT changes have been relatively well diagnosed. A remarkable consistency is observed when reported rates of gain are converted to degrees of gain per week. Despite a wide range of diagnoses, including joint limitation in hemophilia, rheumatoid arthritis, post-traumatic periarticular stiffness, Hansen's disease (post-traumatic finger contractures), closed head injuries, and cerebrovascular accidents (knee contractures), the average rate of gain is 3 degrees per week, with a range of 1 to 9 degrees per week.[54,56–59,61,64–66] As shown in Table 2–1, the rate of gain is more rapid initially, with a gradual falling off.

Overall, these studies suggest that 3 degrees gain in joint motion per week is an acceptable standard for remodeling of DCT for the process of increasing motion.

Mobilization Versus Long-term Positioning

The theoretical assumption that long-term stress is superior to short-term stress is not always confirmed. Clinical studies suggest that different technical applications have different advantages.

TABLE 2–1   Mean Rate of Gain in Motion

| Group | Gain in Motion (degrees/wk after Various Rehabilitation Periods) | | | | |
	4 wk	8 wk	12 wk	16 wk	Average
Traditional physical therapy	0.70	1.50	0.75	0.75	0.93
Traction	5.50	4.20	3.20	2.50	3.85

Source: Data from Rizk, et al.,[63] p. 31.

The assumption that traction and mobilization offer different advantages is supported by four clinical studies.[54,63–65] Rizk and co-workers[63] compared two treatments for adhesive capsulitis. One group was treated with light, balanced traction and transcutaneous electrical nerve stimulation (TENS). Traction was applied for 15-minute periods, with 5-minute rest periods, until a total of 2 hours of traction was completed. The control group was given "traditional" forms of short-term stress including the use of finger ladders and other forms of active and passive stretching. The results of the study are shown in Table 2–1. The average rate of gain in degrees per week is shown for several periods after the initiation of treatment. The gentle traction resulted in faster gain in motion, and also earlier loss of pain, indicating that the traction was less traumatic.

Kolumban[54] also showed the superiority of long-term stress over passive stretching. In a study of finger contractures in Hansen's disease, he found equal rates of gain in patients who performed daily passive stretching (flexion and extension only), underwent paraffin treatments, or had daily or weekly changes of finger cast. The daily treatments turned out to be a waste of time, because weekly cast changes achieved the same result. From the standpoint of cost effectiveness, weekly cast changes were far superior.

The studies of Rizk and co-workers[63] and Kolumban[54] showed the superiority of sustained stress over cyclical forms of active and passive stress provided by finger ladders, wands, and unsophisticated home exercises. One problem with these studies is that they compared well-executed long-term stress with poorly executed cyclical stress. We now recognize that these forms of stretch offer little control of force and do not accurately localize stretch within the capsule. Therefore, despite the results of these reports, additional clinical studies are needed to determine the relative advantages of well-executed forms of short-term and long-term stress.

Sustained, low-intensity forces have been shown to be very effective for the management of DCT contractures at the elbow, knee, and ankle. Hepburn[64] showed, in a multicenter study, that the use of sustained light traction, compared with traditional physical therapy (as defined above), resulted in reduced length of the rehabilitation period, fewer clinical visits, and reduced cost to the patient. The relative effectiveness of sustained light strain is further supported by the fact that the majority of patients had contractures that had either failed to respond or ceased to respond to traditional, cyclical forms of stress.

Each form of treatment has its advantages and limitations. One problem with splints, casts, and traction is that they often fail to localize stress to the target tissues. Restrictions that prevent motion of the articular surfaces may result in excessive strain in adjacent normal tissues. Two examples will be given to illustrate this problem. One form of treatment for adhesive capsulitis is to passively force the distal humerus in the direction of flexion. During this passive stretch, the shortened capsules and ligaments may cause the head of the humerus to wedge against the glenoid labrum, resulting in a sprain of that structure instead of the intended target, the capsule. In addition, the attachments of the rotator cuff muscles may be strained instead of the capsule. Injuries to essential DCTs, that is, ligaments and capsules, have been reported following treatment of adhesive capsulitis in both humans[66] and experimental animals.[67] In mobilization, such injuries can be prevented if stress is applied more accurately to the target tissues. Therefore, mobilization may prove to be a superior mode of treatment in some conditions, as suggested by the following clinical study.

Nicholson[65] reported the rates of gain using manual stretching for treatment of adhesive capsulitis. He used Maitland's oscillatory form of mobilization for total durations of 3 to 6 minutes on each target tissue per session. Treatment was effective despite its brevity. Perhaps this is because the techniques allow accurate localization of force to the restricting tissues. The average rate of gain in degrees per week, averaged over the total rehabilitation period, is shown in Table 2–2.

The rates of gain in Nicholson's study are the highest published. They show that manual therapy alone was superior to the balanced traction in Rizk's study[63] for management of adhesive capsulitis.

Valid comparisons of treatment programs by different investigators are difficult, owing to lack of standardization of treatment methods. The above studies,[54,63–65] however, clearly demonstrate that long-duration light loads, which stimulate the tissue without causing inflammation, are effective and result in a low incidence of trauma. They also indicate that selective tissue stimulation by mobilization can be very effective. Logic suggests that optimal results might be obtained by a judicious combination of these approaches. A clinical examination that clearly establishes which tissues are involved should indicate to the therapist which techniques will result in optimal stimulus of all involved tissues. However, definitive answers about the precise indications for mobilization, stress-relaxation, or combinations of these await further clinical research.

The frequency with which stress-relaxation can be repeated without causing trauma to the cellular components of a tissue may be a function of the percent strain used. When light pressure is used, as described by Hepburn,[62] strain probably remains below 1.5 percent, and collagen denaturation is unlikely. This protocol may be used without interruption. When force is kept within physiologic limits, manual therapy techniques are frequently applied every 2 days, with no adverse effects. Optimal frequency of treatment is another area that is ripe for clinical research.

When stress is used to stimulate remodeling, an immediate post-treatment increase in tissue excursion can be expected. This increase is transient in nature; by the following day, no increase will be noted. However, remodeling will result in permanent increases in excursion that can be detected after a week or 10 days.

TABLE 2–2 Mean Rate of Gain in Motion over Rehabilitation Period

Motion (degrees/wk)	Mobilization	Exercise
Internal rotation	2.8	1.0
External rotation	4.4	3.0
Abduction	6.2	3.5
Mean of total	4.4	2.5

Source: Data from Rizk, et al.,[63] p. 31.

Inflammation

Trauma, whether caused by the initial injury or by treatment, results in inflammation. If the trauma is repeated over 2 or more weeks, chronic inflammation results. Chronic inflammation, in turn, has been shown to have four consequences, two of which are counterproductive. It increases the activity of fibroblasts and accelerates remodeling, which theoretically could lead to more rapid gain in motion, but chronic inflammation also stimulates myofibroblast production and produces pain. The idea of accelerating of remodeling by inflammation was not supported by either Rizk's[63] or Hepburn's[64] studies. In both cases, when more gentle treatments were instituted, chronic inflammation subsided within 2 weeks, and the rate of gain was faster. Perhaps this can be explained by the latter two effects of inflammation. After 2 weeks of chronic inflammation, myofibroblasts appear in DCT and accelerate contracture by active contraction. Myofibroblasts will remain in the tissue as long as chronic inflammation persists, favoring loss rather than gain in motion. Lastly, the clinician is aware that a patient with a painful joint tends to protect the affected part, usually by muscular contractions that lead to myostatic or pseudomyostatic contracture.[68] Overtreatment, resulting in chronic inflammation, therefore, appears to be clearly contraindicated on both theoretical and practical grounds. Well-controlled clinical trials are needed to support this view.

In patients who present with DCT contractures with chronic inflammation, logic indicates that the chronic inflammation should be treated first, followed by treatment of the residual symptoms, namely the limitations of movement. This approach has been proved effective in the clinical studies cited above and in other clinical experience. Finding that optimal results are obtained without hurting the patient has been a welcome relief for therapists and patients alike.

MODALITIES IN THE MANAGEMENT OF DENSE CONNECTIVE TISSUE CONTRACTURES

Heat

Heating DCT to near maximum physiologic limits, 40°C to 45°C, partially melts the bonds between tropocollagen molecules. Melting of these bonds has two important clinical implications when done prior to stress application. First, heating to 40°C makes DCT more ductile. Increased ductility can be an advantage because it allows a more even distribution of force throughout the entire tissue, thus reducing focal points of stress, rupture, and inflammation. This is important when dealing with large or thick tissues, such as large areas of burn scar, or fibrotic adhesions of an entire joint capsule. The second effect of heat poses a serious clinical dilemma. DCT heated 40°C to 45°C allows a greater elongation without structural damage, so long as strain is limited to about 2 percent. This effect could be an advantage, permitting the therapist to produce greater elongation of the tissue without causing damage, but it is not practical because strain cannot be limited to 2 percent in the clinical situation. At 40°C to 45°C, collagen bonds become partially melted, and the tissue becomes much more fragile. As soon as 2 percent strain is exceeded at this temperature, the collagen begins to yield. Tendon heated to 45°C ruptures at only one fourth the force of elongation of unheated tissue.[69,70] Rupture will occur at only 4 percent strain, which allows too small a margin of error for most clinical situations. The decreased strength is a disadvantage when it is desired to remodel but not weaken a tissue. Heating the tissue greatly increases the likelihood of iatrogenic trauma and offers little advantage, if any. There appears to be no evidence that heating the tissue before or during stress accelerates the rate of remodeling in response to stress, by either biologic or physical mechanisms. The use of heat for the treatment of contractures cannot be recommended when integrity of the structure must be preserved.

On the other hand, if the aim of treatment is to destroy a tissue, fragility of the collagen is an advantage, assuming that heat can be localized to the targeted tissues. The advantage is that the levels of force needed to denature the target tissues, being about 25 percent of normal, are obviously much less likely to damage adjacent, nontargeted tissue. Although supported on theoretical grounds, no data have been published to support the advantage of heat for selective denaturing of adhesions. Clinical research is needed to confirm the advantage of heat for collagen destruction.

Ultrasound

Ultasound has been demonstrated to affect the cross bridges of reconstituted collagen.[72] Human collagen that was extracted, reconstituted on grids, and subjected to ultrasound at 0.6 W/cm^2 for 10 minutes increased 9 percent in length. Electron microscopic studies showed that the collagen had increased band widths. Although this reconstituted collagen is not comparable to natural collagen fibers, which are stabilized by proteoglycan and glycoprotein linkages, the study suggests that ultrasound can affect collagen at the level of the intertropocollagen bonding. The disruption of bonding at this level of organization of the collagen fiber may be similar to that found in the stress-relaxation and tissue heating studies, reviewed in Chapter 1. Lengthening occurred in the absence of strain applied to the structure, suggesting that the melting observed would allow even greater lengthening if stress had been applied during application of the ultrasound. Controlled studies demonstrating accelerated degradation of DCT adhesions with the use of ultrasound are needed to confirm this effect.

Because ultrasound can be more focused than diathermy, it may permit a greater effect on the target tissue. More selective focus should make possible the selective denaturing or fracturing of the collagen in the sonated tissues, while preserving the surrounding structures. Combining ultrasound with sustained stress has been a successful strategy in the management of early Dupuytren's contracture.

SUMMARY

1. In nontraumatized tissues, changes in stress or motion result in significant alterations in the compliance, strength, and length of dense connective tissue (DCT).
   A. Immobilization causes significant loss of DCT strength, predisposing patients to injury by excessive stretching forces during rehabilitation. Loss of 80 percent of DCT strength in muscle was found after 4 weeks; 50 percent loss of strength was observed in the collateral ligaments of the knee, and 39 percent loss in the cruciate ligaments, after 8 weeks.

    B. Immobilization causes loss of length and flexibility more slowly than it does loss of strength. Persistent changes in architecture or length, sufficient to limit motion, are not regularly found in nontraumatized DCT that has been immobilized for less than 7 weeks.

    C. Trauma prior to immobilization accelerates shortening of DCT during immobilization. Contractures may occur as early as 4 weeks following immobilization.

    D. Overuse injuries and stress fractures may be prevented by scheduling periods of reduced activity during a build-up in activities such as military training, industrial work, or sports.

2. DCT contractures may be reduced or prevented by:

    A. Placing significant DCT structures in a lengthened position during immobilization.

    B. Introducing stress in immobilized limbs by isometric contractions.

    C. Introducing stress by protected motion during the healing process.

    D. Preventing acceleration of remodeling by reducing acute inflammatory reactions, and by preventing chronic irritation.

    E. Immediate protected mobilization promotes healing of DCT by intrinsic tissues, prevents scar tissue adhesions, and increases the strength of the union.

3. When essential structures such as capsules and major ligaments are shortened, *the only mechanism available for gaining persistent increases in joint motion while preserving the biomechanical properties of these DCTs is remodeling.* Clinical studies confirm that nontraumatic stress achieves the best results.

    A. Splints, casts, and other forms of stress-producing treatment should be applied for 11 hours per day, with force levels set so that the patient remains essentially comfortable for the duration of splinting.

    B. Mobilization and other forms of short-term stress are effective and offer the advantage of precisely localizing stress to the target tissues.

    C. Physical and ischemic trauma causing inflammation are counterproductive. Pain that persists for more than 1 hour following treatment indicates the need to reduce either the intensity or duration of stress.

    D. Optimal rates of gain are 10 degrees during the first week, and 3 to 4 degrees per week thereafter.

4. Destruction of DCT adhesions may be accomplished by denaturing of collagen in the tissue, without inflammatory reaction by:

    A. Elongation of collagen at 1.5 percent for 1 hour, and prevention of recovery by gentle traction for 24 hours.

    B. Heat or ultrasound focused on the adhesion before or during stress may facilitate denaturation of the collagen.

5. We recommend that all future clinical research publications on contractures include the following information:

    A. A clinical, differential diagnosis of contractures.

    B. Full descriptions of treatment protocols:

        (1) Amount of force used;

        (2) Duration of force used;

        (3) Frequency of treatment;

        (4) Intensities and durations of heat or cold;

        (5) Presence and duration of pain or inflammation after treatment; and

        (6) Rates of gain during each week, and averaged rates of pain.

ACKNOWLEDGMENTS

We wish to thank Dr. M.W. Whittle for his editorial comments and Drs. N.I. Speilholz and C.S. Enwemeka for their electron micrographs.

REFERENCES

1. Neuberger, A and Slack, HGB: The metabolism of collagen from liver, bone, skin and tendon in normal rat. Biochemistry 53:47–52, 1953.
2. Madden, JW and Peacock, EE: Studies on the biology of collagen during wound healing: III. Dynamic metabolism of scar collagen and remodeling of dermal wounds. Ann Surg 174:511–520, 1971.
3. Svoboda, ELA, Howlley, TP, and Deporter, DA: Collagen fibril diameter and its relation to collagen turnover in three soft tissue connective tissues in the rat. Connect Tissue Res 12:43–48, 1983.
4. Plaas, AHK and Sandy, JD: Age-related decrease in the link-stability of proteoglycan aggregates formed by articular chondrocytes. Biochemistry 220:337–340, 1984.
5. Noyes, FR, Torvik, PJ, Hyde, WB, et al: Biomechanics of ligament failure. II. An analysis of immobilization, exercise, and reconditioning effects in primates. J Bone Joint Surg [Am] 56:1406–1417, 1974.
6. Maggone, T, DeWitt, MT, Handeley CJ, et al: In vitro response of chondrocytes to mechanical loading: The effect of short term mechanical tension. Connect Tissue Res 12:98–109, 1984.
7. Enwemeka, CS: Ultrastructural changes induced by cast immobilization in the soleus tendon. Presentation at 65th Annual Conference of the American Physical Therapy Association, Anaheim, CA, June 1990.
8. Tabary, JC, Tabary, C, Tardieu, C, et al: Physiological and structural changes in the cat's soleus muscle due to immobilization at different lengths by plaster casts. J Physiol 224:231–244, 1972.
9. Stacy, RJ and Hungerford, RL: A method to reduce work-related injuries during basic recruit training in the New Zealand army. Military Medicine 149:318–320, 1984.
10. Scully, TJ and Besterman, G: Stress fracture: A preventable training injury. Military Medicine 147:285–287, 1982.
11. Videman, T: Connective tissue and immobilization. Clin Orthop 221:26–32, 1987.
12. Finsterbush, A and Friedman, B: Early changes in immobilized rabbit knee joints: A light and electron microscopic study. Clin Orthop 92:305–319, 1972.
13. Reynolds, CA: The Effect of Nontraumatic Immobilization on Ankle Dorsiflexion Stiffness in Rats. 1991. Department of Physical Therapy, Georgia State University, Atlanta, GA, 1991. Thesis.
14. Langenskiold, A, Michelsson, J-R, and Videman, T: Osteoarthritis of the knee in rabbit produced by immobilization. Acta Orthop Scand 50:1–14, 1979.
15. Tardieu, C, Blanchard, O, Tabary, J, et al: Tendon adaptation to bone shortening. Connect Tissue Res 11:35–44, 1983.
16. Flowers, KR and Pheasant, SD: Use of torque angle curves in the assessment of digital PIP stiffness. J Hand Therapy 2:69–74, 1988.
17. Palmoski, MJ and Brandt, KD: The reversal of articular cartilage atrophy which accompanies remobilization of a limb after casting is prevented by exercise. Annals of the Orthopedic Research Society 6:48, 1981.
18. Miura, T: Non-traumatic flexion deformity of the proximal interphalangeal joint, its pathogenesis and treatment. Hand 15:25–34, 1983.
19. Hunt, TK, Banda, MJ, and Silver, IA: Cell interactions in post-traumatic fibrosis. In Fibrosis (Ciba Foundation Symposium 114). Pitman, London, 1985, p 128.
20. Tipton, CM, James, SL, Mergner, W, et al: Influence of exercise on strength of medial collateral knee ligaments of dogs. Am J Physiol 213:894–902, 1970.
21. Vailas, AC, Tipton, CM, Matthes, RD, et al: Physical activity and its influence on the repair process of medial collateral ligaments. Connect Tissue Res 9:25–31, 1981.
22. Rudolph, R: Contraction and the control of contraction. World J Surg 4:279–287, 1980.
23. Nevasier, JS: Adhesive capsulitis of the shoulder: A study of pathologic findings in periarthritis of the shoulder. J Bone Joint Surg [Br] 27:211–222, 1945.
24. Larson, DL: The Prevention and Correction of Burn Scar Contracture and Hypertrophy. Shriners Burns Institute, Univ of Texas Medical Branch, Galveston, TX, 1973.
25. Akeson, WH, Woo, S L-Y, Amiel, D, et al: The connective tissue response to immobility: Biochemical changes in periarticular connective tissue of the immobilized rabbit knee. Clin Orthop 93:356–361, 1973.
26. Gamble, JG, Edwards, CC, and Max, SR: Enzymatic adaption in ligaments during immobilization. Am J Sports Med 12:221–228, 1984.

27. Amiel, D, Frey, C, Woo, S L-Y, et al: Value of hyaluronic acid in the prevention of contracture formation. Clin Orthop 196:306–311, 1985.
28. Buckwalter, JA, Rosenberg, LC, and Tang, L-H: The effect of link protein on proteoglycan aggregate structure. J Biol Chem 259:5361–5363, 1984.
29. Akeson, WH, Amiel, D, Mechanics, GL, et al: Collagen cross-linking alterations in joint contractures: Changes in the reducible cross-links in periarticular connective tissue collagen after nine weeks of immobilization. Connect Tissue Res 5:15–19, 1977.
30. Amiel, D, Akeson, WH, Harwood, FL, et al: Stress deprivation effect on metabolic turnover of the medial collateral ligament collagen. Clin Orthop 172:265–270, 1983.
31. Brody, GS, Peng, STJ, and Landel RE: The etiology of hypertrophic scar contracture: Another view. Plast Reconstr Surg 67:673–684, 1977.
32. Woo, S L-Y, Matthews, JV, Akeson, WH, et al: Connective tissue response to immobility. Arthritis Rheum 18:257–264, 1975.
33. Lavigne, AB and Watkins, RP: Preliminary results on immobilization-induced stiffness of monkey knee joints and posterior capsule. In Kenedi, RM (ed): Perspectives in Medical Engineering. Macmillan, New York, 1973.
34. Frank, C, Amiel, D, Woo, S L-Y, et al: Normal ligament properties and ligament healing. Clin Orthop 196:15–25, 1985.
35. Frank, C, Woo, S L-Y, Amiel, D, et al: Medial collateral ligament healing: A multidisciplinary assessment in rabbits. Am J Sports Med 11:379–389, 1983.
36. Furlow, LT: The role of tendon tissue in tendon healing. Plast Reconstr Surg 57:39–49, 1976.
37. Gelberman, RH, Vande Berg, JS, Lundborg, GN, et al: Flexor tendon healing and restoration of the gliding surface: An ultrastructural study in dogs. J Bone Joint Surg [Am] 65:70–80, 1983.
38. Manske, PR: The flexor tendon. Orthopedics 10:1733–1747, 1987.
39. Slack, C, Flint, MH, and Thompson BM: The effect of tensional load on isolated embryonic chick tendons in organ culture. Connect Tissue Res 12:229–247, 1984.
40. Salter, RD, Simmonds, DF, Malcolm, BW, et al: The biologic effect of continuous passive motion on the healing of full-thickness defects in articular cartilage. J Bone Joint Surg 62-A:1232–1251, 1980.
41. Goldstein, WM and Barmada, R: Early mobilization of rabbit medial collateral ligament repairs: Biologic and histologic study. Arch Phys Med Rehabil 65:239–242, 1984.
42. Madden, JW, DeVore, G, and Arem, AJ: A rational postoperative management program for metacarpophalangeal joint implant arthroplasty. J Hand Surg 2:358–366, 1977.
43. Woo, S L-Y, Gelberman, RH, Cobb, NG, et al: The importance of controlled passive mobilization on flexor tendon healing. Acta Orthop Scand 52:615–622, 1981.
44. Gelberman, RH, Woo, S L-Y, Cobb, N, et al: Flexor tendon healing: The effects of early passive mobilization. Transactions of the 27th Annual Meeting of the Orthopedic Research Society, 6:81, 1981.
45. Gelberman, RH, Woo, S L-Y, Lothringer, K, et al: Effects of early intermittent passive mobilization on healing canine flexor tendons. J Hand Surg 7:170–175, 1982.
46. Carstens, H and Noakes, TD: A study comparing time-to-recovery after functional vs cast management of severe lateral ankle sprains. Presented at the South Africa Sports Medicine Academy Meeting, Cape Town, 1986.
47. Stove, CN: Air-stirrup management of ankle injuries in the athlete. Am J Sports Med 8:360–365, 1980.
48. Salter, RB, Bell, RS, and Keeley, FW: The effect of continuous passive motion on the preservation of articular cartilage in septic arthritis: An experimental investigation in the rabbit. Transactions of the 27th Annual Meeting of the Orthopedic Research Society, 6:23, 1984.
49. O'Driscoll, SW, Kumar, A, and Salter, RB: The effect of continuous passive motion on the clearance of a hemarthrosis from a synovial joint: An experimental investigation in the rabbit. Clin Orthop 176:305–311, 1983.
50. Coutts, RD, Kaita, J, Ball, R, et al: The role of continuous passive motion in the postoperative rehabilitation of the total knee patient. Transactions of the 28th Annual Meeting of the Orthopedic Research Society, 1982.
51. Faso, D and Stills, M: Passive mobilization: An orthothist's view. Clin Prosthet and Orthot 9:7, 1985.
52. Malone, T, Blackburn, TA, and Wallace, LA: Knee rehabilitation. Phys Ther 60:1602–1610, 1980.
53. Brand, P: Clinical Mechanics of the Hand. CV Mosby, St Louis, 1985.
54. Kolumban, SL: The role of static and dynamic splints: Physiotherapy techniques and time in straightening contracted interphalangeal joints. Leprosy India 41:323–328, 1969.
55. Belsole, RJ and Osborn, G: The use of spring-loaded splints in treating wrist-flexion contractures. Plast Reconstr Surg 69:1015–1016, 1982.
56. Becker, AM: Traction for knee flexion contractures. Phys Ther 59:1114, 1979.
57. Green, DP and McCoy, H: Turnbuckle orthotic correction of elbow-flexion contractures after acute injuries. J Bone Joint Surg [Am] 61:1092–1095, 1979.
58. Hepburn, GR: Case studies: Contracture and stiff joint management with dynasplint. Journal of Orthopedic Sports and Physical Therapy 8:498–504, 1987.
59. Savill, D: Evaluation of splinting. Arthritis Rheum 7:585–600, 1964.

60. Reddy, NR and Kolumban, SL: The effects of daily and once per week plaster of paris cylindrical splinting on contracted proximal interphalangeal joints in leprosy. Leprosy India 47:1512–1515, 1975.
61. Becker, AH: Personal communication, 1983.
62. Hepburn, GR and Crivelli, KJ: Use of elbow dynasplint for reduction of elbow flexor contractures: A case study. Journal of Orthopedic Sports and Physical Therapy 5:269–274, 1984.
63. Rizk, TE, Christopher, RP, Penials, RS, et al: Adhesive capsulitis (frozen shoulder): A new approach to its management. Arch Phys Med Rehabil 64:29–33, 1983.
64. Hepburn, GR: Multi-center clinical investigation on the effect of incorporating dynasplint treatment into standard physical therapy practice for restoring range of motion of elbows and knees. Presented at the American Physical Therapy Association State Chapter Meeting, New York, 1985.
65. Nicholson, G: The effects of passive joint mobilization on pain and hypomobility associated with adhesive capsulitis of the shoulder. Division of Physical Therapy, University of Alabama, Birmingham, AL, 1982. Master's Thesis.
66. McLaughlin, HL: The "frozen shoulder." Clin Orthop 20:126–131, 1961.
67. Evans, EB, Eggers, GWN, Butler, JK, et al: Experimental immobilization and remobilization of rat knee joint. J Bone Joint Surg [Am] 42:7373–758, 1960.
68. Cummings, GS, Crutchfield, CA, and Barnes, MR: Orthopedic Physical Therapy, Vol 1. Soft Tissue Changes in Contractures. Stokesville Publishing, Atlanta, GA, 1983.
69. Warren, CG, Lehman, JF, and Koblanski, JN: Heat and stretch procedures: An evaluation using rat tail tendon. Arch Phys Med Rehabil 57:122–126, 1976.
70. Lehman, JF, Masock, AJ, Warren, CG, et al: Effect of therapeutic temperatures on tendon extensibility. Arch Phys Med Rehabil 50:481–487, 1970.
71. Warren, CG, Lehman, JF, and Koblanski, JN: Elongation of rat tail tendon: Effect of load and temperature. Arch Phys Med Rehabil 52:465–484, 1971.
72. Jones, CW: Physical changes in isolated human collagen subjected to clinical dosages of ultrasound. Department of Biology, Midwestern State University, Witchita Fall, TX, 1976. Master's Thesis.

CHAPTER 3

Skeletal Muscle Function

Gary L. Soderberg, Ph.D., P.T., FAPTA

Essential to normal human function is the generation and maintenance of muscular tension for the interval of time required for the intended function. Effective clinical practice requires an understanding of the many factors involved in the performance of even the simplest of muscular contractions. For example, architectural features such as angle of pinnation (line of pull of muscle) and the orientation of sarcomeres play an important role. It is also necessary for the clinician to understand physiologic relations in order to effectively exercise patients with deviations in the normal patterns of tension generation and maintenance. Finally, knowledge of the influence of pathology on normal skeletal muscle function is useful to the clinician. The purpose of this chapter is to present relevant information on these topics and then to discuss clinical implications for the management of patients with disorders affecting skeletal muscle function.

ANATOMIC FEATURES

Fundamentals

The functional musculotendinous unit is composed of several different tissues that form a structure capable of meeting many demands. Each of the components of the structure is discussed in other parts of this book. The reader's attention is specifically directed to those chapters addressing connective tissue, and tendon growth and regeneration. Knowledge of the contents of each of these chapters will enhance the reader's understanding of functional skeletal muscle.

Numerous anatomic features affect the performance of skeletal muscle. Enoka[1] states that there are three major architectural design features that influence tension generation capability. These include (1) the number of sarcomeres per muscle fiber in series, (2) the number of muscle fibers in parallel, and (3) the angle of the fibers relative to the line of pull of the muscle (pinnation).

Sarcomeres/Fiber Arrangement

Numerous works have established that the arrangement of the sarcomeres and fibers are important in determining the functional characteristics of muscle, the most recent being those by Sacks and Roy[2] and by Edgerton and colleagues.[3] Two muscles are diagrammatically presented in Figure 3–1 that have identical mass, fiber angle attachment, and fiber type composition and biochemistry. Twitch contraction and relaxation times are identical for the two muscles. Note, however, that the fiber group labeled A will develop twice as much tension as will group B because of the difference in the cross-sectional area of the muscles. Conversely, fiber group B will produce twice the velocity of shortening per muscle fiber as those fibers in group A because of difference in length. Thus, with simultaneous activation of all the sarcomeres, the force-time characteristics associated with these two groups would be similar. However, the force-velocity and subsequently the muscular power available would be quite different. Figure 3–2 shows that the peak power is of the same magnitude, but the location of the peak shown in fiber group A is reached at twice the velocity as that for fiber group B. Note also that the range of velocities over which power can be produced differs between the two configurations. This performance variation implies that muscles are suited for different functions, the largest in-series sarcomere arrangements[8] being best suited for producing higher velocities of shortening and the in-parallel arrangements (A) being more appropriate for producing higher tension

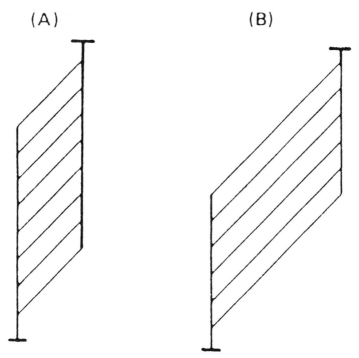

FIGURE 3–1. Two basic designs of muscles showing the effects of architecture on force-velocity properties and isometric contraction time. Whereas both have identical muscle mass and angle of pinnation (as indicated by lines within the muscle), the fiber length in muscle B is twice that of muscle A. The bars (T/⊥) represent tendinous attachments. (From Sacks and Roy,[2] p. 193, with permission.)

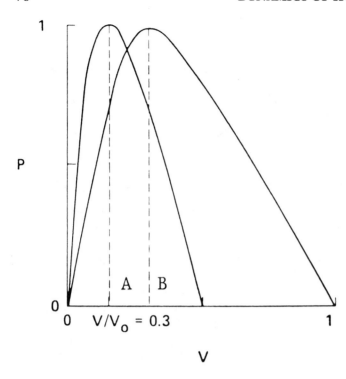

FIGURE 3–2. The theoretic power potentials of conditions A and B from Figure 3–1 are shown. The dashed lines identify the velocity at which peak power was assumed to have occurred relative to the maximum velocity of shortening. (From "Morphological Basis of Skeletal Muscle Power Output" by V.R. Edgerton, R.R. Roy, R.J. Gregor et al. In *Human Muscle Power* (p. 45) by N.L. Jones, N. McCartney, A.J. McComes (Eds.), 1986, Champaign, IL: Human Kinetics Publishers. Reprinted with permission.)

levels. The manifestations and importance of these differences relative to clinical practice will be discussed later in this chapter.

Angle of Pinnation

Observation of muscle structure in cadavers clearly demonstrates that a wide variety of differences exists in the arrangement of muscle fibers within the human body. One characteristic of interest is the angle of pinnation, or the angle that fibers attach to the line of action of the muscle. Gans[4] discusses this factor in detail and describes another way of defining these muscle fiber arrangements: parallel fiber arrangements produce purely translational motion, and pinnate fibered muscles rotate about their origin, changing the angle of pinnation as they shorten. Only arrays of fibers that are responsible for rotation of the muscle should be termed pinnate, even though the fibers may lie parallel to each other within the muscle. However, the individual fibers of the muscle may not always lie parallel to each other. Consequently, fibers of individual muscles will not function collectively, and thereby cause rotation of the segment to which they are attached. Functionally complex muscles show the most complex arrays of pinnation.[4]

There is general agreement that the force generated by muscle fibers attached to tissues is influenced by the angle of fiber attachment. Simply stated, as the angle of attachment increases, the effective force at the attachment site decreases. This concept can also be stated mathematically as

$$F_t = \Sigma \, F_f \cos 0$$

where F_t is tendon force, F_f the force of the individual fibers, and 0 the angle of pinnation. The cosine law establishes that there are marked decreases in the effective force once the angle has exceeded 30 degrees. If the angle exceeds 60 degrees, the effective force will be reduced by 50 percent. Note also that the angle of attachment changes as the muscle shortens, the more change occurring during dynamic (motion) exercise than compared with static (motionless) exercise forms.

Determining the angle of pinnation in human muscles may then be important in understanding the movement of a body segment. Only a few studies in humans have evaluated the actual angle of pinnation and its subsequent influence. Wickiewicz and colleagues[5] are among the few investigators in this field, and they have studied the muscles of the lower extremity of three specimens. They found that while angles of fiber pinnation for most muscles were between 0 and 15 degrees, there were some exceptions. For example, the short head of the biceps femoris muscle had angles between 22 and 25 degrees. Although the soleus muscle values for two specimens ranged from 20 to 30 degrees, the authors noted that one section of the soleus muscle contained fibers of pinnation of up to 60 degrees. Only two other muscles, the semi-membranosus and the medial gastrocnemius, had angles of over 15 degrees. Most angles of fiber pinnation were 5 degrees or less.[5] Thus, there should be only subtle differences across human lower extremity muscles when angle of pinnation is considered. The cat also has angles of fiber pinnation that vary from 0 to 21 degrees, with most being less than 10 degrees.[2] Although Enoka's work summarizes that the angle of fiber pinnation is between 0 and 0.4 radians (22.9 degrees), he provides no reference for the values. He further states that the "advantage of pinnation is that a greater number of fibers and thus sarcomeres in parallel can be packed into a given volume of muscle."[1]

Thus, whereas the importance of the angle of pinnation has been noted in many textbooks and other sources, the real effect of these angles on force production would appear to be minimal because the muscles are mostly attached at rather small angles. As Gans[4] points out, there may be implications for "cost." Included in this context would be radially or multipinnate arrays that could yield an effect such as lateral disposition of the attachment site. Gans and Bock[6] suggested that the pinnate arrangement may compensate for aging, in that as fibers are lost, the fiber arrangement becomes parallel, thus yielding more effective force via the attachment site. In any case, the angle of pinnation needs to be considered relative to other factors associated with muscle architecture in order to determine the total tension available within any given contractile unit.

MECHANICAL BASES FOR FUNCTION

Contracting muscle has been modeled by numerous persons on many occasions. Hill[7] is well known for pioneering work in this area, successfully describing the force-velocity relation more than 40 years ago. The model used makes some difference in the final determination of functional characteristics.

Length-Tension

The models in Figure 3–3 show the basic elements responsible for producing the length-tension relation. The contractile element (CE) designates the contractile com-

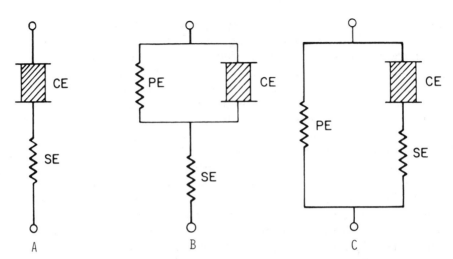

FIGURE 3–3. Models of human muscles. *(A)* According to the Hill model, the series elastic (SE) and the contractile element (CE) are in series. *(B)* In the Voight model, a parallel element (PE) has been added in parallel to CE. *(C)* In the Maxwell model, note that the PE is in parallel with both CE and SE. (Reprinted with permission from Phillips, CA and Petrofsky, JS: The passive elastic force velocity relationship of cat skeletal muscle: Influence upon the maximal contractile element velocity. J Biomech 14. Copyright 1981, Pergamon Press, Inc.)

ponent or the overlap of actin and myosin filaments of muscle fibers. The PE, or parallel elastic component, is made up of the connective tissues surrounding the muscle filaments. The series elastic component is the SE portion of the model and can be considered to be the tendinous portion of the neuromuscular unit. These components exist in every muscle, but exactly how these various elements relate to each other determines the length-tension relation for a given muscle.

To explain the length-tension relation, the contribution of each of the elements must be evaluated. Referring to Figure 3–4, consider an attempt to lengthen muscle.

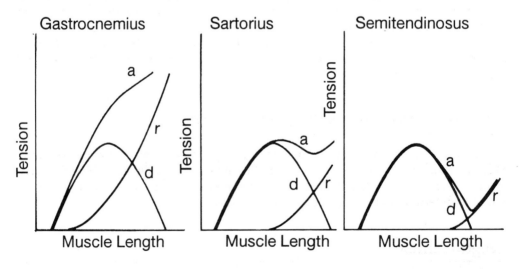

a = Total tension   r = Passive tension   d = Contractile tension

FIGURE 3–4. Length-tension curves for three different muscles. See text for complete description.

To do so, move to the right on the abscissa (x axis). When this is done, passive tension, indicated by the r curve, arises within the muscle. The total tension, shown as a, is available under conditions of contraction of muscle. This total tension represents the combined effect of the passive (r) and the contractile (d) elements. Note that the curve generated by the contractile element (d) is the tension achieved under different lengths by the contractile component, that is, the actin and myosin filaments. However, this contractile element curve is not totally discernible because as contractions are performed at different lengths, the passive elements (r) intervene. Thus, the tension shown by curve a is the result of the passive plus the contractile components, or $a = d + r$.

On review of the length-tension relations for the three different muscles in Figure 3–4, one should readily note the difference in configuration. Differences in the shape of the curve are accounted for by the shifting of the passive element as muscle length is increased; that is, passive tension is a factor earlier in the lengthening process. Since the total tension a is a result of $r + d$, there are concurrent changes in a that are reflective of the shifting of the passive element to the left. Thus, the gastrocnemius muscle would have a much greater total tension-generating capability than the semitendinosus at equivalent lenghts of the respective muscles.[8]

Configuration of the length-tension curve has been shown to vary between species of animals. Goldspink[9] and White[10] have respectively presented length-tension and resting tension diagrams for the bumblebee, locust, frog, and snail. Two factors are apparent from these figures. First, in Figure 3–5 the tension curve of muscle is contained along the vertical axis of the graph. Second, in Figure 3–6 the passive elements have varying degrees of slope. Considering these two factors in relation to the functions performed by each animal, it is not remarkable that the snail pharynx muscle moves slowly, whereas the bumblebee's flight muscle is capable of sustaining wing motions upwards of 600 Hz.[9]

These characteristics vary across muscles, not only in lower animal forms but also in humans. For example, cardiac muscle of humans will more closely simulate the frog gastrocnemius than the frog semitendinosus muscle because of functional requirements related to cardiac output. Intact human muscle has been difficult to evaluate in vivo for obvious reasons, but work published by Ralston and associates[11] indicates that characteristics identified in animals have similar features in humans. Subjects in their experiments were amputees who had undergone a cineplastic procedure, in which the surgeon places a tunnel through the muscle tendon so that a cable or other mechanical mechanism can be permanently attached. Thus, a direct attachment to muscle was possible. Subsequently, Ralston and associates[11] were able to evaluate the passive component and other features associated with tension development at various biceps brachii muscle lengths. When compared across different muscles, the passive components for human muscles vary, as demonstrated and graphically displayed by Yamada[12] (Fig. 3–7).

In vivo force-length relations have not been established,[13] but theoretical and experimental data have been compared for human rectus femoris muscles.[14] The authors speculated that even though the muscle fibers are arranged in parallel, they may reach their optimal length at different muscle lengths. The effect would be a smaller peak force but larger range over which active forces could be expected.

Also of interest is that in 1966 Gordon and associates[15] studied the length-tension curve at the sarcomere level. A schematic summary of the result is shown in Figure 3–8. The arrows along part A represent various stages of overlap portrayed in section

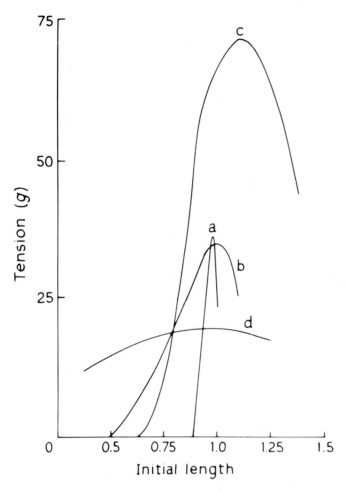

FIGURE 3–5. The length–active tension curves are shown for a variety of muscles. The tensions cannot be directly compared because they are not in g per U cross section. Bumblebee flight muscle is a, b is locust flight muscle, c is frog sartorius muscle, and d is snail pharynx retractor muscle. (From Alexander, RMcN and Goldspink, G: Mechanics and Energetics of Animal Locomotion. New York, John Wiley & Sons, Inc. Copyright 1977. Reprinted with permission.)

B of the figure. Assuming similar findings hold true for all other sarcomeres, a large population of such curves would produce the dome-shaped configuration of the contractile component of the length-tension relation for a total muscle (see Fig. 3–4).

Several specific applications and implications arise from the length-tension relation. The first is the influence of precontraction stretch. Figure 3–9 shows the effect of the passive (elastic) element on muscle action and ultimate tension output. Note, however, that the figure ignores the concept of viscosity, which in fact exists because of the fluid elements within the muscle. This viscosity, influenced by factors such as temperature and amount of body fluids, is difficult to determine. However, for the sake of a more complete model of muscle, inclusion is well warranted. Note that Figure 3–9B shows shortening of the contractile component and stretching of the series elastic component, producing the tension shown on the dial. In Figure 3–9C, a quick stretch has been applied to the muscular unit, while at the same time the contractile component is shortening to the same degree as shown in Figure 3–9B. The ultimate result is an increase in total tension output of the structure. Thus, by applying stretch or by lengthening the muscle and series elastic component during the course of the contraction, a greater amount of tension can be generated. This concept of precontraction stretch is applied in many therapeutic situations and will be elucidated in later chapters.

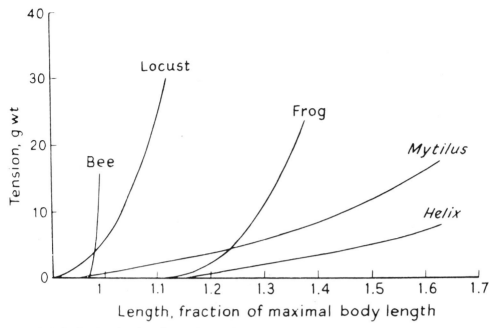

FIGURE 3–6. Resting length–passive tension curves for the muscles shown in Figure 3–5 and the mytilus. The combined curves of Figures 3–5 and 3–6 would form similar active and resting tension curves as for those shown in Figure 3–4, accounting for the mechanics of each of the muscles. (From Alexander, RMcN and Goldspink, G: Mechanics and Energetics of Animal Locomotion. New York, John Wiley & Sons, Inc. Copyright 1977. Reprinted with permission.)

Elastic energy can, in fact, be stored and transformed into kinetic energy. Such was the case illustrated in Figure 3–9, where stretch was applied as the contraction occurred. Other examples can be noted. Goldspink[9] states that flea muscle contains a substance known as resilin. Resilin, a near-perfect rubber material, when stretched or deformed can rapidly return to its original state. Thus, muscle is used to develop tension over a long period of time. Then, with a quick release of tension, the flea performs a tremendous leap.[9]

Asmussen and Bonde-Peterson[16] have evaluated similar characteristics in humans. They compared the squat jump with a jump preceded by a rapid countermovement to stretch the muscle, and with a jump from a height. Their findings showed that the countermovement jump was 22 percent higher than the jump from a static position. Likewise, the jump from a height was 3 to 13 percent higher than from a static position. In other work,[17] these same investigators have calculated that in humans 35 to 53 percent of the energy absorbed during the negative phase is reused during position work. More recently, Komi and co-workers[18–20] have completed similar studies on the stretch-shortening cycle. During a stretch of contracted muscle, mechanical energy is absorbed by the muscle and is subsequently reused if the muscle shortens further immediately after the stretch (e.g., semisquat to vertical jump, or drop to different levels while standing).[20] These studies have reevaluated the stretch-shortening cycle with various activities and by means of electrical and mechanical responses. Their results have indicated that the myoelectrical activity was potentiated during jumps that were preceded by a stretch, attributing the increase in vertical height jumped to both this potentiation and the use of elastic energy.[20] In other work, the

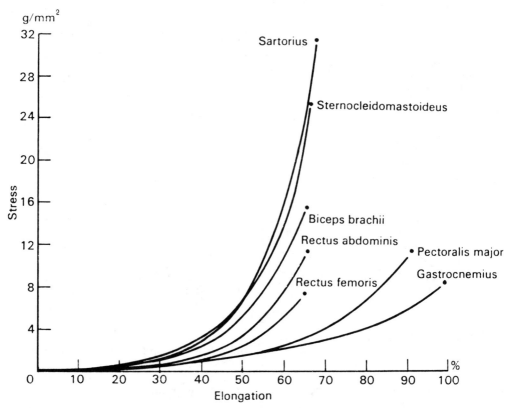

FIGURE 3–7. Stress-elongation curves for tension of skeletal muscle in 29-year-olds. Practically, stress is equivalent to tension and elongation is equal to length of the muscle. Note the variation between muscles. (From Yamada,[12] p. 95, with permission.)

mechanical efficiency of concentric and eccentric exercises performed at different contraction rates was evaluated, revealing that, among other findings, the efficiency was greater for the eccentric than for the concentric contractions. Also, velocity of shortening, as measured indirectly via knee angular velocity, had an influence on the net mechanical efficiency of the eccentrically performed contractions.[19] In general, use of the stretch-shortening cycle invokes both reflex potentiation of muscle and the use of elastic energy.[18] Mention should be made that this cycle is invoked during activities such as walking, but that the velocity of the required performance does not produce the maximum effect in terms of the output of muscle tension. Applications are more relevant when sports or recreational activities are considered to be in the domain of the patient. Thus, these factors become important whenever motion causes the muscle to undergo lengthening prior to contraction.

Force-Velocity

The basic force-velocity relation uncovered by Hill is shown in Figure 3–10. The symbol V_{max} stands for the maximum velocity of shortening, and P_o signifies the maximum load or force. The figure demonstrates that as a load diminishes, the muscle

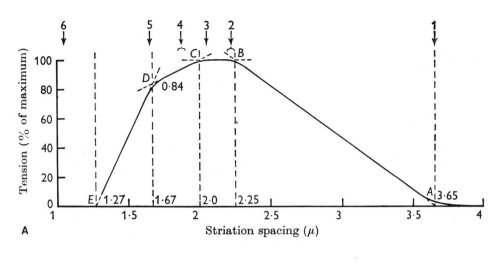

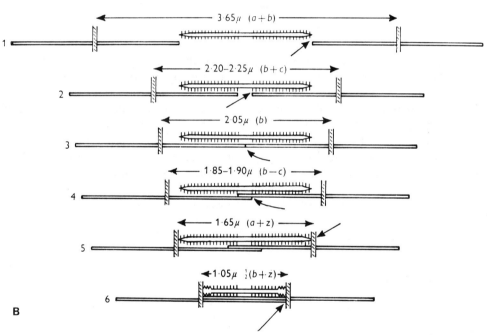

FIGURE 3–8. Composite showing the relationship of sarcomere length to the length-tension curve. Length of the various elements equals 1.60 μm for a, 2.05 for b, 0.15–2 for c, and 0.05 for z. See text for complete explanation. (From Gordon, Huxley, and Julian,[15] p. 185, with permission.)

shortens. That is, heavy loads are moved slower than light loads by muscle. At P_o there is zero velocity, and thus the condition of isometric contraction. The dotted line superimposed on the curve is the mechanical power produced. Such a relation is derived by transforming the formula *Velocity* = d/t into the *Power* = fd/t relation so that $P = FV$; where P is power, F is force, and V is velocity. Note that the maximum mechanical power (the same on the dotted line) is available at the location where the value of one third the maximum velocity would be multiplied by one third the maximum load or force.

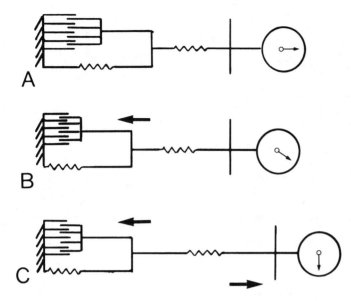

FIGURE 3–9. Influence of elongation on the ultimate tension generated in muscle. *(A)* Model of resting muscle. *(B)* Generation of isometric tension. Note that the two attachments of the muscle have not been separated. *(C)* Contraction of the contractile component with simultaneous lengthening of the muscle increasing the tension available. (From Soderberg, GL: Kinesiology: Application to Pathological Motion. © 1986, the Williams & Wilkins Co., Baltimore.)

The gastrocnemius will produce greater force than the semitendinosus muscle because its cross section is greater than that of the semitendinosus. If velocity of contraction (d/t) were held constant, clearly the greater power would be generated by the gastrocnemius muscle because the force (F) would be greater. Recall also the rate of shortening is influenced by the angle of fiber insertion with a lower velocity of shortening observed for pennate than for fusiform type of muscle. The specific power capabilities of any muscle are, therefore, dependent on the contractile properties and mechanisms that are responsible for the force and the velocity (see Fig. 3–10).

Figure 3–11, from the work of Komi,[21] shows the force-velocity relation for elbow

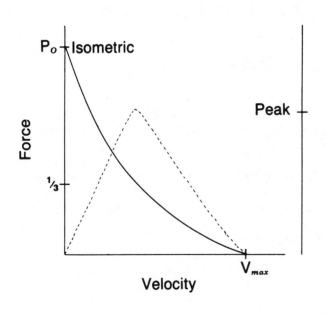

FIGURE 3–10. The force-velocity relationship, based on data from an isolated-muscle preparation. (From Enoka, RM: Neuromechanical Basis of Kinesiology. Human Kinetics Books, Champaign, IL, 1988, p. 169, with permission.)

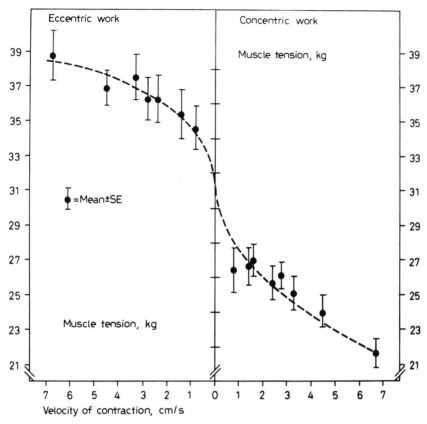

FIGURE 3–11. Force-velocity curve for elbow flexor muscles. Further explanation is contained in the text. (From Komi,[21] p. 227, with permission.)

flexor musculature for concentric and eccentric contractions. Although the tension and velocity scales have been inverted on the graph, as compared with the previous figure, the relation is unaltered. Note that the vertical line in the center of the graph indicates an isometric condition. Concentric work, when the muscle shortens, is to the right of the graph; eccentric contraction is to the left. Observe that at the highest velocity of concentric work, the lowest possible tension is achieved. During the eccentric contraction, the highest tension available is at the highest velocity while the isometric value is shown at approximately 31 kilograms of force (kgf). In retrospect, these data are as we would expect, in that eccentric work is, in fact, stretching the muscle concurrently while a contractile component is attempting to shorten the entire neuromuscular unit. Because we know that humans can move at over 1000 degrees per second, the 7 cm/second velocity (corresponding to approximately 120 degrees/second) represents only a limited range of the velocity available to human muscle.[21]

Other studies of exercise physiology have shown that the energy required by eccentric contractions is far less than that created by concentric exercise.[22] For example, descending stairs is known to be easier than ascending a similar flight of stairs or controlling a specific therapeutic load while lengthening muscle as opposed to doing so while shortening the muscle. These specific examples demonstrate the ability of muscle to use the elastic components during lengthening contractions.

Force-Time

The fundamental relation of force and time is demonstrated in Figure 3–12.[23] This curve applies to isometric contractions and can be explained on the basis of muscle structure. As the contraction is initiated, the contractile component proceeds to stretch the elastic components within the muscle. During that phase, a nonlinear increase in the force production is created. Once the elastic components have been "pulled out," the development of force will reach an essentially linear stage around the point of inflection through which the slope or tangent line has been drawn. The maximum is reached as the contractile component can generate no greater tension by exerting force through the series elastic component. Studies involving training have indicated that maximum tension can be generated to approximately 300 milliseconds.[24]

It is significant that as the joint angle is varied, the force-time curve will vary in P_{100} (maximum tension) reached. At angles of muscle insertion less than 90 degrees, a component of the force will be transmitted to compress the joint.[25] Consequently,

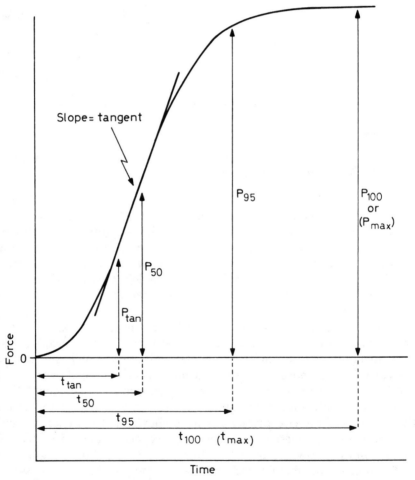

FIGURE 3–12. Force-time curve for human muscle and several common measurements used to evaluate tension generation and maintenance. (From Stothart,[21] p. 212, with permission.)

less tension can go toward creating the turning moment, thus resulting in a lower P_o value measured. Moments are used as the standard and comparative measure within and between patients. Also recall that at greater than 90 degrees a component of the muscular tension is distracting the joint and thereby changing the features of the force-time curve.

Muscle Modeling

Recently Woittiez and associates[26] considered a three-dimensional muscle model, showing that they could closely approximate the actual muscle form and function. Two papers on the topic of modeling were also recently published (Fig. 3–13). DaSilva[27] includes neural elements in using mathematical approaches to the understanding of muscle as an effector organ. Otten[28] focuses on an analysis of muscle models, proposes revision in modeling concepts, and discusses the advantages and rationales of two forms of muscle modeling. Although such models can (1) simulate functional characteristics of muscles that are sometimes hard to measure, and (2) offer analysis of muscle models, there are still some unsolved problems associated with this approach.[28]

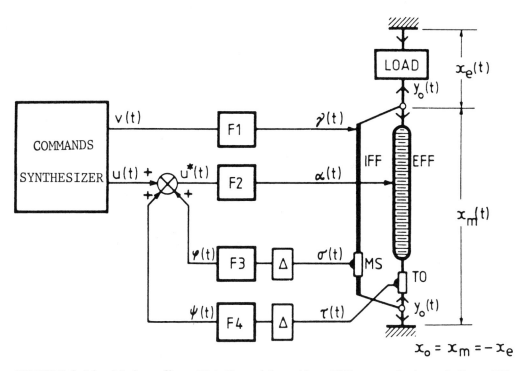

FIGURE 3–13. Mechanoeffector Unit Control Assemblage. EFF = extrafusal muscle fibers; IFF = intrafusal (muscle spindle) muscle fibers; MS = muscle spindle sensor; TO = Golgi tendon organ; F_1, F_2, F_3, F_4 = correcting filters located in the CNS; Δ = propagation delays in the nerve links. Small signal variables: u and v = muscle and fusimotor commands; α and γ = muscle and fusimotor efferent commands; and τ = afferent signals; ϕ and ψ = corrected afferent signals; x_m and x_e = motor and load lengths (or strains); x_o = force developed by (or stress in) the mechanoeffector unit assemblage. (From Berme, N, Engin, AE, and Correia da Silva, KM (eds): Biomechanics of Normal Pathological Human Articulating Joints. Estoril, Portugal, 1983, p. 240, with permission.)

At present there are limited implications for the clinician dealing with patients with muscle dysfunction, but as the models are further developed the modeler will likely consult clinicians to gain insight into function while the model is perturbed.

TENSION GENERATION AND MAINTENANCE

Contraction Types

As is well known, the types of muscle contraction vary. Definitions have not been commonly accepted. The student/clinician must use this observandum against indiscriminate use because the same term may be interpreted differently. The most common terminologic variations are described below.

The most consistently used term is *isometric* (defined below). In this contraction type, constant muscle length is implied because segments remain fixed. However, since there is considerable shortening at the protein filament level in any condition of tension generation, no contraction appears to satisfy isometric conditions.[15]

Isotonic contractions, literally translated as "same tension or force," are typically broken down into two subcategories. They have been defined by O'Connel and Gowitzke[29] as:

Concentric: Sometimes called shortening contraction; a muscle contraction in which the internal force produced by the muscle exceeds the external force of resistance, the muscle shortens, and movement is produced.
Eccentric: A muscle contraction in an already shortened muscle, to which an external force greater than the internal force is added, and the muscle lengthens while continuing to maintain tension.

Bouisset[30] provides another system for definition:

Isometric: External resistance is equal to the internal force developed by the muscle, and there is no external movement.
Isotonic: A muscle contraction when the external force is constant.
Anisotonic: A muscle contraction resulting when external resistance is smaller or greater than the internal muscle force. If smaller, muscle shortens (concentric or positive work); if greater, muscle lengthens (eccentric or negative work).

Some commonalities in definitions are readily recognized. Although Bouisset[30] may have a more sensible form of definition, the most frequently used are those provided by O'Connel and Gowitzke,[29] with the exception that concentric and eccentric contractions are both considered forms of isotonic exercise.

More recently, isokinetic exercises have become a popular exercise mode incorporated in devices. A literal interpretation of the term *isokinetic* is "constant or same speed." In actuality these electromechanical/hydraulic devices enable exercise through a range of motion at a constant angular velocity. Patients, healthy subjects, or both will typically not apply the constant force output implied in the definition of isokinetic exercise. In reality the devices allow individuals to perform at constant velocity, thus making constant force a possibility but not a requirement. In fact, as will be described in subsequent chapters, changes in the forces and resulting torques may be indicative of pathology. Finally, although concentric and eccentric forms of isokinetic exercise may be performed, the eccentric form is more limited by loading requirements and concerns for patient safety than is the concentric form.

Implication of Anatomic and Mechanical Bases

Neural control over contracting muscles is prerequisite to the generation and maintenance of their tension in the appropriate temporal sequence. Without proper neural control, characteristics such as "strength" and endurance cannot be volitionally used. Given that control is possible, then the factors of tension and endurance become important to persons receiving rehabilitation. Each of the factors discussed previously in this chapter play some role in tension generation and maintenance. Both the anatomic and physiologic features are important to normal function.

According to Edgerton and associates,[3] the physiologic cross-sectional area, fiber length, and mass are the primary morphologic determinants of maximal force, velocity, and power, respectively. Of lesser influence are the angle of attachment of fibers and the interfiber connections.[3] Lieber and Boakes[31] support this notion in a study of the frog hindlimb, stating that muscle force and not musculoskeletal anatomy significantly contributed to torque production. In a companion paper that addresses the matter of sarcomere length during torque production in the frog, the authors demonstrated that the sarcomere lengths and the effective lever arms produced rather different effects, although their sum total is dependent on the interaction of both muscular and joint properties.[32]

A more general view of anatomic and mechanical bases may be found in a 1988 paper on mechanical properties of synergistic human muscles. Winters and Stark[33] discuss the importance of geometry, stating that "geometrical parameters such as moment arm, fiber pinnation and length, and muscle size are of greater importance than muscle material properties in determining structural properties." In their discussion, they suggest that moment arm differences of only 1 or 2 cm result in profound effects on the torque produced. Because the torque generated is the factor of primary interest, much of the clinician's attention should be focused on the effect of his or her techniques on this measurable characteristic. Winters and Stark go on to comment that, as should be expected, a muscle with a larger moment arm consistently sacrifices velocity for a greater ability to generate torque. As compensation, muscles with larger moment arms tend to be "faster" muscles with longer muscle fibers and less pinnation. Such an arrangement allows for the muscles around a joint to contract at a similar velocity.[33] Such discussion introduces the issue of muscle synergies (helping or accessory muscles) in human movement. Clearly the human body is designed to invoke simultaneous activity in a number of muscles effecting a torque at a particular joint. This simultaneous muscle activity seems intuitively true from study of the gross anatomy of virtually any joint. The contraction of multiple muscles located in the vicinity of any one joint during various movements of body segments supports such patterns of synergy. Whether these synergies hold true for motions of multiple joints or even entire extremities is still open for discussion. Evidence to answer this type of question needs to be produced before additional credence will be given to this phenomenon as part of normal human movement or as a strategy to treat patients affected by pathology.

Associated with the question of synergy is the issue of the function of superficial versus deep muscles. The deep muscles, often of slow type and considered more useful for postural movements, tend to have less tendon and higher pinnation. Each of these characteristics would tend to make the muscle more effective over a smaller, rather than larger, operating range. Winters and Stark[33] believe that deeper muscles may make significant contribution to faster movements. Probably the superficial muscles are important for all types of movements, tending to be recruited when a need exists for a high initial acceleration of a body segment, or when high resistive loads are applied. In concluding this segment of their discussion, the investigators state that "there is a great need to identify task-specific optimization criteria and then correlate theoretical findings to measured individual muscle activity so as to establish when and why individual synergistic muscles might not contract in unison."[33]

Inherent to any discussion about tension generation and maintenance is the sarcomere. The literature, mostly recent, has provided interesting insights into the role of this contractile unit. While the number of sarcomeres within the muscle is highly adjustable,[34] the length of any sarcomere remains rather constant.[35] Apparently the adjustment in number of sarcomeres allows for the constancy of muscle length, providing the muscle in turn the maximal opportunity (if need be) for force production from the sarcomere.[36] Evidence suggests that the stimulus for control of the sarcomere number is tension within the fiber.[35,36] Thus there is evidence of adaptability within muscle, so that the effective force to be generated can be controlled depending on the circumstances. This concept of muscle adaptability will be elucidated when the effect of immobilization is discussed in a later section of this chapter.

Methods of Measuring Muscle Tension

The determination of in vivo human muscle tension is of great interest, but is difficult to measure.[37] More recently, some researchers have had success in gaining access to animal musculotendinous units for the purpose of measuring tension,[38] but by and large these techniques are available in humans in only isolated instances. Other direct measures have been forthcoming for applications to the human, but their validity and applicability are yet to be determined.[39] Thus indirect measures will continue to be used to assess the level of human muscle tension.

In general, indirect methods consist of two primary forms. One is the determination of the joint moment. This determination is convenient and readily available even to the novice clinician. The force imparted by a motion segment is simply registered by a transducer that can be either manually or mechanically restrained. A hand-held dynamometer and an isokinetic resistive device are respective examples. The resulting force, preferably in the unit of Newtons of force, is then multiplied by the perpendicular distance to the joint center about which the motion is being generated. This procedure results in the calculation of the joint torque and is representative of the tensions from the responsible muscles multiplied by their respective perpendicular distances, or moment arms. Thus, given the appropriate measurement of external joint torques and a set of moment arm data for the musculature, we can satisfactorily derive the muscular tension generated, as shown by the equation

$$F_m = \frac{M}{d}$$

where F_m is muscle force (at angle of insertion of 90 degrees), M is measured moment, and d the moment arm measured as a perpendicular distance from the muscle(s) to the joint axis.

However, several difficulties are inherent in this approach. The first difficulty is that moment arm sets of data for human muscles are not comprehensive or readily available. In addition, the moment arms are known to change as the joint goes through a range of motion. Thus, at best, incomplete data and the dynamic conditions deter the derivation of highly accurate information. Another difficulty is that the clinician cannot ascertain how to distribute the external moment to the contributing muscles, in that there is no method, other than theoretical, to distribute the forces to each of the participating muscles.

The second indirect method of measuring muscle tension is by the use of the electromyograph (EMG). The technique has been used extensively to establish the EMG-tension relation for human muscles. Although information is available that would be of some use in this regard, the matter is complicated by muscle type, difficulties associated with the isolation of recordings from only one muscle, and other technological considerations. Thus there is little immediate prospect that technique will be useful for the accurate determination of muscle force from individual muscles during a contraction that results in tension generation from a number of different muscles acting to produce a moment at a joint.

Hence, the clinician will most commonly resort to indirect methods such as torque measurements to gather an objective measure of patient capability. Although there are some constraints associated with this technique, this alternative is still best for assessing the functional capacity of human muscle.

CLINICAL RELEVANCE AND IMPLICATIONS

During the course of patient care activities, the practitioner must always keep in mind the causes of the muscle dysfunction. Among anatomic and physiologic principles, those addressing function that can be altered should be the focus of concern for patient care. In some studies, exercise training has been shown to have a significant effect on the return of body tissues to normal function. Although the results of various therapeutic interventions are not yet established, evidence is accumulating that segment motion and muscle contraction are desirable during rehabilitation, so that normal function can be assured. This section of the chapter will focus on several key matters, including the effects of rupture and repair of muscle and tendon, the influence of immobilization, and the alteration of mechanics associated with muscle contraction.

Elongation

Many of the injuries seen for clinical care result from excessive elongation of the tissue. These injuries are common in both competitive and recreational athletes and most frequently occur in muscles that have functional capability at more than a single joint. The extreme case is the complete rupture, such as is most frequently found in the gastrocnemius, rectus femoris, and the biceps brachii muscles. Less serious injuries can occur in these and other muscles of the body. These injuries are most likely due to a strong contraction or shortening contraction at one joint while another joint is moving such that an elongation of the muscle is simultaneously occurring. For example, during push-off required for running, the gastrocnemius muscle may be contracting strongly to plantarflex the ankle; simultaneously the knee would be extending, creating the necessary stretch—and the resulting injury.

The nature and mechanisms of tendon strength and healing are discussed more thoroughly elsewhere in this volume. For the purposes of this discussion, the clinician should know that investigators have found tendons are weakest 3 to 14 days post-surgically because the collagen remains relatively soft.[39] Although clinical experience indicates that 3 weeks of postsurgical immobilization is necessary to prevent ruptur-ing, longer than 3 weeks yields adhesions between the tendon, the sheath, and the surrounding soft tissues. Approximately 40 to 50 weeks are necessary to regain normal tendon strength postsurgically.[40] The work of Steiner[41] reveals that after 4 weeks of healing of unsutured rat tendon, 70 percent of the normal stiffness and only 40 percent of the predetermined healthy muscle rupture strength had returned. About 25 percent of the normal tendon strength had returned at 4 weeks. These relatively low per-centages indicate that high loading in the early stages of recovery must be avoided.

To determine the site of rupture in selected muscles of rabbit, Garrett and co-workers[42] examined several muscles following three rates of controlled stretching. Incorporated into the study design were the factors of fiber length and the angle of pinnation in relation to the muscle-tendon axis and line of force generation. For the rabbit tibialis anterior (fusiform), extensor digitorum longus (unipennate), peroneals (fusiform), and the rectus femoris (bipennate) muscles, the rupture occurred at the distal musculotendinous junction in 178 of 180 trials. The exception was the gastroc-nemius (multipennate) muscle, in which case 44.5 percent of the rupture occurred along deeper tendon expansions within each head or between the muscle-tendon junctions separating the two heads. No differences were seen across the rates of strain used, but the rate necessary to create a strain injury in humans has not been exam-ined.[42]

Although injuries to human tendons occur, the usual course of treatment includes stretching rates that elongate tendon very slowly. The extent of allowable tissue elongation, usually measured by clinicians as the joint range of motion, needs con-sideration. This elongation is difficult to determine directly because of inaccessibility of the tissue, but it is well known that as elongation continues, tension in the tissue will rise significantly. On the other hand, motion and tension to the tissue may be the stimulus for promoting repair and return to normal function. Thus the clinician is faced with the proverbial double-edged sword because too little tension may not be a sufficient stimulus to effect healing and too much tension may create another rupture. Studies yielding objective data on the magnitude of forces or moments exerted on joint segments or tissues during the recovery process are needed to deal with this common clinical problem.

Immobilization

Many orthopedic patients who might benefit from treatment have been subjected to immobilization of individual or multiple body segments. The principles associated with changes in muscle as a result of treatment regimens apply to those with fractures, surgeries, and lesions of the neuraxis, such as after cerebrovascular accidents (CVA) or trauma to the head. In all cases, immobilization affects muscle, perhaps within hours of the insult.[43] The result is of great importance to the clinician because unless the changes caused by injury are prevented or reversed, normal function probably cannot ensue. In certain situations, immobilization cannot be avoided; therefore, the focus must be on reversing the changes. These changes have been demonstrated in multiple preparations, as represented in the work of Tabary and co-workers.[44] This classic study showed that when the muscle was immobilized in the shortened position, the number of sarcomeres decreased by as much as 40 percent. Conversely, if the muscle was immobilized in the lengthened position, the number of sarcomeres increased by 19 percent. Other changes were present in the elastic components as well, creating the subsequent changes in the length-tension curve.[44] Further study by the same group of investigators has shown that changes in sarcomere number also occurred after only 12 hours of immobilization when muscle was shortened. This change in sarcomere numbers may be considered equivalent to what occurs in patients immobilized with lesions of the neuraxis, who frequently cannot vary lengths of involved muscles.[43]

The clinician is faced with the problem of reversing these intramuscular changes while also facing the likely prospect of intra-articular changes. Range of motion constraints may result from either or both of the above and may require mutual resolution. Further, the practitioner needs to consider that the altered properties of the involved muscle changes architecture, functional capacity, contractile tissue, and properties of the contralateral muscles.[45] Evidence appears to indicate that the most effective treatment for these intramuscular changes is tension. For example, suppose that changes have been produced by immobilization in the shortened position. Tension should be rendered by elongation so that the sarcomere number can return to normal. This tension can be accomplished by passive stretch or active exercise that will cause muscle elongation, but the temporal aspect should also be considered. Only a few minutes of treatment during a 24-hour period may not provide an adequate stimulus for reversal of the effect of immobilization. Therefore, consideration must be given to a combination of techniques such as continuous passive motion, electrical stimulation, and extensive home exercise programs before treatment will yield effective results. There is growing evidence in the literature that other tissues associated with muscles also benefit from early mobilization. For example, Salter and Bell[46] showed that in a group of animals whose tendons were lacerated and repaired, greater tendon callus formation and breaking strength, as well as a more parallel alignment of collagen, occurred in those animals treated with continuous passive motion, compared with those that were immobilized or allowed limited cage activity.[46] Perhaps the slow time course of recovery is highly related to the stimulus for these intramuscular changes.

Mechanics Associated with Muscular Effort

Changes in muscular function that are produced by pathologic or surgical means are frequently present in clinical settings. Transposition of muscle attachment sites is not an unusual procedure, the results of which need to be managed by the practitioner. Paralytic disorders, neurologic interruptions, and trauma may all require the necessary repair. In cases where temporal sequencing is of concern, such as in muscle transfers to improve gait for the patient with cerebral palsy, the period of activation of the muscle to be transferred should be similar to that of the muscle whose function is to be assumed. Otherwise there may be considerably more difficulty in producing a transfer that is maximally effective.

Transpositions create other types of difficulties for the clinician because the resulting mechanical effect may be quite different from the usual function associated with the muscle. Wickiewicz and associates[5] suggest that the architecture should be similar in fiber length and functional cross-sectional area. Otherwise, inappropriate forces and displacements can result. Thus, less physical therapy treatment would be required to assure that tension generation was adequate to perform the intended task. Further, if other than normal lengths are developed, there will be alterations in the patient's ability to exert appropriate torques at the affected joints.

Finally, comment should be made about measurements commonly performed to assess muscle function in a variety of clinical settings. These procedures typically involve manual muscle testing and a host of different types of equipment that yield more quantifiable information. Although each method has limitations associated with the respective procedure, the clinician must nonetheless be cognizant of the principles of measurement to effectively use any of the data derived from patients. Most crucial to these methods are the principles of validity and reliability; reference to the work of Rothstein[47] should be a common procedure to which clinicians subscribe. One hardly need point out that using invalid and unreliable measurements will lead to erroneous information and incorrect conclusions, something that can hardly be afforded when the quality of patient care is at stake.

SUMMARY

This chapter has discussed the function of muscle. The clinician must understand that the development and maintenance of muscular tension is dependent on a number of factors, including physiologic features such as the length-tension and force-velocity relation, as well as the architecture, the attachment site, and the moment arm of the muscle relative to a joint center of rotation. How the clinician can use these features in determining muscular tension was discussed and possible applications in therapeutic interventions were presented. In particular, evidence seems to be mounting against immobilization regimens when absolute recovery is considered as a measure of the success of treatment intervention. Tension within muscle tissue has now been given considerable credit for facilitating the recovery of muscular function. Problematically, the clinician must attempt to assist healing and recovery through mobilization but yet not be so aggressive as to produce damage to the tissues being stressed.

REFERENCES

1. Enoka, RM: Neuromechanical Basis of Kinesiology. Human Kinetics, Champaign, IL, 1967.
2. Sacks, RD and Roy, RR: Architecture of the hind limb muscles of cats: Functional significance. J Morphol 173:185–195, 1982.
3. Edgerton, VR, Roy, RR, Gregor, RJ, et al: Morphological basis of skeletal muscle power output. In Jones, NL, McCartney, N, and McComas, AJ (eds): Human Muscle Power. Human Kinetics, Champaign, IL, 1986, pp 43–64.
4. Gans, C: Fiber architecture and muscle function. In Terjung, RL (ed): Exercise and Sport Science Reviews, vol 10. The Franklin Institute, Philadelphia, 1982.
5. Wickiewicz, TL, Roy, RR, Powell, PL, et al: Muscle architecture of the human lower limb. Clin Orthop 179:275–283, 1983.

6. Gans, C and Bock, WJ: The functional significance of muscle architecture: A theoretical analysis. Ergeb Anat Entwicklgesch 38:115–142, 1965.
7. Hill, AV: Heat and shortening and the dynamic constants of muscle. Proc R Soc Lond [Biol] 126:136–195, 1938.
8. Wilkie, DR: Muscle. St Martin's Press, New York, 1968.
9. Goldspink, G: Design of muscles in relation to location. In Alexander, RMcN and Goldspink, G: Mechanics and Energetics of Animal Locomotion. Chapman & Hall, London, 1977, pp 1–22.
10. White, DCS: Muscle mechanics. In Alexander, RMcN, Goldspink, G (eds): Mechanics and Energetics of Animal Locomotion. Chapman & Hall, London, 1977, pp 23–56.
11. Ralston, HJ, Inman, VT, Strait, LA, et al: Mechanics of human isolated voluntary muscle. Am J Physiol 151:612–620, 1947.
12. Yamada, H: Mechanical properties of locomotor organs and tissues. In Evans, FG (ed): Strength of Biological Materials. Williams & Wilkins, Baltimore, 1970.
13. Herzog, W and ter Keurs, HEDJ: Force-length relation of in-vivo human rectus femoris muscles. Pflugers Arch 411:642–647, 1988.
14. Herzog, W and ter Keurs, HEDJ: A method for the determination of the force-length relation of selected in-vivo human skeletal muscles. Pflugers Arch 411:637–641, 1988.
15. Gordon, AM, Huxley, AF, and Julian, FT: The variation in isometric tension with sarcomere length in vertebrate muscle fibers. J Physiol (Lond) 184:170–192, 1966.
16. Asmussen, E and Bonde-Petersen, F: Storage of elastic energy in skeletal muscles in man. Acta Physiol Scand 91:385–392, 1972.
17. Asmussen, E and Bonde-Petersen, F: Apparent efficiency and storage of elastic energy in human muscles during exercise. Acta Physiol Scand 92:537–545, 1974.
18. Komi, PV: The stretch-shortening cycle and human power output. In Jones, NL, McCartney, N, and McComas, AJ: Human Muscle Power. Human Kinetics Publishers, Champaign, IL, 1986, pp 27–39.
19. Kaneko, M, Komi, PV, and Aura, O: Mechanical efficiency of concentric and eccentric exercises performed with medium to fast contraction rates. Scandinavian Journal of Sports Science 6:15–20, 1984.
20. Bosco, C, Tarkka, I, and Komi, PV: Effect of elastic energy and myoelectrical potentiation of triceps surae during stretch-shortening cycle exercise. Int J Sports Med 3:137–140, 1982.
21. Komi, PV: Measurement of the force-velocity relationship in human muscle under concentric and eccentric contractions. In Cerquiglini, S (ed): Biomechanics III. Karger, Basel, Switzerland, 1973, pp 224–229.
22. Abbott, BC, Gibland, B, and Ritchie, JM: The physiological cost of negative work. J Physiol 117:380–390, 1952.
23. Stothart, JP: Relationship between selected biomechanical parameters of static and dynamic muscle performance. In Cerquigliani, S (ed): Biomechanics III. Karger, Basel, Switzerland, 1973, pp 210–217.
24. Sukop, J and Nelson, RC: Effects of isometrical training in the force-time characteristics of muscle contractions. In Nelson, RC and Morehouse, CA (eds): Biomechanics IV. University Park Press, Baltimore, 1974, pp 440–447.
25. Soderberg, GL: Kinesiology: Application to Pathological Motion. Williams & Wilkins, Baltimore, 1986.
26. Woittiez, RD, Huijing, PA, Boom, HBK, et al: A three-dimensional muscle model: A quantified relation between form and function of skeletal muscles. J Morphol 182:95–113, 1984.
27. Da Silva, KMC: Biomechanics of muscle. In Berme, N, Engin, AE, and Correia Da Silva, KM (eds): Biomechanics of Normal and Pathological Human Articulating Joints. Esotril, Portugal, 1983.
28. Otten, E: Concepts and models of functional architecture in skeletal muscle. Exercise and Sports Science Reviews, vol 16. Macmillan, New York, 1988, pp 89–121.
29. O'Connel, AL and Gowitzke, B: Understanding the Scientific Bases of Human Movement. Williams & Wilkins, Baltimore, 1972.
30. Bouisset, S: EMG and muscle force in normal motor activities. In Desmedt, JE (ed): New Developments in Electromyography and Clinical Neurophysiology, vol 1. Karger, Basel, Switzerland, 1973.
31. Lieber, RL and Boakes, JL: Muscle force and moment arm contributions to torque production in frog hindlimb. Am J Physiol 254(Cell Physiol 23):C769–C772, 1988.
32. Lieber, RL and Boakes JL: Sarcomere length and joint kinematics during torque production in frog hindlimb. Am J Physiol 254(Cell Physiol 23):C759–C768, 1988.
33. Winters, JM and Stark, L: Estimated mechanical properties of synergistic muscles involved in movements of a variety of human joints. J Biomech 21:1027–1041, 1988.
34. Tardieu, C, Tabary, JC, Tardieu, G, et al: Adaptation of sarcomere numbers to the length imposed on the muscle. Adv Physiol Sci 24:99–114, 1981.
35. Tabary, JC, Tardieu, C, Tardieu, G, et al: Functional adaptation of sarcomere number of normal cat muscle. J Physiol (Paris) 72:277–291, 1976.
36. Williams, PE and Goldspink, G: Changes in sarcomere length and physiology properties in immobilized muscle. J Anat 127:459–468, 1978.
37. Ralston, HJ, Polissow, JJ, Inman, VT, et al: Dynamic features of human isolated voluntary muscle in isolated isometric and free contractions. J Appl Physiol 1:526–633, 1949.

38. Landjevit, B, Maton, B, and Peres, G: In vivo muscular force analysis during the isometric flexion on a monkey's elbow. J Biomech 21:577–584, 1988.
39. Samojla, BG: Surface tendon force measurements in determining muscle contraction properties. J Am Podiatr Med Assn 78:1–10, 1988.
40. Frost, HM: An Introduction to Biomechanics. Charles C Thomas, Springfield IL, 1967.
41. Steiner, M: Biomechanics of tendon healing. J Biomech 15:951–958, 1982.
42. Garrett, WE, Nikolaou, PK, Ribbeck, BM, et al: The effect of muscle architecture on the biomechanical failure properties of skeletal muscle under passive extension. Am J Sports Med 16:7–12, 1988.
43. Tabary, JC, Tardieu, C, Tardieu, G, et al: Experimental rapid sarcomere loss with concomitant hypoextensibility. Muscle Nerve 4:198–203, 1981.
44. Tabary, JC, Tabary, C, Tardieu, C, et al: Physiological and structural changes in the cat's soleus muscle due to immobilization at different lengths by plaster casts. J Physiol (Lond) 224:231–244, 1972.
45. Huijing, PA, Rozendal, RH, Heslinga, H, et al: Skeletal muscle reaction to immobilization. J Rehabil Res Dev 25:247, 1988.
46. Salter, RB and Bell, RS: The effect of continuous passive motion on the healing of partial thickness lacerations of the patellar tendon of the rabbit. Proceedings of the 27th Annual Orthopedic Research Society. Dependable Publishing, Chicago, 1981, p 82.
47. Rothstein, JM (ed): Measurement in Physical Therapy. Churchill Livingstone, New York, 1985.

CHAPTER 4

Force-Frequency Relation in Skeletal Muscle

Stuart A. Binder-Macleod, Ph.D., P.T.

The motor unit (MU) is the smallest functional component for the control of skeletal muscle force. A MU consists of one alpha motoneuron and all of the muscle fibers that are innervated by its peripheral axon. During voluntary contractions synaptic inputs that depolarize the alpha motoneuron initiate a series of action potentials that are propagated down the nerve axon to the muscle fibers. Through chemical transmission across the neuromuscular junction, each nerve action potential results in the initiation of one muscle action potential in each muscle fiber of the MU. The muscle action potential eventually is carried to the interior of the cell via the transverse tubules (T tubules). The T tubule action potential then, through a process known as excitation-contraction coupling, causes the release of calcium ions from the sarcoplasmic reticulum (SR). The calcium ions then initiate the muscle contraction.

A myriad of factors interact to influence the force produced by the contracting skeletal muscle. These factors can be divided into two basic categories: (1) the neural drive that activates the muscle and (2) the characteristics of the muscle at the time of activation.

During voluntary contraction there are two basic mechanisms for modulating the neural drive to muscle: recruitment and rate coding. Analogous to the processes of recruitment and rate coding during voluntary contractions, the neural drive to the muscle can be modulated during electrical stimulation of the motor nerve by varying the amplitude and frequency of the stimulation pulses. The size principle describes a process for the orderly recruitment of MUs during voluntary contractions,[1] that is, the smallest MUs are recruited first and the larger MUs are recruited with successively stronger contractions. During direct electrical stimulation to the motor nerve the recruitment order is reversed; the largest MUs are recruited first, and progressively smaller units are recruited with increasing stimulus amplitude. Interestingly, the recruitment order during transcutaneous neuromuscular electrical stimulation (NMES) appears to be more variable and less orderly than that observed during voluntary contractions or during direct nerve stimulation.[2]

The other mechanism for modulation of the neural drive to the muscle is varying the discharge rate of those motoneurons that have been recruited; this process is called rate coding. The relation between the stimulation frequency and the force output (force-frequency relation) during electrically elicited contractions has generally been described as a sigmoid curve with the contractile characteristics of the muscle (i.e., speed and force-generating capacity) determining the exact characteristics of the curve.[3-8] (Fig. 4–1).

Several problems arise when attempting to use the sigmoid force-frequency relation derived by electrical stimulation to describe the force-frequency relation during voluntary contractions. The discharge frequencies reported during voluntary contractions are far lower than those required to produce similar forces with electrical stimulation.[9,10] Also, a single sigmoid curve cannot accurately portray the true force-frequency relation of any muscle.[3] The force-frequency relation is not unique; it depends on the characteristics of the muscle at the time of stimulation (i.e., the present physical and chemical state of the muscle). The purpose of this chapter is to outline the factors that influence the force-frequency relation and to try to explain how rate coding may be used during voluntary contractions to modulate MU force. Finally, implications for the practice of physical therapy will be discussed.

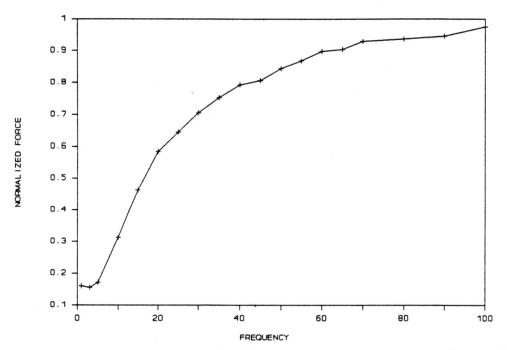

FIGURE 4–1. Isometric force-frequency relationship of human quadriceps femoris muscle. Hip joint in 0° flexion, knee in 90° flexion. Data normalized for each subject (N = 20) by dividing the force produced at each frequency by the maximum force produced at any of the 20 frequencies tested. Test trains were on for 1.5 seconds. Each pulse was a 350-microsecond square wave.

FACTORS THAT INFLUENCE THE FORCE-FREQUENCY RELATION

Factors that influence the force-frequency relation during an isometric contraction include the length, temperature, fatigue state, and degree of potentiation of the muscle. During nonisometric contraction, the force-velocity relation also plays an important role; however, it will not be discussed in the present chapter. Because of methodologic problems, very little data are available regarding the force-frequency relation in skeletal muscle during voluntary contractions. As noted above, force is graded by both recruitment and rate coding. This combination of mechanisms makes it very difficult to separate out the force-frequency relation from changes in force output because of recruitment. In addition, until recently, single MU discharge characteristics had been very difficult to analyze during all but the weakest contractions.[11] Most studies have therefore used electrical stimulation of skeletal muscle to investigate factors that affect the force-frequency relation.

Each of the above factors (i.e., length, temperature, fatigue state, and degree of potentiation) affect the force-frequency relation by altering a muscle's force-generating ability or contractile rate, or both. The contractile rate of a muscle is a function of the characteristics of the muscle fibers that make up that muscle. The differences in the contractile rates of the different muscle fibers is a function of the rate of release and reuptake of Ca^{2+} from the sarcoplasmic reticulum and the rates of formation and breaking of cross-bridges.[12] The faster the contractile rate of a muscle, the greater the frequency needed to produce the maximum tetanic force. That is, based solely on the contractile rate of a muscle, the faster the contractile rate, the further to the right the force-frequency relation should lie.

Alterations in the force-generating ability of a muscle will also affect the position of the force-frequency curve. Decreasing the force-generating ability causes a downward shift in the force-frequency relation. If the force depression is not uniform across frequencies, as is usually the case, this depression may appear as a shift to the right. Similarly, increasing the force output over selected frequencies (as is seen during post-tetanic potentiation) makes the curve appear to shift to the left. Most studies that have tried to quantify the force-frequency relation have used the frequency needed to produce a set percentage of maximum force (e.g., 50 percent of maximum) to identify the location of the curve.[4,6] During most physiologic activities, both the force-generating capacity of a muscle and its contractile rate may change simultaneously.

Muscle Length

Changes in muscle length may affect the force-frequency relation by altering both the force-generating capacity and activation rate of the muscle. Variations in the maximum isometric tension that skeletal muscle could generate at different muscle lengths have been well studied.[13–16] The classic graph of the length-tension relation (Fig. 4–2) can be divided into four segments: (1) an initial steep portion of the ascending limb corresponding to very short sarcomere lengths, (2) a shallow portion of the ascending limb corresponding to sarcomere lengths that are shorter than optimum, (3) a plateau corresponding to optimum sarcomere lengths, and (4) a descending limb

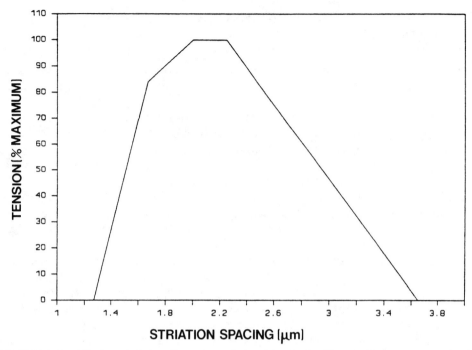

FIGURE 4–2. The isometric length-tension relationship of a frog muscle fiber. (Based on the data of Gordon et al.[13])

corresponding to sarcomere lengths that are longer than optimum.[13] At any length other than optimum, less than maximum forces can be generated by the muscle.

The sliding filament theory of muscle contraction has long been used to explain the observed length-tension relation.[13,17] In good agreement with the sliding filament theory of muscle contraction, virtually all investigators have found peak force at lengths that allowed maximum overlap of the thin and thick filaments, with a nearly linear decline at longer and shorter lengths. There is general agreement that the decline in force at muscle lengths beyond optimum (descending limb of the length-tension curve) can be attributed to a decrease in the amount of overlap between the thin and thick filaments.[13,18] The basis for the ascending limb, corresponding to muscle lengths shorter than optimum, remains a subject of controversy.[14] It has been suggested that the shallow ascending portion is a result of the increasing overlap of the thin filaments from opposite ends of the sarcomere interfering with cross-bridge attachments as the sarcomere length was decreased. The steep portion of the relation was thought to result from the compression of the ends of the thick filaments against the Z-lines. Other investigators have suggested that at short sarcomere lengths activation may be length dependent,[14] with the amount of Ca^{2+} released during tetanic stimulation a function of the sarcomere length. Recently, Allen and Moss[14] concluded that at high Ca^{2+} levels the shape of the ascending limb of the length-tension curve is most likely determined by filament overlap. However, during low Ca^{2+} (low excitation frequencies) the increased filament spacing produced at short lengths probably reduces the normal cooperative activation of the thin filaments. The length-tension relation is therefore also a function of the frequency of stimulation of the muscle.

Changes in muscle length also appear to change the contractile rate of the muscle.

In 1969, Rack and Westbury[16] showed that the rate of rise of isometric tension depended on the muscle length as well as the rate of stimulation. The contractile machinery has been suggested to be more effectively activated at long than at short lengths. From recent data presented by Gandevia and McKenzie,[15] it can be calculated that for human abductor digiti minimi muscle (ADM), elbow flexors, and tibialis anterior muscle, the rate of rise of tension and the rate of relaxation both decrease when the muscle is in a shortened versus an anatomically neutral position. Despite this contractile slowing, because the twitch force was markedly decreased at the shortened length, the twitch contraction times (CT, time from the onset of force to the peak force) and the half relation times (RT, time from the peak force to half of peak force) both significantly decreased for all muscles. These decreases in twitch characteristics were shown to produce a shift in the force-frequency relation of the ADM to the right (see Gandevia and McKenzie,[15] Fig. 2). For muscle lengths significantly less than optimum, we would, therefore, predict a shift in the force-frequency relation to the right. This shift in relation would require, compared with the neutral or optimum length of a muscle, application of higher frequencies to produce comparable forces.

Muscle Temperature

Changes in muscle temperature affect the contractile rate of the muscle.[8,19] The time to peak and the time to half-relaxation of the isometric twitch increase during cooling of the muscle. Maximum tetanic tension has been shown to decrease only slightly within the range of temperatures normally experienced during physiologic situations (temperature range of 35°C to 25°C).[8] This slowing of the contractile process, without a concurrent decrease in the twitch amplitude, has been shown to produce a shift in the force-frequency relation toward lower frequencies (to the left) as the muscle is cooled (see Ranatunga,[8] Fig. 2). Cooling, therefore, allows lower frequencies to be used to generate the maximum tetanic force, with greater forces produced at all subtetanic frequencies.

Muscle Fatigue

As a muscle begins to fatigue, there is a slowing of the rate of contraction and relaxation as well as a decline in its force-generating capacity.[11,20,21] Bigland-Ritchie and associates[11] have shown for human adductor pollicis muscle that following fatigue, the twitch CT decreased slightly and the half RT markedly increased. Based on these findings and the fact that MU firing frequencies were shown to decrease markedly during sustained, fatiguing, maximum voluntary contractions, Bigland-Ritchie and associates suggested that the force-frequency relation should shift to the left as a muscle begins to fatigue. Recent work appears to disprove this assumption.[22,23,23a] In several different human muscles, the force-frequency relation is shifted to the right when the muscle is fatigued by electrically or volitionally induced contractions. The shift in the force-frequency relation (as measured by changes in the frequency needed to produce 50 percent of the muscle maximum tetanic force) is the result of a greater attenuation of the twitch force than the tetanic force (i.e., a decrease in the twitch:tetanus ratio) with fatigue; a similar observation of a disproportionate depression of force generated in response to low-frequency stimulation (20 pps) has been made by others during many different types of fatiguing exercises.[24,25] This twitch attenuation has been termed low-frequency fatigue and may result from impaired electrical transmission within the T tubular system or a reduction in the amount of Ca^{2+} released from the sarcoplasmic reticulum.[24] During fatigue, although there is a reduction in Ca^{2+} released per impulse, high-frequency stimulation (50 pps) would allow sufficient Ca^{2+} release to permit full cross-bridge interaction to occur. This case could not occur during low-frequency stimulation.

Muscle Potentiation

The final factor to be discussed is the degree of potentiation of the muscle. Posttetanic potentiation (PTP) is the increase in the twitch and subtetanic tension seen following tetanic stimulation.[26-28] PTP has no effect on the maximum tetanic tension. Similar to PTP is the process of postactivation potentiation, where an increase in twitch and submaximum tetanic forces are seen following subtetanic stimulation.[28] As a muscle becomes potentiated, the force-frequency curve will appear to shift to the left.

In 1972, Close[28a] suggested that the mechanism for PTP involved an increased release of activator Ca^{2+}. At present, this mechanism is not strongly accepted.[29,30] One strong argument against an increased release of Ca^{2+} is that the aequorin response, an indicator of Ca^{2+} concentration, becomes reduced during repetitive stimulation. This aequorin response suggests a decrease, rather than an increase, in the amount of Ca^{2+} being released. More recent findings have shown that the amount of phosphate incorporated into the fast phosphorylatable light chain (P-light chain) of myosin in animal skeletal muscle can be temporally correlated with PTP.[31,32] Based on these findings, Sweeney and Stull[33] have suggested that P-light chain phosphorylation may increase the number of actin-bound myosin cross-bridges under conditions of suboptimal Ca^{2+} activation to produce PTP. To argue against this theory, Stuart and co-workers[29] recently noted that no similar correlation between PTP and P-light chain phosphorylation could be made for human muscle. The role of myosin P-chain phosphorylation, as well as the mechanism for PTP, therefore, remains unclear.

FORCE-FREQUENCY RELATION DURING ELECTRICAL STIMULATION

When electrical stimulation is used to produce muscle contractions, the stimuli are generally delivered in brief pulses, each lasting 200 to 300 microseconds. The pulses are grouped together to form a train.[33,34] Clinically, trains of pulses lasting from several tenths of a second (for functioned electrical stimulation [FES] during ambulation) up to tens of seconds (for muscle strengthening) are used. If the pulses are separated by regular intervals, a particular pulse rate or frequency can be assigned to the train. The interpulse interval (IPI) is the amount of time between successive pulses. The reciprocal of the IPI can be used to calculate the train frequency. If pulses are occurring at irregular intervals, the IPI between any two successive pulses can be used to determine the instantaneous frequency for that pair of pulses. The stimulation frequency helps to determine the rate of rise of force,[36–38] strength of the contraction,[4,5,7,37] and rate of force fatigue.[39,40] Successive trains of stimuli are separated by periods of rest also lasting from tenths to tens of seconds. The pulse train along with the rest time between trains forms the cycle period.

Constant Rate Stimulation

Considering the recent popularity of electrical stimulation, the dearth of information on the actual force-frequency relation of human skeletal muscle is surprising. We are presently investigating the force-frequency relation in human quadriceps femoris muscle at different joint angles (for a preliminary report, see Binder-Macleod and Johnson[41]). Results to date support previous findings that electrical stimulation is less effective in generating force at low frequencies when the muscle is in a shortened position than when the muscle is positioned at its optimum length.[16] Our findings have shown that (1) at shorter muscle lengths (15 degrees of knee flexion), higher frequencies are needed to produce submaximum forces (i.e., <80 percent of maximum tetanic force) than are required at optimum lengths (90 degrees of knee flexion); (2) there is no difference in the frequencies needed to produce near maximum forces (>80 percent of maximum tetanic force) at different muscle lengths; and (3) there is no difference in the position or shape of the force-frequency relation with the knee positioned in 90 degrees or 130 degrees of flexion (Fig. 4–3).

We are also attempting to identify characteristics of the muscle twitch that can

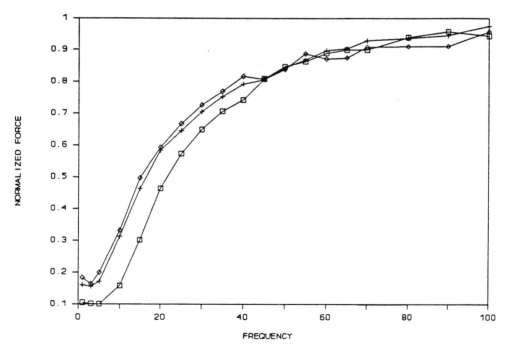

FIGURE 4–3. Comparison of isometric force-frequency relationship of human quadriceps femoris muscle at three different knee joint angles (15° = boxes, 90° = crosses, 130° = diamonds). All other parameters are the same as described for Figure 4–1.

be used to help predict the force-frequency relation. The most obvious characteristic would appear to be the muscle's twitch CT and half RT. In 1983, Kernell and colleagues[6] showed in the peroneus longus muscle of cat, that the stimulus interval needed to produce half maximum force in single MUs was strongly correlated to both the twitch CT and half RT of each unit. Pulse intervals of 1.5 times the CT were needed in fast MUs and 2 times the CT in slow units. For both types of units, the stimulus rates corresponded to pulse intervals 1.4 times the unit's half RT of the twitch. In a more recent study, Botterman and colleagues[4] used the integrated twitch time (ITT, the tension-time area divided by the peak amplitude) to study the relation between the contractile rate of cat flexor carpi radialis MUs and the force-frequncy relation. The ITT was used as a measure of twitch duration, because it takes into account both the contraction and relaxation phases of the twitch. The ITT is highly correlated with both the twitch CT and half RT.[4] For both fast and slow twitch units, a highly significant, linear relation between the frequency needed for each unit to produce 50 percent maximum force and its ITT was found. The stimulus interval needed to produce 50 percent force corresponded to ~70 percent of the ITT or ~1.25 times the twitch CT and ~1.30 times the half RT. Botterman and colleagues point out that when their results are compared with those of Kernell and colleagues, they can conclude that twitch CT and half RT cannot be related in some simple way to the normalized force-frequency curves of units isolated from different muscles.[4] Different muscles show both different degrees of potentiation and different viscoelastic properties. These differences effect how successive twitches summate and hence the position and shape of the force-frequency relation. Our laboratory hopes to soon look at similar characteristics using whole muscles (versus single MUs) in both human and animal models.

Variable Rate Stimulation

The discharge rate during voluntary contractions does not remain constant but varies even within brief bursts of activity.[42,43] With this in mind, several authors have investigated the force output of skeletal muscle during trains of stimuli where the interpulse intervals were not kept constant.[3,28,44-52] One significant finding is the catchlike property of skeletal muscle.[44,47,51] As originally outlined by Burke and colleagues,[44] the catchlike property of skeletal muscle is the tension enhancement seen when an extra pulse is delivered at a short interval at the beginning of a subtetanic constant-rate stimulus train. The tension enhancement seen is greater than that which would be expected from the additional stimulus alone. In a recent paper, we extended this definition to include the fact that once a muscle is stimulated with a higher frequency, the catchlike property allows the unit to "hold" the maximum possible force at each subsequent lower frequency.[3]

Burke suggests the catchlike property (as originally proposed) and PTP share a common mechanism because the two phenomena occlude each other.[44] A time-dependent rate of tension development and decay may also contribute to this catchlike property. Because the rate of rise of force is a function of the stimulation frequency, when skeletal muscle is stimulated with a subtetanic rate a considerable amount of time may be required for the muscles to plateau.[5,37,38] In contrast, a higher frequency burst will produce a rapid rate of force development. If the higher frequency burst is of an appropriate duration to produce a force output which is less than or equal to the maximum force that the subtetanic train is capable of producing, and if the subtetanic train is begun before the force declines, the subtetanic train will maintain the maximum force for the duration of the train. This phenomenon is demonstrated in Figure 4–4 for rat soleus muscle.

Another significant finding is the marked dependence of the force-frequency relation on the immediate past discharge history of the muscle. If skeletal muscle is stimulated with trains in which the frequency is varied either sinusoidally or linearly, there is a tension hysteresis with greater forces produced when the frequency is decreasing than when it is increasing.[3,47,48,53] That is, marked differences exist in the force-frequency relation, depending on whether the muscle was experiencing a higher or lower force level at the time of arrival of the stimulus. This tension hysteresis helps to demonstrate why a single sigmoidal curve cannot fully explain the force-frequency relation in skeletal muscle. We have shown that a time-dependent rate of tension development and decay, along with a catchlike property, can account for all of the properties of hysteresis in cat single MUs and appears to be the primary factor in the production of hysteresis in fully potentiated units.[3,36] This observation of a tension hysteresis has been used to theorize how rate coding may be employed during voluntary contractions.[3]

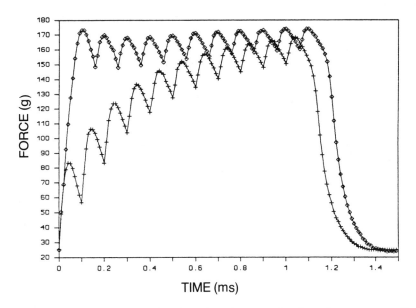

FIGURE 4–4. The force output produced by the soleus muscle of a rat in response to direct nerve stimulation. Top trace *(diamonds)* is the response to a variable-frequency train consisting of an initial frequency burst of 4 pulses at 50 pps followed by a train of 10 pulses at 20 pps. Bottom trace *(crosses)* is the response to a constant-frequency train of 11 pulses at 20 pps. The top trace demonstrates a marked catchlike property by this muscle.

FORCE-FREQUENCY RELATION DURING VOLUNTARY CONTRACTIONS

The relative role of rate coding for the modulation of MU force has been somewhat controversial since it was originally described by Adrian and Bronk.[54] Recruitment has been suggested to be the major mechanism at low force levels, whereas rate coding becomes prominent at high forces.[55] Kukulka and Clamann[56] suggest that the relative contribution each process makes may also vary with the muscle being tested. They showed that in humans, MU recruitment was a factor for grading force from 0 to 90 percent of maximum voluntary contraction (MVC) in the biceps brachii muscle. In contrast, for the adductor pollicis muscle, recruitment was not used to modulate force beyond 50 percent MVC, with the major recruitment occurring below 30 percent MVC. A similar pattern, where force is largely controlled by rate coding, has also been reported for the human first dorsal interosseous muscle[55,57] and the cat soleus muscle.[58] These results suggest that rate coding may play different roles in different muscles based on the muscle's function or fiber type composition.

Rate Coding During Voluntary Contractions

As previously noted, several problems arise when one is attempting to use the simple force-frequency relation found during neuromuscular electrical stimulation (NMES) of skeletal muscle to explain the force-frequency relation during voluntary contractions.[3] First, the reported sigmoid force-frequency relation[4,5,8,37,59] tends to overestimate the discharge rates seen during voluntary contractions.[42,43,60,61] In human adductor pollicis muscle, Bellemare and colleagues[9] have shown that 30 pps is sufficient to produce a maximum voluntary contraction, whereas others have shown that NMES of the same muscle required 50 to 80 pps to produce maximum force.[10] Second, as noted above, the force-frequency relation is multivalued, with force depending on stimulation history as well as on the stimulation frequency. This lack of a unique force-frequency relation can produce major control problems for the central nervous system (CNS) because the short-term alterations (e.g., alterations in successive IPIs) happen too quickly to allow for compensation by feedback mechanisms. Effective rate coding strategies must therefore compensate for these short-term alterations directly.

Several observations may help to explain the discrepancies in frequency between volitional and electrically elicited contractions. First, during voluntary contractions the active MUs do not fire synchronously. This asynchronous discharge serves to smooth the contraction (at low forces and discharge rates) and allows greater forces to be produced at each stimulation frequency than is possible with synchronous stimulation.[16,62] Second, in many of the previous studies that described the force-frequency relation during NMES, the burst or train of pulses used at each frequency was kept on for a relatively brief period (300 to 1000 milliseconds) to avoid fatigue. Close inspection of the presented data shows that the force output often continued to increase throughout the period of stimulation, particularly at subtetanic frequencies, allowing the force produced at each subtetanic frequency to be underestimated.[4-6,37,63] This fact has been acknowledged by previous investigators.[37,64]

As previously noted, varying the discharge rate by beginning a train with a higher frequency and then dropping the frequency to a lower rate can take advantage of the rapid rate of force development at the higher discharge rate[38] and the catchlike property of skeletal muscle.[3,44] Varying the stimulation rate allows the lower frequency to produce the maximum force that it is capable of producing. A declining discharge rate, with an initial doublet or triplet (two or three discharges of a single MU separated by very short IPIs as seen on electromyograms) has been reported in the literature to occur often during voluntary contractions.[43,65-68] This "high to low" discharge rate strategy (a high initial frequency followed by a lower frequency), along with the known asynchronous discharge of MUs, can begin to explain the discrepancy in observed discharge rates between volitional and electrically induced contractions.[3]

This same "high to low" strategy can also explain how the CNS can compensate for the short-term activation history of each MU. Such a strategy would allow each unit to produce the maximum force at each frequency. By producing the maximum force at each frequency, a single sigmoid curve can then be used to describe the force-frequency relation, provided that there are no changes in any of the other factors identified that would produce longer-term alterations (minutes to hours—e.g., fatigue or PTP) in the force-frequency relation. Feedback is used to compensate for any of these long-term alterations in the force-frequency relation.

Thus rate coding appears to be an important mechanism for modulation of MU force. While the force-frequency relation plotted during synchronous electrical stimulation does not give us the true force-frequency relation during voluntary contractions, it has provided us with many important insights into the factors that affect this relation. By better understanding how rate coding is used during voluntary contractions, perhaps we can design muscle stimulators that more effectively activate skeletal muscle.

CLINICAL DECISION MAKING

NMES has long been used by physical therapists to delay muscle atrophy,[69-72] improve strength,[73-80] maintain range of motion,[87-89] and produce functional movement patterns. The last of these applications is commonly known as functional electrical stimulation (FES). Examples of its use include stimulation of the ankle dorsiflexors to help treat foot-drop in hemiplegic patients,[90-93] and computer-controlled stimulation of lower extremity muscles to help paraplegic patients stand or walk.[94,95] Each application requires a unique set of force output requirements. Given that the stimulation rate helps to determine the rate of force fatigue,[39,96-98] the rate of rise of force,[37,38] and the amount of force generated, it behooves clinicians to select the optimum stimulation frequency for each application.

In all published clinical studies, the IPI has remained constant both within each train (constant rate train) and across trains throughout the entire treatment. In general, clinicians have used the lowest stimulation frequency that produced the desired response. The use of the lowest frequency may be a logical approach. Using any single frequency may not, however, be the "best" way to stimulate muscle. Two examples will be presented that will show that decreasing the stimulation frequency, either within or across trains of pulses, may produce a superior response to any single frequency.

Electrical Stimulation for Muscle Strengthening

Electrical stimulation for muscle strengthening requires the use of trains of relatively long duration (measured in seconds), which are used to produce repeated, near maximum contractions. The rate of rise of force is not important, and in fact, many commercially available stimulators incorporate a gradual increase in stimulation amplitude (ramping) to allow the contraction to build gradually. To maximize the force and minimize the fatigue, using the lowest stimulation frequency that produces the maximum force appears appropriate.

There is considerable evidence to suggest that decreasing the pulse rate as muscle begins to fatigue will slow the rate of fatigue and produce a greater force output than maintaining the initial rate of stimulation.[39,96,98] It has been well documented that MU discharge rates decrease during fatiguing voluntary contractions, and that this decrease in discharge rate probably delays the onset of force fatigue.[9,40,99] In 1979, Jones and associates[39] and Marsden and co-workers[96] studied the human adductor pollicis muscle and found that, while a 60 pps constant rate train initially produced as great a force as a maximum voluntary contraction, during a sustained contraction (60 to 95 seconds) the rate of fatigue was much greater during the electrically elicited contraction than during the voluntary contraction.[39,96] However, if the rate of stimulation was progressively decreased during the contraction, nearly the same rate of fatigue as a voluntary contraction was seen.

Recently we conducted experiments to determine the effects of a progressive reduction in the pulse frequency of NMES delivered to human quadriceps femoris muscle during intermittent, fatiguing contractions.[98] Twelve normal subjects each attended two experimental sessions. A stimulus/rest cycle of 8 seconds on and 12 seconds off was used. Thirty cycles were applied during each session. During one of the sessions, a frequency of 60 pps was used for all 30 trains. During the other session, the subjects were stimulated with 60 pps for the first train. The stimulating frequency of each train was then progressively reduced, in 5-pps steps for contractions 2, 3, 5, 8, 12, and 20, until 30 pps was reached. By the 11th contraction the difference between the 60-pps train and the reduced rate train was significant ($p<.05$) with the difference continuing to increase over time. By the last contraction, a 46 percent increase in force was produced by the reduced rate train (30 pps) versus the 60-pps train ($p<.01$). These results show that, compared with a constant pulse frequency, reducing the pulse frequency during a fatiguing contraction can markedly increase the force output of skeletal muscle. The next step is to determine if the enhanced force output seen with a progressive reduction in stimulation frequency results in an increased ability to strengthen muscle.

Functional Electrical Stimulation

In contrast to the findings for muscle strengthening, FES generally requires short trains that are capable of producing targeted levels of force with a rapid rate of rise. As an example, stimulation of weak ankle dorsiflexors at heel strike would require relatively large forces that are rapidly developed and last just several tenths of a second. To produce such a contraction a brief, higher frequency train could be used (e.g., a 60-pps, 300-millisecond duration train). Lower frequency trains produce less than maximum forces and slower rates of rise of force than do higher frequency trains.[37] Repetitive application of a higher frequency train produces a rapid rate of fatigue, caused in part by failure of the muscle to transmit the electrical signal.[21,25,100,101] This type of fatigue has been termed high-frequency fatigue and is not seen during voluntary contractions.[21,100,102,103]

An alternative to higher frequency stimulation would be to use a variable frequency train similar to that shown in Figure 4–4. The initial higher frequency burst would produce the rapid rate of rise of force needed, and the catchlike property would allow the lower frequency to maintain the force. This variable frequency train should produce less force fatigue than the higher frequency train.

Recently we tested this assumption.[97] A study was designed to compare the force output produced by a constant rate, short duration train with that produced by a variable rate, short duration train. Twelve healthy subjects participated in the study. A constant voltage stimulator (Grass SD-9), controlled by an IBM PC computer, was used to stimulate the quadriceps femoris muscle for 300-msec trains once every second for 180 seconds. Each subject participated in four experimental sessions. During three sessions a constant rate train of 80, 40, or 20 pps was used. During the fourth session a variable rate train, which consisted of two IPIs at an instantaneous frequency of 80 pps, one IPI at 40 pps, and five IPIs at 20 pps, was used. The results showed that, compared with the constant rate trains, after 180 seconds of stimulation the variable rate train produced (1) the most rapid rate of force development, (2) the greatest average force, and (3) the least force fatigue. These results may have significant implications for the stimulation patterns used by physical therapists for the activation of skeletal muscle during FES.

SUMMARY

In summary, we have shown that the force-frequency relation of any given muscle is not a static relation but depends on a myriad of factors that influence the muscle. These factors include the length, temperature, fatigue state, degree of potentiation, and the immediate past discharge history of the muscle. In addition, even under similar circumstances, different muscles may show markedly different force-frequency relations because of differences in their inherent contractile rates and viscoelastic properties. Because the frequency of stimulation of skeletal muscle affects not only the force production but also the rates of force development and fatigue, a thorough understanding of the force-frequency relation has significant clinical implications. We have identified some recent work that suggests modulation of stimulation frequency during NMES may have some advantages over the presently used constant rate patterns of stimulation. Additional research is necessary to determine if functional outcomes can actually be improved by modulating the stimulation frequency in ways that were discussed. Now is certainly an exciting time for both the clinicians and researchers who use NMES.

REFERENCES

1. Lüscher, H-R, Ruenzel, P, and Henneman, E: How the size of the motoneurons determines their susceptibility to discharge. Nature (Lond) 282:859–869, 1979.
2. Knaflitz, M, Merletti, R, and DeLuca, CJ: Inference of motor unit recruitment order in voluntary and electrically elicited contractions. J Appl Physiol 68:1657–1667, 1990.

3. Binder-Macleod, SA and Clamann, HP: Force output of cat motor units stimulated with trains of linearly varying frequency. J Neurophysiol 61:208–217, 1989.

4. Botterman, BR, Iwamoto, GA, and Gonyea, WJ: Gradation of isometric tension by different activation rates in motor units of cat flexor carpi radialis muscle. J Neurophysiol 56:494–506, 1986.

5. Cooper, S and Eccles, JC: The isometric response of mammalian muscles. J Physiol 69:377–385, 1930.

6. Kernell, D, Eerbeek, O, and Verhey, BA: Relation between isometric force and stimulation rate in cat's hindlimb motor units of different twitch contraction times. Exp Brain Res 50:220–227, 1983.

7. Mannard, A and Stein, RB: Determination of the frequency response of isometric soleus muscle in the cat using random nerve stimulation. J Physiol (Lond) 229:275–296, 1973.

8. Ranatunga, KW: Temperature-dependence of shortening velocity and rate of isometric tension development in rat skeletal muscle. J Physiol (Lond) 329:465–483, 1982.

9. Bellemare, F, Woods, JJ, Johansson, R, et al: Motor-unit discharge rates in maximal voluntary contractions of three human muscles. J Neurophysiol 50:1380–1392, 1983.

10. Bigland-Ritchie, B and Woods, JJ: Changes in muscle contractile properties and neural control during muscular fatigue. Muscle Nerve 7:691–699, 1984.

11. Bigland-Ritchie, B, Johansson, R, Lippold, OCJ, et al: Changes in motoneuron firing rates during sustained maximal voluntary contractions. J Physiol (Lond) 340:335–346, 1983.

12. Peachey, LD: Excitation-contraction coupling: The link between the surface and the interior of a muscle cell. J Exp Biol 115:91–98, 1985.

13. Gordon, AM, Huxley, AF, and Julian, FJ: The variation in isometric tension with sarcomere length in vertebrate muscle fibres. J Physiol (Lond) 184:170–192, 1966.

14. Allen, JD and Moss, RL: Factors influencing the ascending limb of the sarcomere length-tension relationship in rabbit skinned muscle fibres. J Physiol (Lond) 390:119–136, 1987.

15. Gandevia, SC and McKenzie, DK: Activation of human muscles at short muscle lengths during maximal static efforts. J Physiol (Lond) 407:599–613, 1988.

16. Rack, PMH and Westbury, PR: The effects of length and stimulus rate on tension in the isometric cat soleus muscle. J Physiol (Lond) 204:443–460, 1969.

17. Huxley, AF and Niedergerke, R: Structural changes in muscle during contraction. Interference microscopy of living muscle fibres. Nature (Lond) 173:971–973, 1954.

18. terKeurs, HEDJ, Luff, AR, and Luff, SE: Force-sarcomere-length relation and filament length in rat extensor digitorum muscle. In GH Pollack, H Sugi, editors: Advances in Experimental Medicine and Biology. Contractile Mechanisms in Muscle, vol 170. New York, Plenum Press, 1984, pp 511–522.

19. Close, R and Hoh, JFY: The after-effects of repetitive stimulation on the isometric twitch contraction of rat skeletal muscle. J Physiol (Lond) 197:461–477, 1968.

20. Dubose, L, Schelhorn, TB, and Clamann, HP: Changes in contractile speed of cat motor units during activity. Muscle Nerve 10:744–752, 1987.

21. Edwards, RHT: Human muscle function and fatigue. Ciba Found Symp 82:1–18, 1981.

22. Cooper, RG, Edwards, RHT, Gibson, H, et al: Human muscle fatigue: Frequency dependence of excitation and force generation. J Physiol (Lond) 397:585–599, 1988.

23. Jones, DA, Newham, DJ, and Torgan, C: Mechanical influences on long-lasting human muscle fatigue and delayed-onset pain. J Physiol (Lond) 412:415–427, 1989.

23a. Binder-Macleod, SA and McDermond, LR: Changes in the force-frequency relationship of the human quadriceps femoris muscle following electrically and voluntarily induced fatigue. Phys Ther 72:97–104, 1992.

24. Bigland-Ritchie, B, Cafarelli, E, and Vollestad, NK: Fatigue of submaximal static contractions. Acta Physiol Scand 128:137–148, 1986.

25. Edwards, RHT, Hill, DK, Jones, DA, et al: Fatigue of long duration in human skeletal muscle after exercise. J Physiol (Lond) 272:769–778, 1977.

26. Bagust, J, Lewis, DM, and Luck, JC: Post-tetanic effects in motor units of fast and slow twitch muscles of the cat. J Physiol (Lond) 237:115–121, 1974.

27. Brown, GI and vonEuler, US: The after effects of a tetanus on mammalian muscle. J Physiol (Lond) 93:39–60, 1938.

28. Burke, RE, Rudomin, P, and Zajac, FE: Catch properties in single mammalian motor units. Science 168:212–214, 1970.

28a. Close, RI: Dynamic properties of mammalian skeletal muscles. Physiol Rev 52:129–197, 1972.

29. Stuart, DS, Lingley, MD, Grange, RW, et al: Myosin light chain phosphorylation and contractile performance of human skeletal muscle. Can J Physiol Pharmacol 66:49–54, 1988.

30. Vandervoort, AA, Quinlan, J, and McComas, AJ: Twitch potentiation after voluntary contraction. Exp Neurol 81:141–152, 1983.

31. Manning, DR and Stull, JT: Myosin light chain phosphorylation in mammalian skeletal muscle. Am J Physiol 242:c234–c241, 1982.

32. Moore RL and Stull JT: Myosin light chain phosphorylation in fast and slow skeletal muscles in situ. Am J Physiol 240:c462–c471, 1984.

33. Sweeney, HL and Stull, JT: Phosphorylation of myosin in permeabilized mammalian cardiac and skeletal muscle cells. Am J Physiol 250:c657–c660, 1986.

34. Binder, SA: Applications of low and high voltage electrotherapeutic currents. In Wolf, SL (ed): Electrotherapy. Churchill Livingstone, New York, 1981, pp 1–24.
35. Cook, TM: Instrumentation. In Nelson, RM and Currier, DP (eds): Clinical Electrotherapy. Appleton & Lange, Norwalk, CT, 1987, pp 11–28.
36. Binder-Macleod, SA: Force-frequency relations of cat motor units during linearly varying dynamic stimulation. Department of Physiology, Medical College of Virginia, Richmond, VA 1987. Doctoral Dissertation.
37. Buller, AJ and Lewis, DM: The rate of tension development in isometric tetanic contractions of mammalian fast and slow skeletal muscle. J Physiol (Lond) 176:337–354, 1965.
38. Miller, RG, Mirka, A, and Maxfield, M: Rate of tension development in isometric contractions of a human hand muscle. Exp Neurol 73:267–285, 1981.
39. Jones, DA, Bigland-Ritchie, B, and Edwards, RHT: Excitation frequency and muscle fatigue: Mechanical responses during voluntary and stimulated contractions. Exp Neurol 64:401–413, 1979.
40. Marsden, CD, Meadows, JC, and Merton, PA: Isolated single motor units in human muscle and their rate of discharge during maximal voluntary effort. J Physiol (Lond) 217:12p–13p, 1971.
41. Binder-Macleod, SA and Johnson, TL: Effects of muscle length on the force-frequency relationship in human quadriceps femoris muscle. Abstracts of Platform and Poster Presentations, 65th Annual Conference of the American Physical Therapy Association, 1990, p 49.
42. Andreassen, S and Rosenfalck, A: Regulation of the firing pattern of single motor units. J Neurol Neurosurg Psychiatr 43:897–906, 1980.
43. Zajac, FE and Young, JL: Discharge properties of hindlimb motoneurons in decerebrate cats during locomotion induced by mesencephalic stimulation. J Neurophysiol 43:1221–1235, 1980.
44. Burke, RE, Rudomin, P, and Zajac, FE: The effect of activation history on tension production by individual muscle units. Brain Res 109:515–529, 1976.
45. Parmiggiani, F and Stein, RB: Nonlinear summation of contractions in cat muscle. II. Later facilitation and stiffness changes. J Gen Physiol 78:295–311, 1981.
46. Partridge, LD: Modification of neural output signals by muscles: A frequency response study. J Appl Physiol 20:150–156, 1965.
47. Partridge, LD: Signal-handling characteristics of load-moving skeletal muscle. Am J Physiol 210:1178–1191, 1966.
48. Partridge, LD: Interrelationships studied in a semibiological "reflex." Am J Physiol 223:144–158, 1972.
49. Stein, RB and Parmiggiani, F: Optimal motor patterns for activating mammalian muscle. Brain Res 175:372–376, 1979.
50. Stein, RB and Parmiggiani, F: Nonlinear summation of contractions in cat muscles. I. Early depression. J Gen Physiol 78:277–293, 1981.
51. Wilson, DM and Larimer, JL: The catch properties of ordinary muscle. Proc Natl Acad Sci U S A 61:909–916, 1968.
52. Zajac, FE and Young, JL: Properties of stimulus trains producing maximum tension-time area per pulse from single motor units in medial gastrocnemius muscle of the cat. J Neurophysiol 43:1206–1220, 1980.
53. Wilson, DM, Smith, DO, and Dempster, P: Length and tension hysteresis during the sinusoidal and step function stimulation of arthropod muscle. Am J Physiol 218:916–922, 1970.
54. Adrian, ED and Bronk, DW: The discharge of impulses in motor nerve fibres. Part II. The frequency of discharge in reflex and voluntary contractions. J Physiol (Lond) 66:119–151, 1928.
55. Milner-Brown, HS, Stein, RB, and Yemm, R: Changes in firing rate of human motor units during linearly changing voluntary contractions. J Physiol (Lond) 230:371–390, 1973.
56. Kukulka, CG and Clamann, HP: Comparison of the recruitment and discharge properties of motor units in human brachial biceps and adductor pollicis during isometric contractions. Brain Res 219:45–55, 1981.
57. Monster, AW, Chan, HC, and O'Conner, C: Activity patterns of human skeletal muscle: Relation to fiber type composition. Science 200:314–317, 1978.
58. Grillner, S and Udo, M: Recruitment in the tonic stretch reflex. Acta Physiol Scand 81:571–573, 1971.
59. Mannard, A and Stein, RB: Determination of the frequency response of isometric soleus msucle in the cat using random nerve stimulation. J Physiol 229:275–296, 1973.
60. Bigland, B and Lippold, OCJ: Motor unit activity in the voluntary contraction of human muscle. J Physiol (Lond) 125:322–335, 1954.
61. Hoffer, JA, Sugano, N, Loeb, GE, et al: Cat hindlimb motoneurons during locomtion. II. Normal activity patterns. J Neurophysiol 57:530–553, 1987.
62. Lind, AR and Petrofsky, JS: Isometric tension from rotary stimulation of fast and slow cat muscles. Muscle Nerve 1:213–218, 1978.
63. Wuerker, RB, McPhedran, AM, and Henneman, E: Properties of motor units in a heterogeneous pale muscle (m. gastrocnemius) of the cat. J Neurophysiol 28:85–99, 1965.
64. Burke, RE: Motor units: Anatomy, physiology, and functional organization. In Handbook of Physiology, sect 1: The Nervous System. vol 2, Motor Control, part 1. American Physiological Society, Bethesda, MD, 1981, pp 345–422.

65. Bawa, P and Calanchie, B: Repetitive doublets in human flexor carpi radialis muscle. J Physiol (Lond) 339:123–132, 1983.
66. Cordo, PJ and Rymer, WZ: Motor-unit activation patterns in lengthening and isometric contractions of hindlimb extensor muscles in the decerebrate cat. J Neurophysiol 47:782–796, 1982.
67. Denslow, JS: Doublet discharges in human motor units. J Neurophysiol 11:209–215, 1948.
68. Gurfinkel, VS, Mirsky, ML, Tarko, AM, et al: Function of human motor units on initiation of muscle tension. Biofizika 17:303–310, 1972.
69. Eriksson, E and Häggmark, T: Comparison of isometric muscle training and electrical stimulation supplementing isometric muscle training in the recovery after major knee ligament surgery. Am J Sports Med 7:169–171, 1979.
70. Liu, CT and Lewey, FH: The effect of surging currents of low frequency in man on atrophy of denervated muscles. J Nerv Ment Dis 105:571–581, 1947.
71. Morrissey, MC, Brewster, CE, Shields, CL, et al: The effects of electrical stimulation on the quadriceps during post-operative knee immobilization. Am J Sports Med 13:40–45, 1985.
72. Wigerstad-Lossing, I, Grimby, G, Jonsson, T, et al: Effects of electrical muscle stimulation combined with voluntary contractions after knee ligament surgery. Med Sci Sports Exerc 20:93–98, 1988.
73. Boutelle, D, Smith, B, and Malone, T: A strength study utilizing the electro-stim 180. Journal of Orthopedic Sports and Physical Therapy 7:50–53, 1985.
74. Currier, DP, Lehman, J, and Lightfoot, P: Electrical stimulation in exercise of the quadriceps femoris muscle. Phys Ther 59:1508–1512, 1979.
75. Currier DP and Mann R: Muscular strength development by electrical stimulation in healthy individuals. Phys Ther 63:915–921, 1983.
76. Delitto A, Rose SJ, McKowen JM, et al: Electrical stimulation versus voluntary exercise in strengthening thigh musculature after anterior cruciate ligament surgery. Phys Ther 68:660–663, 1988.
77. Duchateau, J and Hainaut, K: Training effects of sub-maximal electrostimulation in a human muscle. Med Sci Sports Exerc 20:99–104, 1988.
78. Halbach, JW and Straus, D: Comparison of electro-myo stimulation to isokinetic training in increasing power of the knee extensor mechanism. Journal of Orthopedic Sports and Physical Therapy 2:20–24, 1980.
79. Kramer, JF and Mendyrk, SW: Electrical stimulation as a strength improvement technique: A review. J Orthop Sports Phys Ther 4:91–98, 1982.
80. Laughman, RK, Youdas, JW, Garrett, TR, et al: Strength changes in the normal quadriceps femoris muscle as a result of electrical stimulation. Phys Ther 63:494–499, 1983.
81. McMiken, DF, Todd-Smith, M, and Thompson, C: Strengthening of human quadriceps muscles by cutaneous electrical stimulation. Scand J Rehab Med 15:25–28, 1983.
82. Mohr, T, Carlson, B, Sulentic, C, et al: Comparison of isometric exercise and high volt galvanic stimulation on quadriceps femoris muscle strength. Phys Ther 65:606–611, 1985.
83. Romero, JA, Sanford, TL, Schroeder, RV, et al: The effects of electrical stimulation of normal quadriceps on strength and girth. Med Sci Sports Exerc 14:194–197, 1982.
84. Selkowitz, DM: Improvement in isometric strength of the quadriceps femoris muscle after training with electrical stimulation. Phys Ther 65:186–196, 1985.
85. Soo, C-L, Currier, DP, and Threlkeld, AJ: Augmenting voluntary torque of healthy muscle by optimization of electrical stimulation. Phys Ther 68:333–337, 1988.
86. Stefanovska, A and Vodovnik, L: Changes in muscle force following electrical stimulation: Dependence on stimulation waveform and frequency. Scand J Rehab Med 17:141–146, 1985.
87. Baker, LL, Yeh, C, Wilson, D, et al: Electrical stimulation of wrist and fingers for hemiplegic patients. Phys Ther 59:1495–1499, 1979.
88. Bowman, BR, Baker, LL, and Waters, RL: Positional feedback and electrical stimulation: An automated treatment for the hemiplegic wrist. Arch Phys Med Rehabil 60:497–502, 1979.
89. Munsat, TL, McNeal, D, and Waters, R: Effects of nerve stimulation on human muscle. Arch Neurol 23:608–617, 1976.
90. Liberson, WT, Holmquest, HJ, Scot, D, et al: Functional electrotherapy: Stimulation of the peroneal nerve synchronized with the swing phase of gait of hemiplegic patients. Arch Phys Med Rehabil 42:101–105, 1961.
91. Merletti, R, Zelaschi, F, Latella, D, et al: A control study of muscle force recovery in hemiparetic patients during treatment with functional electrical stimulation. Scand J Rehab Med 10:147–154, 1978.
92. Takebe, K, Kukulka, C, Narayan, M, et al: Peroneal nerve stimulator in rehabilitation of hemiplegic patients. Arch Phys Med Rehabil 56:237–240, 1975.
93. Waters, RL, Mcneal, D, and Perry, J: Experimental correction of footdrop by electrical stimulation of the peroneal nerve. J Bone Joint Surg 57:1047–1054, 1975.
94. Bajd, T and Kralj, A: Standing-up of a healthy subject and a paraplegic patient. J Biomech 15:1–10, 1982.
95. Bajd, T, Kralj, A, Sega, J, et al: Use of a two-channel functional electrical stimulator to stand paraplegic patients. Phys Ther 61:526–528, 1981.
96. Marsden, DC, Meadows, JC, and Merton, PA: "Muscular wisdom" that minimizes fatigue during

prolonged effort in man: Peak rates of motoneuron discharge and slowing of discharge during fatigue. Adv Neurol 39:169–211, 1983.

97. Binder-Macleod, SA and Barker, CB: Use of a catchlike property of human skeletal muscle to reduce fatigue. Muscle Nerve 14:850–857, 1991.

98. Binder-Macleod, SA and Guerin, T: Preservation of force output through progressive reduction of stimulation frequency in the human quadriceps femoris muscle. Phys Ther 70:619–625, 1990.

99. Grimby, L, Hannerz, J, and Hedman, B: Firing properties of single human motor units on maintained maximal voluntary effort. Ciba Found Symp 82:157–177, 1981.

100. Bigland-Ritchie, B, Jones, DA, and Woods, JJ: Excitation frequency and muscle fatigue: Electrical responses during human voluntary and stimulated contractions. Exp Neurol 64:414–427, 1979.

101. Clamann, HP and Robinson, AJ: A comparison of electromyographic and mechanical fatigue properties in motor units of the cat hindlimb. Brain Res 327:203–219, 1985.

102. Bigland-Ritchie, B, Kukulka, CG, and Lippold, OCJ: The absence of neuromuscular transmission failure in sustained maximal voluntary contractions. J Physiol 330:265–278, 1982.

103. Kukulka, CG, Russell, AG, and Moore, MA: Electrical and mechanical changes in human soleus muscle during sustained maximum isometric contraction. Brain Res 362:47–54, 1986.

CHAPTER 5

Effects of Neuromuscular Electrical Stimulation on Skeletal Muscle Ultrastructure

David G. Greathouse, Ph.D, P.T.
Daniel H. Matulionis, Ph.D.

The use of neuromuscular electrical stimulation (NMES) as a treatment modality in physical therapy has increased in the recent past. NMES has been claimed to relieve pain in injured areas, increase local blood flow, strengthen muscles, cause muscle hypertrophy, and facilitate muscle contraction.[1-5] As impressive as these observations are, there is a paucity of information concerning the effects of short-term (less than 6 weeks) NMES on structure of skeletal muscle. Further, the existing literature on NMES is incomplete and often conflicting.

With the development of different types of electrical stimulators that use various waveforms and frequencies and the increased interest of NMES therapy, there is a need for the basic understanding of the structural changes that may occur as a result of this type of treatment. The purpose of this chapter is to provide an overview of the effects of NMES on structure of skeletal muscle. Knowledge of skeletal muscle ultrastructure following NMES is important to clinicians who use this type of modality in their patients' treatment programs, in that it gives insight as to the true condition of muscle. A brief review of normal skeletal muscle ultrastructure components that have been reported to change subsequent to NMES is provided as a basis for discussing the changes produced by NMES.

The literature regarding the effects of long-term (greater than 6 weeks) and continued NMES on skeletal muscle ultrastructure is extensive, but will be only briefly described in this chapter. In addition, the effects of NMES on denervated and partially denervated skeletal muscle ultrastructure will also be considered and discussed. Clinical application of current and waveform when using NMES to prevent atrophy of denervated muscle should be based on scientific rationale.

SUBCELLULAR SKELETAL MUSCLE

The cell membrane (Fig. 5–1) or sarcolemma of skeletal muscle is 7 to 11 nanometers (nm) in thickness, and is composed of 60 percent protein, 35 percent lipid, and 5 percent carbohydrate.[6] The sarcolemma's structure is typical of all cellular plasma membranes. The fluid mosaic model of the cell membranes has been described as a composition of glycerol and fatty acid groups intermingled with integral proteins and additional peripheral proteins along the exterior and interior of the membrane structure.[7] The sarcolemma limits and confines the contents of the muscle cell, to allow selective movement of substances into and out of the cell, and may serve as a receptor site for neurotransmitters, hormones, and enzymes.

The smallest independent cellular units of mature skeletal muscle are called fibers or muscle cells. Muscle fibers are cylindrical, multinucleate, cellular structures that vary greatly in length.[6] Myofibrils, cross-striated contractile organelles, occupy the largest volume of each muscle fiber. Surrounding the myofibrils and located near the nuclei are the remaining cytoplasmic components of the fiber, collectively called the sarcoplasm.[6] Examination of skeletal muscle by light microscopy shows that these myofibrils are arranged across each fiber or "cross-striated." The cross-striations result from an internal structure of repeating subunits, called sarcomeres.[6] A sarcomere is the fundamental structural and functional unit of contraction. The sarcomeres of each myofibril are viewed as an orderly three-dimensional assembly of many fiber filaments, called myofilaments.[6] Actin and myosin (thin and thick filaments, respectively) are the contractile proteins of the muscle cell, and the interaction of the actin and

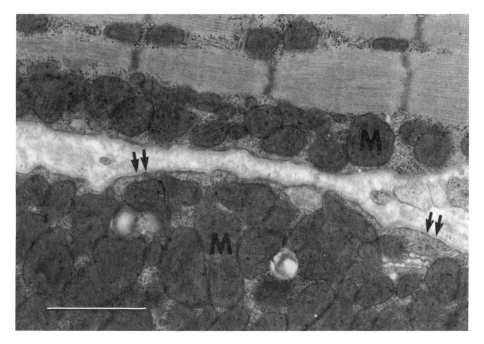

FIGURE 5–1. Sarcolemma of tibialis anterior muscle of a control animal. Sarcolemma *(double arrowhead)* is characterized by an even appearance with numerous mitochondria (M) located subjacent to the membrane. In this and subsequent electron micrographs, the calibration bar located in the lower left corner is equal to 1 μm (magnification ×21,000).

myosin results in the generation of contractile force via the sliding filament mechanism of muscle contraction.

The sarcoplasm is the cytoplasm of the muscle cell and is confined within the sarcolemma. The sarcoplasm consists of a matrix material, organelles, and inclusion bodies. The cell matrix or cytosol is an intracellular substance composed of water and proteoglycan ground substance. The sarcoplasm should not be thought of as a structureless fluid phase in which the contractile myofilaments, actin and myosin, are suspended. Instead it should be considered as a complex assembly of organelles that provide structural and energetic support for the contractile apparatus, in addition to serving the metabolic requirements of the muscle cell.[6] The organelles, suspended within the cytosol, are structures that perform the metabolic functions within the cell, whereas the inclusion bodies are nonliving structures that serve as storage areas of substances (lipid, glycogen, water) that will be used by the cell. Several organelles of the muscle cell respond to neuromuscular electrical stimulation and will be detailed below.

Of all the organelles in the skeletal muscle cell, mitochondria are perhaps most numerous. They are of great importance to cell function. Mitochondria are found beneath the sarcolemma (see Fig. 5–1) around the nuclei, and in the sarcoplasm between the myofibrils (Fig. 5–2). The mitochondria measure 0.2 to 1 μm in diameter and 2 to 12 μm in length. Each mitochondrion is bound by two membranes, an outer and an inner membrane, which lie in close opposition. The inner membrane is thrown into folds called cristae, which function to increase the surface area for enzymatic reactions. The interior of the mitochondria, not occupied by cristae, is filled with a mitochondrial matrix in which are located highly dense matrix granules that serve as binding sites for Ca^{2+}. Deoxyribonucleic acid (DNA) and ribonucleic acid (RNA) are also found in the mitochondria. The production of phosphate bond energy by adenosine triphosphate (ATP) within the muscle cell is the major function of mitochondria. There are specific loci for the chemical reactions involved in intracellular energy production and transfer. The inner membrane is the site of electron transport and oxidative phosphorylation processes, and the energy freed in oxidation is converted into phosphate bond energy (ATP).[8]

Another organelle within the skeletal muscle cell affected by NMES is the sarcoplasmic reticulum (SR) (see Fig. 5–2), which is a network of cisterns or membranous tubules that course between and around the myofibril. The SR is the storage site for calcium, which is used in the excitation-contraction of skeletal muscle. The SR expands into terminal cisterns in the vicinity of the I band or Z disc, and these terminal cisterns are arranged in pairs that flank a transverse tubule (Tt), a tubular membranous structure (see Fig. 5–2). The Tt are narrow, regularly arranged invaginations of the sarcolemma. An action potential travels along the Tt, causing release of calcium from the terminal cisterna. A Tt and its two closely opposed terminal cisterns constitute a triad.

Nonorganelle inclusions (inclusion bodies) such as glycogen are also affected by NMES. Glycogen particles (see Fig. 5–2) function as storage sites for glucose. These small, dense particles, 15 to 40 nm in diameter, are located throughout the sarcoplasm but tend to congregate near the I band.

A prominent structure within the muscle cell is the Z disc or Z line. The Z disc is a filamentous network that serves to link actin filaments of one sarcomere to those of the adjoining sarcomere. Z disc filaments are reinforced with a dense sarcoplasmic matrix, which gives them their characteristic dark appearance on electron micro-

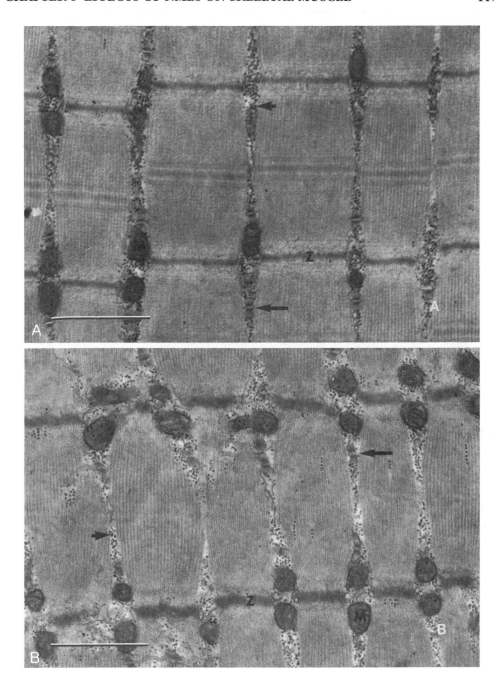

FIGURE 5–2. Electron micrograph of *(A)* rat tibialis anterior and *(B)* soleus muscles from a control animal. Note the differences in number of mitochondria (M) triads *(arrow)*, glycogen particles *(arrowhead)*, and size of the Z-line (Z) in the two muscles (magnification ×27,000; bar = 1µm).

graphs. The Z disc is a distinguishing feature between tonic (slow) and phasic (fast) twitch skeletal muscle. Slow-twitch muscle displays a broad, dense Z disc (0.12 μm) (see Fig. 5–2) and fast-twitch muscle is characterized by an irregular Z disc that is narrow (0.07 μm) (see Fig. 5–2A) when compared with the Z disc of the slow-twitch fiber.

Distribution of different muscle fiber types determined by myosin ATPase histochemical procedures has been documented in human muscles. Johnson and associates[9] discussed the distribution of muscle fiber types in 36 human muscles. Two distinct types of muscle fiber can be classified by their contractile and metabolic characteristics. Slow- (type I) and fast- (type II) twitch muscle fibers have been identified. The proportion of muscle fiber types in human muscle probably remains constant throughout life.[10] Slow-twitch (ST) fibers are predominantly aerobic, with a relatively slow speed of contraction. The fast-twitch (FT) muscle fiber has three basic subdivisions (type IIa, fast-oxidative glycolytic; type IIb, fast-glycolytic; and type IIc, undifferentiated fiber that may be involved in re-innervation or motor unit transformation) and possesses a high capability for the anaerobic production of ATP during glycolysis.[8] When a person is exercising at near maximum aerobic and anaerobic levels, as in running or swimming, which require a blend of aerobic and anaerobic energy, both muscle fiber types are activated.[11]

Slow- and fast-twitch muscle fibers can be structurally differentiated by other ultrastructural characteristics. The former (see Fig. 5–2B) have a large number of mitochondria, a smaller volume of sarcoplasmic reticulum, and a smaller volume of glycogen compared with the fast-twitch (phasic) muscle fibers (Fig. 5–A). Fast-twitch muscle fibers have fewer mitochondria, a larger volume of sarcoplasmic reticulum, and a larger volume of glycogen than slow-twitch fiber. Identification of differences in muscle fiber type is routinely made with histochemical staining (myosin ATPase), although differences in subcellular structure have also been described as a reliable method to differentiate slow- from fast-twitch fibers.[6]

Effects of Short-term Neuromuscular Electrical Stimulation on Muscle Ultrastructure

Effects of short-term (less than 6 weeks) neuromuscular electrical stimulation on the ultrastructure of muscle must be related to the specific waveform and current produced by the electrical generator in mind. Redanna and co-workers[12] showed that short-term NMES of frog skeletal muscle resulted in a decrease in glycogen and a reduction in the total muscle protein content. Eriksson and associates[13] assessed the effects of short-term, low-frequency NMES on the human quadriceps femoris muscle. These researchers studied the effects of NMES in human vastus lateralis muscles using surface electrodes and 10 milliampere (ma) amplitude for 0.5 millisecond duration in a square waveform and a frequency of 200 pps (Hz). The treatment cycle was 15 seconds on/off for 6 minutes, four to five times per week for 5 weeks. An active depletion of phosphagen and glycogen stores occurred, but no changes in muscle enzyme activities, fiber type characteristics, and volume fraction and number of mitochondria were noted.[13] In a study analyzing the combined effects of exercise and short-term NMES by means of prodding on rat skeletal muscle, Ogilvie and Rhein[14] noted a disruption of the A and I band and Z disc.[14] Taylor and colleagues[15] reported that 10-minute faradic current NMES for 10 successive days did not alter muscle fiber composition or the cross-sectional area in the vastus lateralis muscle. The current and method of application were not described. In a recent study, Horacek and co-workers[16] stimulated the thighs of adult female rabbits using a 400-pps current and noted a strength increase after 3 weeks. They found that both the type IIA and type IIB fibers hypertrophied in the vastus lateralis muscles of the treated animals when compared with the same muscles in control animals. In addition, these researchers noted type I fibers were rarely observed in the vastus lateralis muscle in the rabbit, and that no changes in muscle ultrastructure were reported.[16]

A study by Greathouse and colleagues[17] has evaluated the effects of 2500-pps carrier frequency electrical stimulation (using the Electrostim 180-2) on subcellular components in quadriceps femoris and hamstring muscle cells of normal rats. The Electrostim 180-2, an electrical generator developed in Canada, is used in orthopedic and sports medicine to increase strength in normal skeletal muscles in humans. This type of electrical stimulation modality, especially in humans, had not hitherto been studied to determine its effect in skeletal muscle ultrastructure. The Electrostim 180-2 is a specific generator that delivers 15-second trains of electrical pulses that repeat at 50 bursts per second (bps). The shape of each pulse within the train is a sine wave with a peak amplitude of the train maintained for 10 seconds. The current train of stimulation applied for 15 seconds was followed by a 50-second rest period producing an on/off treatment cycle of 15/50 seconds. A similar study to determine the effects of NMES on quadriceps femoris muscle strength had been performed in humans; however, the effect of this type of NMES on the skeletal muscle ultrastructure was not evaluated.[18] Following 3 weeks (5 days per week) of treatment, Greathouse and colleagues,[17] using the rat model, observed an increase in the number and volume fraction of mitochondria (quadriceps femoris and hamstring muscles) but a decrease in the number and volume fraction of triads (hamstrings) and glycogen particles (hamstrings). Houston and co-workers[19] also reported a decrease in glycogen content in both fast- and slow-twitch fiber types in the human quadriceps femoris muscles following a 60-minute, 50-pps electrical stimulation treatment. The electrical generator used in this study produced a square wave pulse of 0.6 milliseconds duration, delivered at 50 pps stimulation with the on/off cycle at 12 seconds stimulation/48 seconds recovery.[19]

Other studies by Greathouse and colleagues[20,21] evaluated the effects of short-term NMES on the subcellular components in fast-twitch tibialis anterior and slow-twitch soleus muscle cells of normal rats. Again, the Electrostim 180-2 electrical generator was used to produce the NMES. The leg muscles of the rats were treated daily 5 days per week for 4 weeks. In addition to the muscle ultrastructure, muscle function, neural conduction/electromyography, muscle cell cross-sectional area, and muscle cell fiber type in these animals were also assessed. Distinction between fast- and slow-twitch muscle fibers was based on the width of the Z disc of the myofibrils. The width of the Z disc in control soleus (primarily slow-twitch) and tibialis anterior (fast-twitch) muscles measured 0.12 μm and 0.07 μm, respectively. The muscle fiber type within these muscles, evaluated by histochemical procedure (myosin ATPase staining), was not altered. The Z discs in the NMES tibialis anterior and soleus muscles were likewise unaltered in dimension when compared to control values.

Two weeks of NMES of the tibialis anterior and soleus muscles in healthy animals did not alter the morphology of the mitochondria. However, after 3 weeks of NMES, the mitochondria (Fig. 5–3) in both muscles increased in size (volume fraction) when compared with those of controls and NMES weeks 1 and 2. These authors likewise

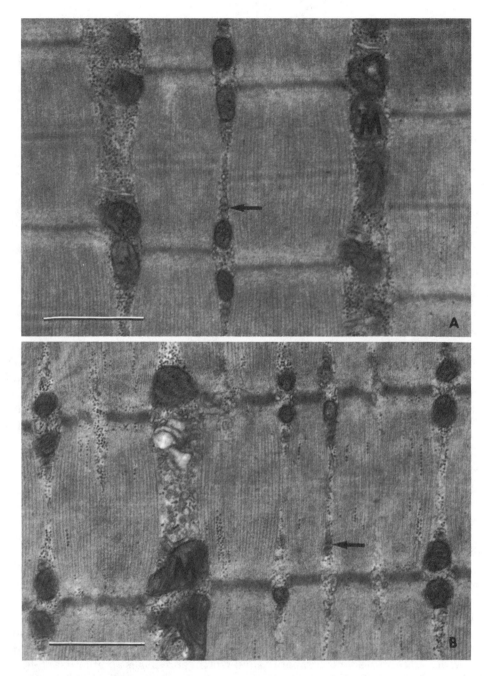

FIGURE 5–3. Electron micrograph of *(A)* tibialis anterior and *(B)* soleus muscles in a normal, healthy animal whose leg was treated for 3 weeks with NMES. Mitochondria (M) appear larger and triads *(arrow)* relatively small compared to control animal tissue (see Fig. 5–2) (magnification ×27,000; bar = 1 μm).

evaluated the effects of the Electrostim 180-2 on another organelle of the rat skeletal muscle. The triads, which are functionally involved in the storage and release of calcium during the excitation-contraction of skeletal muscle, decreased in size and number per area and volume fraction in tibialis anterior muscles (Fig. 5–3A) electrically stimulated for 4 weeks. The mean volume fraction of triads in the soleus muscle (Fig. 5–3B) of normal animals decreased following 3 and 4 weeks of NMES when compared with controls; however, the size and number per area were not altered. Volume fraction (percent volume) of glycogen decreased following 1, 3, and 4 weeks of NMES in the tibialis anterior muscle (Fig. 5–3A) when compared with that of controls (see Fig. 5–2A). Glycogen of the predominantly slow-twitch soleus muscle (Fig. 5–3B) was unaltered compared with controls (see Fig. 5–2B) after 4 weeks of NMES.[20,21]

These authors concluded that the Electrostim 180-2, used as a NMES treatment modality for 4 weeks (following clinical treatment parameters), would change the ultrastructure of the rat tibialis anterior and soleus muscles to resemble that of slow-twitch muscles. However, width of the Z discs in the myofibrils was unaltered as a result of the NMES. Although muscle enzyme activity was not quantified in this study, fiber type characteristics were unaltered as a result of NMES. The unaltered state of fiber types indicates that short-term, 50-bps frequency NMES does not change the contractile properties in muscle. Thus this type of electrical current and waveform may be used in the clinic to strengthen healthy, normal muscle without changing the fiber type of these muscles.[20,21]

Many electrical generators are available to the clinician that provide a specific waveform and current. However, the effects of the different types of waveforms and currents on skeletal muscle ultrastructure are not known. Further research on the effects of short-term NMES on skeletal muscle structure and function is needed to provide the clinician a scientific basis with which to choose an appropriate electrical generator.

Correlation of Changes in Subcellular Components of Skeletal Muscle with Clinical Effects of Neuromuscular Electrical Stimulation

Evidence exists in the literature to indicate that short-term NMES using different waveforms and frequencies affects the size and strength of skeletal muscle.[3,22,23] In contrast, other studies using short-term NMES have not supported the claims of increased muscular strength.[24,25] Reports of increased strength in healthy muscle have been provided by Kots and his associates (unpublished studies) via a current and waveform that could produce a maximum muscle contraction without causing pain and skin irritation.[1,26,27] When used for 2 weeks in treating human thigh muscle, this type of NMES increased muscle strength by 20 percent. Kots reported that 20 NMES treatment sessions produced a subsequent 30 to 40 percent increase in muscle strength. He also stated that this type of NMES would increase muscle strength of healthy individuals at a greater rate than would exercise regimens eliciting maximum tetanic contraction. Kots further reported an increase in cross-sectional area of individual muscle fibers after 3 weeks of NMES. He attributed this finding to an increase in the density of myofibrils at the expense of sarcoplasm within the cell.[1,26,27] Currier and Mann[18] studied human quadriceps femoris muscles stimulated by the Electrostim 180-2 stimulator and found increased strength in subjects trained with isometric exercises. However, Owens and Malone[28] did not demonstrate a significant strength gain following NMES with the Electrostim 180-2.

Increases in size (girth) in extremities has been reported following NMES.[3,22,23,29] After 2 weeks of treatment with the "Russian wave" NMES, Kots[26,27] showed, in human thigh muscles, an increase in muscle girth (as measured by ultrasonic waves) but a decrease in subcutaneous fat. Significant increases in girth measurements of the treated thighs of rats stimulated for 3 weeks (15 sessions) with the Electrostim 180-2 have been reported.[17]

Use of clinical NMES has been shown to increase the size of skeletal muscle fibers in animals. Horacek and colleagues[16] used NMES (4000 pps, triweekly, 3 months) to treat adult rabbit thigh muscles and noted a significant hypertrophy in the type IIA and IIB muscle fibers of the vastus lateralis when compared with the contralateral nonstimulated side. Greathouse and colleagues[20,21] treated the leg muscles of rats with the Electrostim 180-2 5 days a week for 4 weeks and found significant increases in leg girth of rats treated for 4 weeks with NMES when compared with the contralateral nonstimulated side and with the controls. These authors reported that fast- and slow-twitch muscle fibers of the tibialis anterior (TA) muscle appeared to increase in size and diameter. However, when the mean areas and diameters of TA fast- and slow-twitch fibers were analyzed, no significant difference was found over time (NMES over weeks) or because of NMES (NMES normal versus controls). Significant increases in fiber size (cross-sectional area) and diameter were observed in the fast- and slow-twitch fibers in the soleus muscle of animals that received NMES for 4 weeks.[20,21] The differences in the size of the fast-twitch muscles between the hypertrophied vastus lateralis muscle of the rabbit (Horacek and colleagues[16]) and the nonhypertrophied tibialis anterior muscle of the rat (Greathouse and colleagues[20,21]) may be due to the electrical stimulator used in each study, the difference in current and waveform, length of treatment days (3 months versus 4 weeks), or the species response of muscle tissue (rabbit versus rat) to the NMES.

Response of Normal Muscle to Long-term Electrical Stimulation

Although they are not a focus of this chapter, the changes in skeletal muscle following long-term or continuous NMES will be briefly described. There is little documented use of continuous long-term NMES in the treatment of orthopedic and sports problems. The muscle alterations noted following long-term stimulation are not in complete accord with those observed after short-term electrical stimulation. Several investigators stimulated predominantly fast-twitch muscles for extended periods (greater than 6 weeks) and observed increases in width of the Z disc in fast-twitch fibers, but no disruption of A band or I band was noted.[34-36] In addition to the change in Z disc width, an increase in the volume fraction and number of mitochondria following long-term electrical stimulation was observed.[34-36] However, following similar treatment, the number and volume fraction of T tubule systems of fast-twitch muscle fibers were reduced.[36] Impressive as these ultrastructural changes are following long-term NMES, Streter and associates[37] demonstrated that changing ultrastructural characteristics of fast-twitch to slow-twitch muscle by long-term electrical stimulation was produced not only by continuous stimulation using trains of impulses at a low frequency, but also by stimulation using trains at a higher frequency.[37] The studies indicate that ultrastructural changes from fast-twitch to slow-twitch characteristics depends more on the total contractile activity of the muscle than on the pattern of stimulation. Histochemical analysis of muscle subjected to long-term electrical stimulation has shown a significant decline in calcium-activated myosin ATPase activity starting after 3 weeks of stimulation and progressing through subsequent months to levels characteristic of slow muscle.[38] Long-term and continuous NMES is sometimes used as an electrical modality in rehabilitation medicine, for example, spinal cord injuries. There is little or no use of continuous NMES in the treatment of patients with orthopedic or sports-related disorders.

EFFECTS OF SHORT-TERM NEUROMUSCULAR ELECTRICAL STIMULATION ON THE ULTRASTRUCTURE OF IMMOBILIZED MUSCLE

NMES has an effect on muscles that have been insulted. Skeletal muscle structure is altered by cast or splint immobilization.[31] A decrease in succinate dehydrogenase (SDH) has been prevented by using short-term stimulation of immobilized muscles.[31] In addition, it was reported that stimulation of muscles of limbs that had undergone knee ligament surgery and had been immobilized for weeks did not alter glycogen content when compared with untreated, immobilized muscles.[31] In another study, Eriksson and associates,[13] assessing the effects of short-term, low-frequency NMES on normal human quadriceps femoris muscles, found that there was no change in muscle enzyme activities (magnesium-stimulated ATPase and SDH) or fast- and slow-twitch fiber type characteristics. This information suggests that muscle enzyme activity, which is affected in immobilized muscle, may be altered by NMES, but that NMES has no effect on enzyme activity in normal muscles. Curwin and co-workers[32] studied the effects of NMES on immobilized muscles and found that myofibrillar ATPase enzyme activity decreased in immobilized muscles; however, following treatment with NMES, myofibrillar ATPase enzyme activity was maintained at a normal level. Stanish and colleagues,[33] in a similar study, confirmed these results for myofibrillar ATPase and glycogen responses to NMES. They proposed that the stimulation used did not have sufficient current to produce maximal contraction necessary to elicit any structural changes.

EFFECTS OF SHORT-TERM NEUROMUSCULAR ELECTRICAL STIMULATION ON THE ULTRASTRUCTURE OF DENERVATED MUSCLE

Denervation of muscles results in changes in the muscle ultrastructure. Such muscles undergo functional, electrophysiologic, structural, and biochemical alterations.[39] The most obvious fine structural change following denervation is loss of myofilaments resulting in shrinkage or atrophy of the muscle fibers. In general, atrophy occurs throughout the period of denervation, although the rate of atrophy is most rapid during the first 2 weeks.[39] Niederle and Mayr[40] showed in rats that atrophy occurs earlier and to a greater extent in predominantly fast-twitch than in slow-twitch muscles. Following nerve transection, degenerative autolysis with loss of striation in the areas of soleus and gastrocnemius muscle fibers was detected as early as the eighth day; the maximum loss striation was observed at the 14th day; and Z lines became disrupted first, followed by disorder in the alignment of filaments.[41] Stonnington and Engel[42] showed that during the first few days after denervation there was an increase in mitochondrial volume fraction and sarcotubular surface area. One week after denervation the volume fraction of the former organelles decreased, but returned to normal values 1 month after denervation. Subsequent to denervation mitochondrial profiles changed from elongated to round configuration, and at the same time, the sarcotubular profiles continued to increase in surface area and become more prominent and dilated as the time of denervation progressed.[42] Denervation of rat and rabbit skeletal muscle by nerve transection was shown to have no effect on the glycogen content in either fast- or slow-twitch muscle.[43-45] Contrary to changes of other organelles, glycogen appeared not to be affected by denervation.

NERVE TRANSECTION AND NEUROMUSCULAR ELECTRICAL STIMULATION

The clinical use of NMES in the treatment of denervated skeletal muscle has been well documented.[46-51] Neuromuscular electrical stimulation retards muscle atrophy following denervation by providing a stimulus to cause the muscle to contract artificially. The effect of the electrotherapy depends on pulse duration, frequency and amplitude of the current, and number of treatment sessions.[52,53]

Pulsed current of less than 20 pps is capable of stimulating denervated muscle and delays atrophy significantly.[54-62] Monophasic pulsed current is used most frequently by physical therapists in an effort to reduce or prevent atrophic changes and subsequent degeneration in muscle following lesions of a peripheral nerve.[39]

Pachter, Oberstein, and Goodgold[63] evaluated the effects of NMES on denervated (nerve transection) rat extensor digitorum longus muscle (EDL). They found that both type I and II fibers atrophied following denervation of skeletal muscle that was not treated with NMES. Atrophy was greater in fast-twitch than in slow-twitch fibers. However, when denervated rat EDL muscle was subjected to NMES, denervation atrophy was retarded in both types of fibers. Glycogen complexes were found to be in greater proportion in fast-twitch stimulated fibers but were observed infrequently in denervated nonstimulated muscles. The authors postulated that the glycogen might be expressions of sarcoplasmic reticulum anabolic functions.[63] These functions are thought to be indications of a high degree of regenerative metabolic activity in NMES-treated fibers.

Conflicting information exists, however, concerning the effects of pulsed NMES on atrophy. Jaweed and associates[60] found that pulsed stimulation may impair the mechanism of isometric twitch development in denervated slow-twitch muscle of the rat. Impairment of the isometric twitch might impede contraction of the muscle, which is necessary in preventing atrophy. Schimrigk, McLaughlin, and Gruniger[64] found no benefit of pulsed NMES in retarding the effect of atrophy in denervated (nerve transect and crush) rat quadriceps femoris muscle. These investigators postulated that NMES may not delay atrophy in denervated muscle as previously thought.

Current of the faradic type delays muscle atrophy for a period up to 2 weeks following nerve transection.[55,56,65] However, after 2 weeks, chronically denervated muscle was unresponsive to faradic current. Therefore, this current was considered useless as a treatment modality to prevent or retard atrophy.[58-60] There is little evidence to support the hypothesis that faradic electric stimulation may improve the rate and extent of reinnervation of denervated skeletal muscle.[61] As much as the faradic current was being used, it is surprising that no information exists in the literature that describes its effects on the ultrastructure of denervated, partially denervated, and immobilized skeletal muscle.

Greathouse and colleagues[66] studied the effects of short-term NMES on the ultrastructure of denervated skeletal muscle, subsequent to transection of the sciatic nerve in the hind limb of rats. There were clear alterations in the denervated muscle ultrastructure. Two weeks following nerve transection, the mitochondria in the tibialis anterior (TA) muscle appeared larger and more elongated (Fig. 5–4A) compared with those of control tissue. The elongated mitochondria in soleus muscle (Fig. 5–4B) were reduced in number, slightly smaller, and disoriented within the fiber compared with those of control tissue. The triads in both TA and soleus muscles of animals with transected sciatic nerves seemed larger and dilated. Furthermore, there were disruptions in the Z discs and a loss of myofilaments with resultant disruptions in the I and A bands in both muscles.[66]

At 4 and 6 weeks following sciatic nerve transection, these authors found that the mitochondria in the TA muscle became smaller in relation to those at week 2, and appeared more like those of controls. At the same time, mitochondria in soleus muscles in animals whose sciatic nerve had been transected seemed reduced in number, but their size increased to those of controls. The increased size and dilated shape of the triads in the TA and soleus muscles continued at 4 and 6 weeks following nerve injury. Glycogen content increased in both TA and soleus muscles. Loss of myofilaments and disorientation of Z discs in both TA and soleus were still observed, although the degree was reduced at 4-week and 6-week sampling points. There were no apparent changes in muscle fiber area, mitochondria, triads, or glycogen content in either TA or soleus muscle in animals whose sciatic nerve had been transected and followed by 4 weeks of NMES (Electrostim 180-2) when compared with the same muscles in the group of animals that did not receive NMES. Likewise, there were no apparent changes in regard to loss of myofilaments or disorientation in Z discs in animals whose sciatic nerves had been transected and whose muscles were treated with 4 weeks of NMES. These authors concluded that the type of electrical stimulus used in that study did not produce a current and waveform necessary to deter the effects of muscle subcellular alteration that resulted from nerve transection.[66]

NERVE CRUSH AND NMES

Another method of injury to nerve with resultant denervation to muscle is that of crushing the nerve. Jaweed, Herbison, and Ditunno[60] crushed the sciatic nerve of rats and subjected the soleus muscle to NMES. They determined, using nerve conduction tests, that reinnervation of rat soleus muscle occurs between 2 and 3 weeks after crushing the nerve. Reinnervation of the exterior digitorum longus (EDL) muscle in mice was indicated at 9 days after sciatic nerve crush by the presence of miniature end plate potentials.[67] Greathouse and associates[66] crushed the sciatic nerve in rat hind limbs, which resulted in denervation in the tibialis anterior (TA) and soleus muscles. There was a decrease in TA and soleus muscle fiber area at 2 and 4 weeks postinjury. By the sixth week following nerve injury, the fiber area of both muscles approached that of controls. The crush nerve injury also produced alterations in the

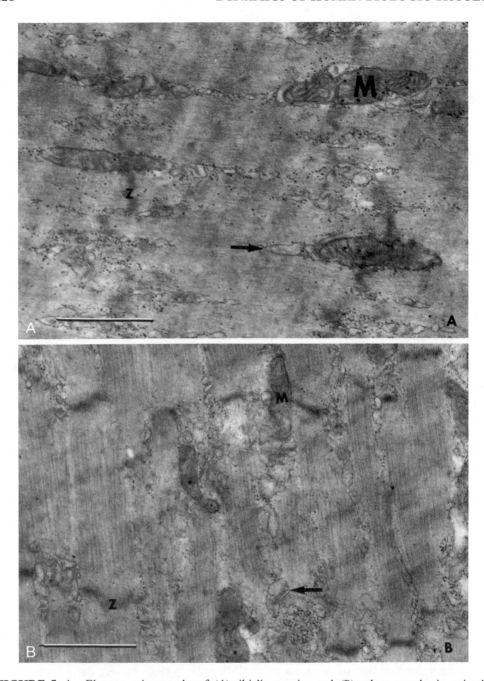

FIGURE 5–4. Electron micrographs of *(A)* tibialis anterior and *(B)* soleus muscles in animals whose sciatic nerves were transected 2 weeks prior to sacrifice. Note the disruptions in Z-lines and loss of myofilaments in both tibialis anterior and soleus muscles compared with control tissue. Elongated mitochondria (M) are noted in the tibialis anterior, *A*, and an increased size and dilation of triads *(arrow)* is depicted in the tibialis anterior and soleus muscles (magnification ×27,000; bar = 1 μm).

ultrastructure of muscle innervated by that nerve. At 2 weeks postinjury, some animals had alterations in muscle structure (Fig. 5–5A). In these muscles, the mitochondria were smaller and fewer, and the triads were larger and dilated. Consequently there was a disruption of the Z line and a loss of myofilament. The altered muscles in animals whose nerves had been crushed resembled those muscles that were subjected to nerve transection (see Fig. 5–4A). There were also animals in the nerve crush group (Fig. 5–5B) whose muscle ultrastructure did not appear to be affected by the nerve manipulation, and appeared to be similar to that of controls (see Fig. 5–2B).[66]

Four weeks following sciatic nerve crush, the mitochondria and triads in TA and soleus muscles appeared normal in shape and size to that of control tissue. However, elongated mitochondria were still noted occasionally. The amount of glycogen particles (percent volume) in both muscles increased when compared with that in animals at 2 weeks and those in the control group. No alteration was observed in Z discs, A or I bands, or myofilaments in TA or soleus muscles at this time. Six weeks following sciatic nerve crush, the fine structure in the TA and soleus muscles was similar to that of controls. Neuromuscular electrical stimulation of TA and soleus muscles in animals whose sciatic nerve had been crushed did not appear to have an effect on the ultrastructure of these muscles when compared with subcellular structures in TA and soleus muscles in animals (nerve crush) that did not receive NMES. The authors concluded that the type of electrical stimulator used in that study did not produce a current and waveform necessary to deter the effects of muscle subcellular alteration that resulted from nerve crush injury.[66]

COMPRESSION NERVE INJURY AND NEUROMUSCULAR ELECTRICAL STIMULATION

Nerve damage can occur as a result of tourniquet usage during limb surgery. The effect of pressure on the nerve and muscle ischemia as a result of pneumatic tourniquet applied to the thigh of rats was evaluated by Makitie and Teravainen.[68] They studied the ultrastructure of TA muscles whose thighs had undergone pneumatic tourniquet application for 1, 2, 3, 4, and 6 hours at 300 mm Hg. No ultrastructural alterations were seen after 1 hour of tourniquet application. Muscle glycogen was absent, and swelling mitochondria were noted 2 hours following tourniquet application. Application of tourniquet for 3 hours or longer resulted in disappearance of Z disc, disruption of cell membrane, and vacuolation of mitochondria. Autolysis of the fibers was observed in muscles undergoing tourniquet application for 6 hours. By the 18th day following tourniquet application, the fine structure of the muscle fibers had returned to normal appearance, indicating that the damage to the muscle was reversible. Other studies confirmed the findings of Makitie and Teravainen concerning ultrastructural changes in skeletal muscles following tourniquet pressure.[69–72]

Studies by Nitz and Matulionis[73,74] determined that tourniquet pressure (200 mm Hg) applied for 2 hours to the thigh of the rat was sufficient to cause sciatic nerve injury and subsequent partial denervation of musculature innervated by that nerve. Electromyographic assessment revealed that the sciatic nerve of animals was most affected 1 week after tourniquet compression. During the next 6 weeks, progressive improvement toward normal electrical activity was observed. However, the nerves still had abnormal electrical characteristics 6 weeks post-treatment. The ultrastructural

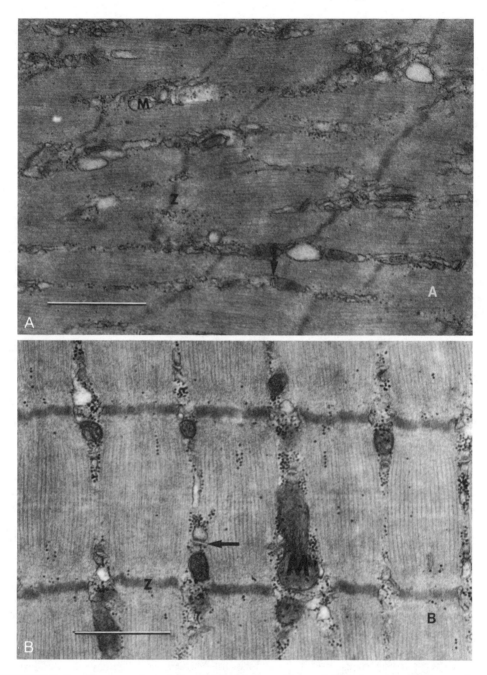

FIGURE 5–5. Electron micrographs of *(A)* tibialis anterior and *(B)* soleus muscles in rats whose sciatic nerve was crushed 2 weeks prior to sacrifice. Note disrupted state of tibialis anterior muscle, *A*, when compared with normal appearing soleus muscle, *B*. M = mitochondria; arrow = triads; Z = Z-line (magnification ×27,000).

changes of the sciatic nerves subjected to tourniquet compression were examined; however, the fine structure changes of the resultant injured musculature were not evaluated.[73,74]

Greathouse and colleagues[66] applied a tourniquet pressure (200 mm Hg/2 hours) to the thigh of rats to cause sciatic nerve insult resembling crush or partial denervation injury. No significant differences in mean muscle fiber areas of fast- and slow-twitch fibers in TA and soleus muscles were observed at 1, 2, 3, 4, and 5 weeks following tourniquet application. Furthermore, no difference as a result of NMES in mean muscle fiber area (tourniquet pressure animals) for both TA and soleus muscles was noted following 1, 2, 3, and 4 weeks of NMES (Electrostim 180-2). No alterations were observed at 1, 2, 3, and 4 weeks for the mitochondria, triads, or glycogen content in TA or soleus muscles in animals whose limb underwent tourniquet application. The Z discs were intact, and the A and I bands were not disrupted. The myofilaments were present and appeared to be unaltered because of the tourniquet pressure on the sciatic nerve. The results of this study differ from those of Makitie and Teravainen[68] with regard to normal mitochondria, glycogen, and Z lines. Makitie and Teravainen found swollen mitochondria and absent glycogen following 1 hour of tourniquet application. However, these authors examined the muscle tissue on the first day following tourniquet application, whereas Greathouse and colleagues waited until the seventh post-tourniquet day to examine the tissue. Perhaps changes in the mitochondria and glycogen occurred in the time between tourniquet applications and seven days post-tourniquet. Furthermore, Greathouse and colleagues studied the effects of tourniquet application on muscle for a period of 2 hours, whereas Makitie and Teravainen found disruptions in the Z lines and a loss of myofilaments following 3 hours of tourniquet application.[68]

The animals whose limbs had undergone tourniquet pressure followed by neuromuscular electrical stimulation to the TA and soleus muscles did not appear to have any fine structural changes after 4 weeks when compared with animals whose limbs were subjected to only tourniquet pressure but not NMES. Again, there were no alterations in A or I bands or Z discs as a result of the NMES.[66]

The results of the study by Greathouse and colleagues revealed that the three types of nerve injuries (i.e., sciatic nerve transection, crush, and tourniquet application) produced adverse alterations of varying degrees in muscle function, EMG activity, and structure.[66] The reported observations clearly indicated that the type of NMES produced by the Electrostim 180-2 does not rectify the adverse muscle alterations resulting from the above injuries. Apparently the nerve supply to the muscle must be intact for the electrical current and waveform generated by the Electrostim 180 stimulator to be effective. For this reason, clinical use of this type of stimulation should not be used to treat partially or completely denervated muscle.

SUMMARY

The purpose of this chapter was to provide an overview of NMES effects on structure of skeletal muscle. A brief review of normal skeletal muscle ultrastructure components that have been reported to change subsequent to NMES was provided. In addition, the ultrastructural differences between fast- and slow-twitch muscle fiber components were reviewed; these served as a basis for discussing the changes produced by neuromuscular electrical stimulation in skeletal muscle.

The effects of long-term (greater than 6 weeks) and continuous neuromuscular electrical stimulation are well documented. Investigators have shown that following continuous long-term NMES, fast-twitch muscle fiber might acquire the characteristics of slow-twitch fibers, that is, wide Z disc, increase in mitochondrial number and size, and reduced size and number of T tubule systems. This type of NMES is sometimes used as an electrical modality in rehabilitation medicine, but there is little use of continuous NMES in orthopedic or sports medicine.

The use of short-term NMES as an electrical treatment modality in physical therapy has increased in the recent past. Short-term NMES has been shown to decrease pain, increase local blood flow, strengthen skeletal muscle, and facilitate muscle contraction. Numerous studies substantiate these findings; however, there is no one type of electrical generator (producing a specific current and waveform) that is common to all the different types of electrical treatments available to physical therapists. Furthermore, there are few studies that examine the effects of these different electrical generators on the structure of skeletal muscle.

Neuromuscular electrical stimulation from a specific type of electrical generator that produces a 2500-pps carrier wave interrupted by 50 bursts per second appears capable of increasing girth in extremities of normal, healthy animals. Concomitant with the increase in leg girth, muscle fiber areas in muscles treated with the specific type of NMES also increased. The use of a specific type of NMES (2500-pps carrier wave interrupted by 50 bursts per second) on normal, healthy muscles of animals alters the subcellular components in those muscles. The number and size of mitochondria increase, while the volume of sarcoplasmic reticulum decreases. The volume and size of mitochondria and triads in NMES-treated muscles have been reported to change from fast- to slow-twitch proportions following this specific type of NMES. Glycogen content and the width of the Z lines in myofibrils were, however, unaltered as a result of the NMES.

Even though several muscle parameters were altered following this type of NMES, electrophysiology and volume fraction of fast- and slow-twitch fibers in muscles treated were unchanged. This finding indicates that a 2500-pps carrier wave interrupted by 50 bursts per second NMES does not change the contractile properties in muscle and may be used in the clinic to strengthen healthy, normal muscle without changing the fiber types of those muscles.

Nerve injuries (i.e., nerve transection, crush, and tourniquet application) produce adverse alterations of varying degrees in muscle function, electrophysiologic properties, and structure. There is conflicting information concerning the effects of NMES on retarding muscle denervation following nerve insult; however, there are few studies that evaluate the effects of short-term NMES on ultrastructure of denervated and partially denervated skeletal muscle. Recent studies have shown that 2500-pps carrier waves interrupted by 50 bursts per second NMES does not rectify muscle alterations resulting from denervation. Likewise, clinical studies indicate that the nerve supply to the muscle must be intact for this type of NMES to be effective. For these reasons this type of electrical current and wave should not be used clinically to treat partially or completely denervated muscles. Research is warranted to study the effects on denervated skeletal muscle of additional types of electrical generators that produce other waveforms and currents.

REFERENCES

1. Babkin, D and Timtsenko, N: Notes from Dr. Kots' (USSR) lectures and laboratory periods. Canadian-Soviet Exchange Symposium on Electro-stimulation of Skeletal Muscles. Concordia University, Montreal, Quebec, Canada, December 6–15, 1977.
2. Cummings, G: Physiological basis of electrical stimulation in skeletal muscle. Certified Athletic Trainers Association Journal 3:7–12, 1980.
3. Johnson, DH, Thurston, P, and Ashcroft, PJ: The Russian technique of faradism in the treatment of chondromalacia patella. Physiotherapy Canada 29:266–268, 1977.
4. Nelson, RM and Currier, DP: Clinical Electrotherapy. Appleton & Lange, Norwalk, CT, 1987.
5. Snyder-Mackler, L and Robinson, AJ: Clinical Electrophysiology: Electrotherapy and Electrophysiologic Testing. Williams & Wilkins, Baltimore, 1989.
6. Kelly, DE, Wood, RL, and Enders, AC: Bailey's Textbook of Microscopic Anatomy, ed 18. Williams & Wilkins, Baltimore, 1984.
7. Singer, SJ and Nicholson, GL: The fluid mosaic model of the structure of cell membranes. Science 175:720–731, 1972.
8. McArdle, WD, Katch, FI, and Katch, VL: Exercise Physiology: Energy, Nutrition, and Human Performance. Lea & Febiger, Philadelphia, 1985.
9. Johnson, MA, Polgar, J, Weightman, D, et al: Data on the distribution of fiber types in thirty-six human muscles. J Neurol Sci 18:111–129, 1973.
10. Grimby, G: Muscle morphology and function in 67–81 year old men and women (abstr). Med Sci Sports Exerc 72–95, 1980.
11. Gollnick, PD, Parsons, D, Riedy, M, et al: Fiber number and size in overloaded chicken anterior latissimus dorsi mucle. J Appl Physiol 54:1292–1297, 1983.
12. Redanna, P, Moorthy, CV, and Govidappa, S: Pattern of skeletal muscle chemical composition during in vivo electrical stimulation. Indian J Physiol Pharmacol 25:33–40, 1981.
13. Eriksson, E, Haggmark, T, Kiessling, KH, et al: Effect of electrical stimulation on human skeletal muscle. Int J Sports Med 2:18–22, 1981.
14. Ogilvie, RE and Rhein, GA: Exercise and electrical current related microscopic changes in skeletal muscle. Proceedings of The Annual Conference of the American Association of Anatomists, Atlanta, GA, April 3–7, 1983.
15. Taylor, AW, Kots, YM, and Lavoie, M: The effects of faradic stimulation on skeletal muscle fiber area. Can J Sport Sci 3:185, 1978.
16. Horacek, MJ, Earle, AM, and Metcalf, WK: Morphologic and physiologic consequences of transcutaneous medium frequency current on rabbit skeletal muscle and peripheral nerve tissue. Anat Rec 218:64A, 1987.
17. Greathouse, DG, Nitz, AJ, Matulionis, DH, et al: Effects of short-term electrical stimulation on the ultrastructure of rat skeletal muscles. Phys Ther 66:946–953, 1986.
18. Currier, DP and Mann, R: Muscular strength development by electrical stimulation in healthy individuals. Phys Ther 63:915–921, 1983.
19. Houston, ME, Farrance, BW, and Wight, RI: Metabolic effects of two frequencies of short term surface electrical stimulation on human muscle. Can J Physiol Pharmacol 60:727–731, 1982.
20. Greathouse, DG: Effects of short-term, medium frequency electrical stimulation on normal, partially denervated, and denervated rat skeletal muscle. University of Kentucky, Lexington, KY, 1985. Dissertation.
21. Greathouse, DG, Matulionis, DH, Currier, DP, et al: Response of normal rat skeletal muscle to electrical stimulation. Anat Rec 214:44A, 1986.
22. Godfrey, CM, Jawawardena, H, Quance, TA, et al: Comparison of electrostimulation and isometric exercise in strengthening the quadriceps muscle. Physiotherapy Canada 31:265–267, 1979.
23. Halbach, JW and Straus, D: Comparison of electromyostimulation to isokinetic training in increasing power of knee extensor mechanism. Journal of Orthopedics and Sports Physical Therapy 2:20–24, 1980.
24. Eriksson, E: Sports injuries of the knee ligament: Their diagnosis, treatment, rehabilitation, and prevention. Med Sci Sports Exerc 8:133–144, 1976.
25. Massey, BH, Nelson, RC, Sharkey, BC, et al: Effects of high frequency electrical stimulation on the size and strength of skeletal muscle. J Sports Med Phys Fitness 5:136–144, 1965.
26. Kots, YM and Chulion, VA: The training of muscular power by method of electrical stimulation. State Central Institute of Physical Culture. Moscow, USSR, 1975.
27. Kots, YM: Methods of investigation of muscular aparatus. State Central Institute of Physical Culture. Moscow, USSR, 1976.
28. Owens, J and Malone, T: Treatment parameters of high frequency electrical stimulation as established on the electrostim 180. Journal of Orthopedics and Sports Physical Therapy 4:162–168, 1983.
29. Williams JGP and Street, M: Sequential faradism in quadriceps rehabilitation. Physiotherapy 62:252–254, 1976.

30. Laughman, RK, Youdas, JW, Garrett, TF, et al: Strength changes in normal quadriceps femoris muscle as a result of electrical stimulation. Phys Ther 63:494, 1983.
31. Eriksson, E and Haggmark, T: Comparison of isometric muscle training and electrical stimulation supplementing isometric muscle training in the recovery after major knee ligament surgery. Am J Sports Med 7:169–171, 1979.
32. Curwin, S, Standish, WD, and Valliant, G: Clinical applications and biochemical effects of high frequency electrical stimulation. Canadian Athletic Therapy Association Journal 7:15–16, 1980.
33. Stanish, WD, Valiant, GA, Bonen, A, et al: The effects of immobilization and of electrical stimulation on muscle glycogen and myofibrillar ATP-ase. Canadian Journal of Applied Sport Science 7:266–271, 1982.
34. Salmons, S: Functional adaptation in skeletal muscle. Trends Neurosci 3:134–137, 1980.
35. Salmons, S, Gale, DR, and Streter, FA: Ultrastructural aspects of the transformatin of muscle fiber type by long-term stimulation: Changes in Z-disc and mitochondria. J Anat 127:17–31, 1978.
36. Eisenberg, BR and Salmons, S: Stereological analysis of sequential ultrastructural changes in the adaptive response of fast skeletal muscle to chronic stimulation. Muscle Nerve 3:277, 1980.
37. Streter, FA, Pinter, K, Jolesz, F, et al: Fast to slow transformation of fast muscles in response to long term phasic stimulation. Exp Neurol 75:95–102, 1982.
38. Streter, FA, Romanul, FCA, Salmons, S, et al: The effect of a changed pattern of activity on some biochemical characteristics of muscle. Excerpta Medica 2:338–343, 1974.
39. Davis, HL: Is electrostimulation beneficial to denervated muscles? A review of results from basic research. Physiotherapy Canada 35:306–312, 1983.
40. Niederle, B and Mayr, R: Course of denervation atrophy in type I and type II fibres of rat extensor digitorum longus muscle. Anat Embrol 153:9–21, 1981.
41. Pelligrino, C and Franzini, C: An electron microscopic study of denervation atrophy in red and white skeletal muscle fibers. J Cell Biol 14:327–349, 1963.
42. Stonnington, HH and Engel, AG: Normal and denervated muscle: A morphometric study of fine structure. Neurology 23:714–724, 1973.
43. Pitchey, EL and Smith, PB: Denervation and developmental alteration of glycogen synthase and glycogen phosphorylase in mammalian skeletal muscle. Exp Neurol 65:118–130, 1979.
44. Stankiewicz-Niczyporowicz, J and Gorski, J: Effect of tenotomy and denervation on the early post-exercise glycogen recovery in skeletal muscles of the rat. Acta Physiol Pol 32:450–454, 1981.
45. Dubois, DC and Max, SR: Effect of denervation and reinnervation on oxidation of [6-14 C] glucose by rat skeletal muscle homogenates. J Neurochem 40:727–733, 1983.
46. Park, HW and Watkins, AL: Facial paralysis. Analysis of 500 cases. Arch Phys Med Rehabil 30:749, 1949.
47. Mosforth, J and Taverner, D: Physiotherapy for Bell's palsy. BMJ 2:675, 1958.
48. Ghiora, A and Winter, ST: The conservative treatment of Bell's palsy. Am J Phys Med Rehabil 41:213, 1962.
49. Eng, GD: Brachial plexus palsy in newborn infants. Pediatrics, 48:18, 1971.
50. Merletti, R, Andina, A, Galante, M, et al: Clinical experience of electronic peroneal stimulators in 50 hemiparetic patients. Scand J Rehabil Med 11:111, 1979.
51. Merletti, R and Pinelli, P: A critical appraisal of neuromuscular stimulation and electrotherapy in neurorehabilitation. Eur Neurol 19:30, 1980.
52. Sunderland, S: Factors influencing onset, development and severity of atrophy in striated muscle due to denervation. In Sunderland, S (ed): Nerves and Nerve Injuries, ed 2. Churchill Livingstone, New York, 1978, pp 298–311.
53. Stillwell, GK: Therapeutic Electricity and Ultraviolet Radiation. Williams & Wilkins, Baltimore, 1983, pp 157–158.
54. Fischer, E: Effect of faradic and galvanic stimulation upon on the course of atrophy in denervated skeletal muscles. Am J Physiol 127:605, 1939.
55. Wermacher, WH, Thomson, JD, and Hines, HM: Effects of electrical stimulation on denervated skeletal muscle. Arch Phys Med Rehabil 26:261–266, 1945.
56. Kosman, AJ, Osborn, SL, and Ivy, AC: Importance of current form and frequency in electrical stimulation of muscles. Arch Phys Med Rehabil 29:559–562, 1948.
57. Melichna, J and Gutmann, E: Stimulation and immobilization effects on contractile and histochemical properties of denervated muscle. Pflugers Arch 352:165–178, 1974.
58. Herbison, GJ, Teng, C, Reyes, T, et al: Effect of electrical stimulation on denervated muscle of rat. Arch Phys Med Rehabil 52:526–522, 1971.
59. Jaweed, MM, Alam, I, Herbison, GJ, et al: Prostaglandins in denervated skeletal muscle of rat: Effect of direct electrical stimulation. Neuroscience 6:2787–2792, 1981.
60. Jaweed, MM and Herbison, GJ: Direct electrical stimulation of rat soleus during denervation-reinnervation. Exp Neurol 75:589–599, 1982.
61. Girlanda, P, Dattola, R, Vita, G, et al: Effect of electrotherapy on denervated muscles in rabbits: An electrophysiological and morphological study. Exp Neurol 77:483–491, 1982.

62. Cole, BG and Gardiner, PF: Does electrical stimulation of denervated muscle, continued after rein-
    nervation, influence recovery of contractile function? Exp Neurol 85:52–62, 1984.
63. Pachter, BR, Eberstein, A, and Goodgold, J: Electrical stimulation effect on denervated skeletal myofi-
    bers in rats: A light and electron microscopic study. Arch Phys Med Rehabil 63:427–430, 1982.
64. Schimrigk, K, McLaughlin, J, and Cruninger, W: The effect of electrical stimulation on the experi-
    mentally denervated rat muscle. Scand J Rehabil Med 9:55–60, 1977.
65. Stolov, WC, Riddell, WW, and Shrier, KP: Metabolism of immobilized innervated and denervated rat
    gastrocnemius muscle. Arch Phys Med Rehabil 52:589–590, 1971.
66. Greathouse, DG, Currier, DP, Nitz, AJ, et al: Effects of moderate frequency electrical stimulation in
    partially denervated and denervated rat skeletal muscle. Anat Rec 218:52A, 1987.
67. Sellin, LC, Libelius, R, Lundquist, I, et al: Membrane and biochemical alterations after denervation
    and during reinnervation of mouse skeletal muscle. Acta Physiol Scand 110:181–186, 1980.
68. Makitie, J and Teravainen, H: Ultrastructure of striated muscle of the rat after temporary ischemia.
    Acta Neuropathol (Berl) 37:237–245, 1977.
69. Kirucki, T: Electron microscopic observations of experimental ischemia of muscle. Orthop Surg (Tokyo),
    20:1385, 1969.
70. Scully, RE, Shannon, TM, and Dickerson, GR: Factors involved in recovery from experimental skeletal
    muscle ischemia produced in dogs. Am J Pathol 39:721, 1961.
71. Dahlback, LO and Rais, O: Morphologic changes in striated muscle following ischemia: Immediate
    post-ischemic phase. Acta Chir Scand 131:430, 1966.
72. Tountas, CP and Bergman, RA: Tournament ischemia: Ultrastructural and histochemical observations
    of ischemic human muscle and of monkey muscle and nerve. J Hand Surg 2:31–37, 1977.
73. Nitz, AJ and Matulionis, DH: Ultrastructural changes in rat peripheral nerve following pneumatic
    tourniquet compression. J Neurosurg 57:660–666, 1982.
74. Nitz, AJ and Matulionis, DH: Assessment of nerve injury resulting from tourniquet application. Anat
    Rec 208:473–474, 1984.

CHAPTER 6

Peripheral Vascular Effects of Electrical Stimulation

Brian V. Reed, Ph.D., P.T.

Electrical stimulation (ES) has been used for a number of years to treat various vascular disorders. Although it would appear from some studies that ES can be tremendously beneficial for conditions such as vasospastic disorders, soft tissue wounds, and edema and for prevention of deep vein thrombosis, there is also evidence in the literature to refute such conclusions. Indeed there is a large, bewildering volume of literature on the vascular effects of ES. The findings and the proposed explanations have been diverse, and to date there is no clear consensus about ES effects for many of the vascular syndromes in which it has been used. Consequently there is no "standard" electrotherapy treatment for most of the syndromes. This chapter will attempt to put the literature into perspective, to crystallize our present understanding about ES as a treatment for vascular disorders, to present rationales for treatment, and to suggest directions for future research.

To achieve these goals, a theoretical foundation is essential as a basis for considering the vascular effects of ES. Hence, key physiologic mechanisms known to regulate the peripheral vascular system will first be reviewed, and then the variables which can affect treatment outcome will be considered.

FUNDAMENTALS

Physiologic Regulation of the Peripheral Vascular System: A Brief Review

The peripheral vascular system consists of arterial vessels, venous vessels, and the exchange vessels (capillaries, postcapillary venules) that connect the arterial and venous vessels. Oxygen-rich blood flows from the heart through the arterial vessels to the exchange vessels, where oxygen and nutrients are exchanged for carbon dioxide and waste products. The blood then flows through the veins back to the right side of the heart. The driving force for the circulation is the blood pressure gradient from the left side to the right side of the heart.

The arteries and veins are invested with vascular smooth muscle, and this tissue mediates the control of peripheral blood flow. Vascular smooth muscle contraction causes vessel constriction, which, in turn, affects the local pressure gradient for blood flow. Because of their geometry and high proportion of vascular smooth muscle, the small arteries and the arterioles create most of the resistance to peripheral blood flow; consequently these vessels are known as the resistance vessels. The degree of constriction of the resistance vessels determines the perfusion pressure (and therefore the amount of blood flow) at each of the various vascular beds. By contrast, the primary effect of venous vessel constriction is enhanced return of blood to the right side of the heart. Remember that rhythmic contraction of skeletal muscles creates a pumping effect on the veins, which also assists return of venous blood to the right heart chambers. The degree of vascular smooth muscle contraction at any given time is the net result of influences from two major control systems: extrinsic and intrinsic.

The Extrinsic Control System

The extrinsic control system is made up of neural and humoral components. The *neural component* is the sympathetic nervous system. Central to the sympathetic nervous system is a vasomotor area in the medulla and lower pons that determines the amount of tonic activity in the sympathetic nerves innervating the arteries, arterioles, and veins (most blood vessels have no parasympathetic innervation). The capillaries and venules are not contractile and receive no innervation. The sympathetic nervous system is primarily an adrenergic system, the postganglionic neurotransmitter being norepinephrine. Whereas sympathetic stimulation causes vascular smooth muscle constriction in most blood vessels, it is important to realize that *some* sympathetic nerves in vascular smooth muscle release acetylcholine and thereby induce vasodilation. The function of these sympathetic cholinergic fibers is presumed to be associated with control of the body's response to exercise. It has also been proposed that some other type of sympathetic vasodilator fibers supplies the vessels of the skin, but this hypothesis is not universally accepted. The neural input and output of the vasomotor center is diagrammed in Figure 6–1.

The *humoral component* of the extrinsic control system consists of a variety of circulating substances such as epinephrine, vasopressin, serotonin, and angiotension. In general the response to these hormones is vasoconstriction, although vasoactive intestinal polypeptide (VIP) is a vasodilator and is suspected of playing a role in the vascular response to some forms of electrical stimulation. Plasma concentrations of the vasoactive hormones are determined by complex mechanisms (which are beyond the scope of this review).

Catecholamines are amine compounds (norepinephrine and epinephrine) derived from the adrenal medulla that affect neural transmission, vascular tone, and many metabolic activities. Catecholamines (neural or humoral) affect vascular smooth muscle through receptor operated mechanisms. There are two types of receptors, alpha and beta. Norepinephrine excites mainly alpha receptors that vasoconstrict blood

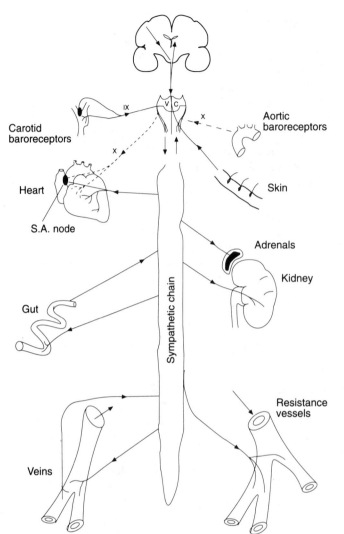

FIGURE 6–1. Neural input and output of the vasomotor center (VC). IX, glossopharyngeal nerve; X, vagus nerve. Note that sympathetic nerves to skeletal muscle resistance vessels may be either vasoconstrictor or vasodilator fibers. (Reproduced by permission from Berne, Robert M., and Levy, Matthew N.: Cardiovascular Physiology, ed. 5, St. Louis, 1986, The C.V. Mosby Co.)

vessels but also excites beta receptors to a small extent. The beta receptors mediate vasodilation of blood vessels.

The extrinsic controls can be thought of as being reflex in nature. Through baroreceptors they help to buffer sudden changes in blood pressure. In addition a generalized sympathetic response to exercise or sudden stress causes vasodilation in some vascular beds (heart, exercising skeletal muscle), vasoconstriction in others (kidneys, splanchnic organs), resulting in a redistribution of the cardiac output.

Finally, it is important to remember that sympathetic activity determines the degree of tonus in the veins. Veins are sometimes called capacitance vessels, because when tonus is low they dilate and store blood. This storage of blood, along with other factors such as varicosities or decreased skeletal muscle activity, can contribute to venous stasis.

The Intrinsic Control System

The intrinsic control system is less a system than a number of local factors that influence peripheral blood flow. Prominent among these are metabolic factors, prostaglandins, and the myogenic properties of the vascular smooth muscle concerned.

The conditions that result from cellular metabolism—decreased PO_2; increased PCO_2, adenosine, and hydrogen ions (H^+)—have a potent vasodilatory effect. These metabolic factors help the vascular bed to match blood supply to metabolic demand. Skeletal muscle blood flow is especially influenced by metabolic control.

Myogenicity is the tendency for resistance vessels to constrict when stretch on the vascular smooth muscle is increased (increased perfusion pressure) and to dilate when stretched less (decreased perfusion pressure). Other factors aside, this property helps local tissues to maintain a relatively constant blood flow despite changes in perfusion pressure.

Prostaglandins are a specialized group of hormonelike, fatty acid compounds that serve as chemical messengers in nearly all tissues. Prostaglandins are capable of influencing a number of physiologic functions including vasodilation and constriction. Although prostaglandins are potent vasoactive substances, their effect on local blood flow is difficult to predict because of the number of prostaglandins and the fact that some cause vasodilation whereas others cause vasoconstriction.

The local control factors are better suited for maintaining local blood flow over time than for providing a rapid reflex response to stress. In many cases, their effect is actually to counteract the extrinsic influences. As with extrinsic control, the relative potency of the intrinsic factors varies among the various vascular beds.

Integrated Function of Intrinsic and Extrinsic Controls

The essence of peripheral vascular control (arterial) is that it is the result of the degree of balance between the central (extrinsic) and local (intrinsic) factors. The response of the resistance vessels is the algebraic sum of the opposing inputs.[1] For example, during prolonged exercise, decreased blood flow to the kidneys caused by sympathetically induced vasoconstriction can be counteracted by a buildup of metabolites and other local factors. The major factors affecting arteriolar radius are summarized in Figure 6–2.

Microvascular Exchange

Exchange of nutrients and waste products takes place between the plasma and the interstitial fluid at the level of the capillaries and postcapillary venules; these vessels are known, therefore, as the exchange vessels. Although it is primarily diffusion that permits this exchange, filtration and reabsorption of fluid also take place, and this plays an important role in fluid balance.

The nature of this fluid balance is determined primarily by *Starling forces*, and by the action of lymphatic vessels. Four forces are described in the Starling hypothesis: (1) capillary hydrostatic pressure (P_c), (2) interstitial oncotic pressure (Π_i), (3) interstitial hydrostatic pressure (P_i), and (4) colloid oncotic pressure (Π_c). The first two

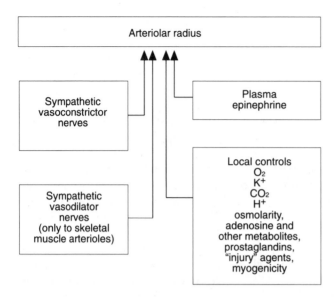

FIGURE 6–2. Major factors affecting arteriolar radius. (From Vander, AJ and Luciano, DS: Human Physiology: The Mechanics of Body Function. New York, McGraw Hill, Copyright 1980. Reproduced with permission of McGraw Hill, Inc.)

forces tend to drive fluid out of the exchange vessels (filtration); the latter two forces tend to drive fluid into the exchange vessels (reabsorption). An equilibrium of fluid exchange will be reached according to the algebraic sum of these forces. If the outward forces become greater than the inward forces, there will be net filtration. If the inward forces become greater than the outward forces, there will be net reabsorption. The concept of this balance of forces is schematized in Figure 6–3.

Lymphatic vessels also play an important role in determining compartment fluid volume. The lymphatics are capable of returning modest amounts of fluid and leaked plasma proteins to the vascular system. The lymphatic vessels are lined by endothelial cells with very loose, overlapping junctions. This structure allows entry of fluid and proteins but prevents their escape back into the interstitium. The lymphatic vessels return their contents to the vascular system near the superior vena cava. The lymphatic

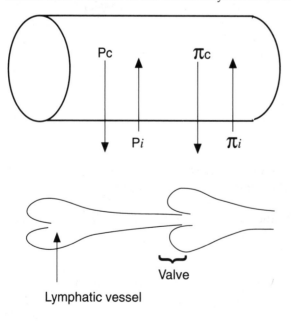

FIGURE 6–3. The balance of Starling forces. Direction of arrows indicate direction of force; arrow size indicates relative contribution of each force under normal circumstances. P_c = capillary hydrostatic pressure; P_i = interstitial hydrostatic pressure; π_c = capillary oncotic pressure; π_i = interstitial oncotic pressure.

fluid is moved there by rhythmic contraction of the lymphatic vessels and by external compression from skeletal muscle contraction. Reflux of the fluid is prevented by valves in the lymphatic vessels.

Peripheral edema, one of the most common fluid balance problems, is often caused by shifts in oncotic pressure. This edema may be due to changes in the exchange vessels or malfunction of the lymphatic vessels, or both. For example, acute injury causes inflammation, and this, in turn, causes increased permeability of the micro-vessels. Plasma proteins and other macromolecules leak out, increasing interstitial oncotic pressure and decreasing colloid oncotic pressure. Because the proteins are osmotically active (hydrophilic), fluid follows them into the interstitium. If the volume of fluid and macromolecules overwhelms the ability of the lympathics to carry them away, edema results. Even if the balance of Starling forces is unchanged, pathology or surgical resection of the lymphatics alone is enough to cause edema, as evidenced following a radical mastectomy.

Variables Affecting the Vascular Response to Electrical Stimulation

Given the complexity of peripheral vascular control, it is not surprising that ES can elicit a myriad of *vascular responses*. The variables that can affect the vascular response can be divided into at least two major categories, (1) the stimulation site, and (2) the stimulus characteristics. Consideration of these variables is important for establishing a perspective on the existing literature.

STIMULATION SITE

Assuming an adequate electrical stimulus, extrinsic or intrinsic control factors, or both, may be brought into play depending on where the current is applied. For example, electrical stimulation may affect autonomic nerves (extrinsic control). Theoretically, if ES decreased sympathetic nerve activity to an area, blood flow would be increased. At present there is no convincing evidence that sympathetic activity can be blocked by ES. Another potential mechanism for increasing blood flow is stimulation of sympathetic cholinergic fibers in vascular smooth muscle. Increased activity in these special fibers would presumably result in vasodilation.

Electrical stimulation is commonly used to elicit contraction in skeletal muscle and may also thereby enhance intrinsic regulation of local blood flow. Contraction of muscle is triggered either by stimulation of the motor nerve or by direct stimulation of denervated muscle. So long as the stimulus does not cause a prolonged tetanic contraction, which would mechanically impede blood flow, it is logical that an increase in blood flow should occur in response to accumulating metabolites, by-products of elevated metabolism induced by ES. If rhythmic contraction is produced, ES would also be expected to assist venous and lymphatic flow.

Another theoretical mechanism by which ES may increase blood flow is an *axon reflex*. In an axon reflex, stimulation of cutaneous afferent (somatic) nerve fibers causes impulses which travel centrally, but also antidromically, down branches of the afferent nerve. The antidromic stimulation causes vasodilation of the arterioles adjacent to the site of stimulation. The axon reflex has been described primarily in skin, although skeletal muscle may also be affected. The pathway of the axon reflex is diagrammed in Figure 6–4.

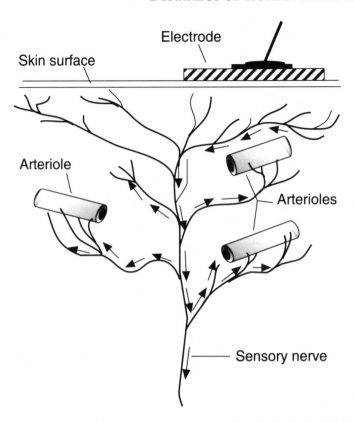

FIGURE 6–4. The axon reflex in response to cutaneous electrical stimulation. Arrows indicate the pathways of impulses in a sensory nerve from the site of stimulation to adjacent arterioles to produce local vasodilation (flare). (Reproduced by permission from Berne, Robert M., and Levy, Matthew N.: Cardiovascular Physiology, ed. 5, St. Louis, 1986, The C.V. Mosby Co.)

Stimulation of key points on the body may also cause reflex vasodilation in distant areas of the body. Both *percutaneous* and *transcutaneous* (acupuncturelike) ES are now accepted treatment for chronic pain syndromes. Although the observations are difficult to explain in terms of known physiologic mechanisms, the literature suggests that increased arterial blood flow may accompany, or even be partially responsible for, the pain relief.[2,3]

Finally, it is conceivable that ES might affect vascular smooth muscle directly. Stimulation of isolated resistance vessels in vitro is known to cause constriction, and one component of that constriction is attributable to direct activation of the vascular smooth muscle.[4,5] Electrical stimulation of noncontractile soft tissues could possibly result in decreased blood flow by such a mechanism.

Not all the determinants of blood flow associated with ES at specific sites are clear at this time. Increased blood flow associated with electrical stimulation of skeletal muscle probably is, at least in part, the result of metabolic demands for oxygen and possibly of vasodilation by sympathetic cholinergic fibers. Whereas some research has demonstrated increased blood flow associated with ES in tissues other than skeletal muscle, it is presently unknown whether the mechanism(s) involved was sympathetic blockage, an axon reflex, or some other central or spinal level reflex.

STIMULUS CHARACTERISTICS

The other major variable that probably affects the peripheral vascular response to ES is the electrical stimulus itself. *Electrical stimuli* can be characterized by their pulse duration, pulse charge, peak current, total current, on/off times, and polarity. Further, electrical stimuli can be *pulsed* or *cycled* over a wide range of frequencies. A great variety of waveforms were used in past studies, and the findings were inconsistent. Recent research seems to suggest that some of these characteristics are critical determinants of the vascular response and others are not.

Types of Vascular Problems Treated with Electrical Stimulation

The vascular problems that can be treated with ES are arterial disorders, venous disorders, and microcirculatory disorders (i.e., edema).

ARTERIAL DISORDERS

Arterial disorders include certain chronic, acute, arterial occlusive diseases. The chronic occlusive diseases are degenerative in nature and include arteriosclerosis obliterans and thromboangiitis obliterans (Buerger's disease). The acute arterial occlusive diseases are vasospastic in nature and include Raynaud's disease, Raynaud's syndrome, and causalgia. Decreased peripheral pulses, pallor, coldness, loss of hair, intermittent claudication, ischemic ulcers, and dysesthesia are common signs and symptoms of chronic arterial occlusion. The signs and symptoms associated with vasospastic disorders are pain, pallor, and, rarely, ischemic lesions. In both the acute and chronic disorders, rubor may be seen as a result of inflammation secondary to the ischemia.

There is no apparent rationale for using ES to treat arterial inflammatory disease (arteritis) or degenerative diseases such as aneurysm, and consequently there are no reports on such uses of ES.

VENOUS DISORDERS

Venous problems of interest are chronic venous insufficiency, thrombophlebitis, and orthostatic hypotension. With both venous insufficiency and thrombophlebitis, there is pooling of venous blood in the lower extremities. This pooling is associated with blue-brown discoloration of the skin, pitting edema, perceived heaviness and achiness, and "venous stasis ulcers." *Orthostatic hypotension* is a special (acute) type of venous insufficiency, which can be controlled with ES. Other venous disorders, such as varicose veins, have not been treated with ES.

LOCALIZED EDEMA

Localized peripheral edema is a common clinical problem, and one which may benefit from electrotherapy. Examples are lymphedema secondary to a radical mastectomy or edema associated with acute injury. Generalized edema resulting from systemic diseases such as congestive heart failure or nephrotic syndrome has not been successfully treated with ES.

REVIEW OF RELEVANT LITERATURE

The Effects of Electrical Stimulation on Arterial Blood Flow

SKELETAL MUSCLE

Most but not all investigators who have stimulated muscle at its motor point or more proximally on the motor nerve have reported increased blood flow to the muscle.[6-14]

Studies on animal models provide evidence of the strong influence of local controlling factors in determining blood flow with ES of skeletal muscle. Kjellmer[15] found that even the vasoconstrictor effect of direct sympathetic chain stimulation could not override the increased blood flow associated with muscle contraction induced by ES in cats. This inability to override effects of muscle contraction indicates that the resistance vessels were more sensitive to local control than to sympathetic control (the opposite relation was found for venous vessels). Whereas sustained contraction is thought to impede blood flow by compressing blood vessels[9,16] or otherwise altering their geometry,[17] several investigators have demonstrated increased blood flow even with isometric contractions.[9-11,18] Crayton and associates[10] found that neither alpha receptor blockade nor section of the lumbar spinal nerve dorsal roots altered this response in the exercised muscle, indicating that the vascular response was not reflexly controlled, but locally controlled. Thus it seems certain that *the skeletal muscle vascular response to ES is largely the result of metabolic and myogenic factors in the stimulated tissue.*

Kniffki and colleagues[19] and Kalia and associates[20] argued that extrinsic factors may also play a role in determining blood flow with ES of skeletal muscle. Kniffki's group reviewed research regarding recorded activity in group III (A delta) and IV (C) fibers in response to ES induced muscle contraction and to other factors (chemical, thermal stimuli) associated with muscle contraction. Kalia and associates[20] provided anatomic as well as physiologic evidence that the group III fibers and fibers from muscles are responsible for the cardiopulmonary response to exercise. Both groups of investigators hypothesized that these muscle afferents were ergoreceptors, intimately involved with the circulatory changes that occur with muscle contraction.[19,20]

These group III and IV fibers, then, may provide afferent input for the reflex sympathetic response to exercise, whether the exercise is physiologic or induced by ES. This proposed *ergoreceptor mechanism* should be seen as distinct from the *axon reflex*, a phenomenon which is presumably mediated at local level.

There is additional evidence that ES can increase arterial blood flow in skeletal muscle via extrinsic control mechanisms. In 1901, Bayliss[21] reported that stimulation of lumbosacral spinal nerve dorsal roots caused increased tissue volume in the skinned hindlimb of the dog, which he interpreted as vasodilation in skeletal muscle. Bayliss proposed that some of the dorsal root sensory afferent fibers in the lumbosacral area also functioned as vasodilator fibers. He hypothesized that the mechanism involved was *antidromic excitation of the afferent fibers*, an explanation that persists to this day. Bayliss thought that centrally induced antidromic excitation of these "vasodilator" fibers might be a physiologic mechanism for controlling peripheral blood flow, but such a function has never been proved. Later animal research confirmed the findings of Bayliss, although some investigators concluded that dorsal root stimulation caused increased blood flow only in skin, not in skeletal muscle,[22] whereas others concluded that skeletal muscle was affected.[23] Recently both *epidural stimulation* and *transcutaneous stimulation* of spinal nerve dorsal roots in patients have been associated with increased limb volumes as measured by plethysmography;[24–26] increased resting blood flow as measured by ^{133}Xe washout;[2] and improved muscular function in relation to blood flow: increased claudication distance and increased exercise tolerance.[2] Cook and associates[24] asserted that dorsal root stimulation was, in fact, more effective than sympathectomy in relieving the clinical symptoms of ischemia.

It is unclear whether the increased blood flow associated with dorsal root stimulation is simply "upstream" activation of an axon reflex, or if it is some other mechanism. *Antidromic stimulation* should logically activate the axon collaterals responsible for the axon reflex equally as well as when the stimulus is through the peripheral receptors.[22] Thus the axon reflex would seem to be a good explanation; however, it has been argued that the axon reflex is functional only in skin, not in skeletal muscle.[22] An alternative explanation can be found in the fact that the fibers responsible for the changes in blood flow are group IV (C) fibers.[22,24,27] Presuming spinal stimulation causes orthodromic as well as antidromic excitation in the C fibers, the ergoreceptor function of muscle afferents proposed by Kniffki and co-workers may play a role.[19] Dorsal root stimulation would involve the central sympathetic response associated with exercise in this case. Another explanation is that stimulation of the small afferents somehow causes production of prostaglandins in skeletal muscle, and that the prostaglandins induce vasodilation. Hilton and Marshall[23] proposed this mechanism based on their finding that vasodilation resulting from dorsal root stimulation could be greatly reduced by the prostaglandin synthetase inhibitors indomethacin or acetylsalicylic acid. A final mechanism that has been postulated for the increased muscle blood flow associated with dorsal root stimulation is that vasoconstriction secondary to pain may be reduced as a result of ES-induced pain relief.[2,3]

In neuromuscular electrical stimulation, both the pulse frequency and the pulse waveform characteristics may be critical determinants of the arterial blood flow response.

In general, studies in animals or humans that have used a spectrum of pulse rates have found that increased blood flow can be demonstrated with frequencies from 1 up to about 50 pps.[7–9,14,28] Higher frequencies do not seem to be as effective.[28] One of these studies used a carrier frequency of 2500 Hz alternating current (AC) modulated at 50 bursts per second. It seems that in this case, then, the critical determinant of blood flow response was the burst frequency rather than the faster carrier frequency.

Without doubt, this optimal frequency range is at least partially due to the mechanical constraints imposed by muscle contraction. Tetanic muscle contraction impedes arterial blood flow by compression or twisting of the blood vessels, or both.[16,17] Thus, increased rates of stimulation frequencies will tend to produce increased metabolites and increase blood flow, but, conversely, the higher the frequency of stimulation, the less time there is for blood flow during contractions. The findings produced by bursts of AC can be explained in this context because it is the bursts of current that are associated with action potentials and thereby muscle contraction.[7] Studies of the effects of interference current (IFC) on muscle blood flow have not been reported, but one would expect the beats of IFC to produce effects similar to bursts of 2500-Hz AC, with the *beat frequency* being the critical determinant. Whether the increased blood flows observed with 1- to 50-pps frequencies reported in the previously cited studies were also a result of extrinsic effects (such as direct or indirect stimulation of ergoreceptors) is unknown.

The electrical *pulse waveform* may be another critical determinant of vascular response. For example, there have been at least three published reports that blood flow did not increase in humans in response to "high voltage" pulsed current (HVPC) stimulation.[29–31] The HVPC waveform is a monophasic twin peaked waveform of very short duration (in the range of 20 to 60 microseconds), low pulse charge, and low total current (<2.0 mA), although peak current may be high. Even though different modes of stimulation were used in the studies (Walker and associates[31] induced motor responses, whereas Hecker and co-workers[30] and Alon[29] used sensory stimulation to determine stimulus amplitude), a question that arises is whether the unique HVPC waveform was responsible for the negative results.[14,28]

The lack of an effect with HVPC in the work of Walker and associates[31] is difficult to explain in terms of local control. Since HVPC was stimulation of sufficient amplitude to elicit muscle contraction, metabolic factors should have played a role. One is forced to speculate that HVPC might have activated an extrinsic mechanism(s) such as sympathetic vasoconstriction, which counteracted the vasodilatory effects of metabolites.

In any case, HVPC has been shown to increase arterial blood flow in the rat hindlimb. Blood flow was found to increase in proportion to voltage, and a pulse frequency of 20 pps was found to be optimal.[6] These findings are consistent with those of the aforementioned basic studies that used more conventional waveforms. Conceivably, species differences are responsible for the different findings in the human and the animal studies; perhaps low pulse charge may not recruit sufficient numbers of motor units in humans to result in inci eased blood flow.

The relative importance of frequency versus waveform in determining muscle blood flow was addressed recently by Tracy and co-workers.[14] Experiments on human subjects were performed in which contractions of the quadriceps femoris muscle were induced with two different waveforms (sinusoidal and symmetrical rectangular) at several frequencies. Blood flow increased with frequencies of 10, 20, and 50 pps regardless of which waveform was used. These results indicate that in this case blood flow was dependent on frequency but not waveform.[14] Additional research is needed to clarify the role of waveform in determining skeletal muscle blood flow.

In summary, although the physiologic mechanisms are not totally clear, the weight of the literature does indicate that *some ES waveforms can increase arterial blood flow to skeletal muscle when applied at frequencies between 1 and 50 Hz, pulses, bursts, or beats per second and at an amplitude strong enough to elicit contraction.* The increased blood flow is mediated through local and possibly reflex controlling factors.

There are certain circumstances in which ES does not appear to increase skeletal-muscle blood flow. Flow does not increase greatly when the frequency is less than 1 per second or much greater than 50 per second. Furthermore, the ability of ES to increase skeletal-muscle blood flow when current amplitude is subthreshold for contraction has not been demonstrated. Finally, at least one waveform, HVPC, is not optimal for increasing skeletal-muscle blood flow. The ability of this waveform to increase flow in humans is dubious.

To be of therapeutic value (in terms of increasing blood flow), ES must induce greater blood flow than required for metabolism alone. One must hope, therefore, that reflex control mechanisms such as the axon reflex or activation of ergoreceptor responses do play a significant role in the observed increases in skeletal muscle blood flow. Whether or not ES can cause "extra" blood flow with resulting clinical benefits is a question that awaits further clarification in basic and clinical research studies.

SKIN

For some time, ES has been known to affect *cutaneous blood flow*. Foerster[32] found that dorsal root stimulation caused noticeable hyperemia in the area of skin innervated by the sensory afferent concerned, and in 1933 he used this phenomenon to map the human dermatomes. In animal models, direct antidromic stimulation of pain afferents[22] and direct stimulation of sympathetic afferent fibers have been associated with vasodilation in skin specifically.[33-39] In humans, percutaneous ES of cervical and thoracic levels of the spinal cord with invasive electrodes has been associated with increased cutaneous blood flow as suggested by increased skin temperature[24,40,41] and fluorescence measurements,[42] although Tallis[2] observed only an equivocal increase in cutaneous blood flow using ^{133}Xe clearance measurements with this type of epidural stimulation. Epidural stimulation[24,26,41] and transcutaneous stimulation have been reported to have the clinical benefit of improved wound healing, and this might be related to increased cutaneous blood flow.

Vascular responses to *transcutaneous electrical nerve stimulation* (TENS) vary according to stimulation amplitude and electrode placement. Unlike epidural ES, "conventional" TENS over dorsal roots is seldom associated with hyperemia in dermatomes. However, TENS applied at distal locations can apparently affect skin circulation. Skin temperature of whole extremities was increased with *acupuncturelike TENS* in patients with Raynaud's disease or diabetic polyneuropathy, indicating improved blood flow.[39,48-50] Various stimulation modes of TENS have also been reported to be of benefit in other vasospastic disorders (e.g., reflex sympathetic dystrophy) which involve skin as well as deeper tissues.[41,42,51,52]

As with skeletal muscle, the physiologic mechanisms by which skin blood flow is increased are only partially known. Dorsal root stimulation of pain afferents or of the proposed sympathetic vasodilator fibers may have been responsible for the results observed in the animal preparations or the percutaneous ES studies on humans, but it seems unlikely that this occurs with dorsal root stimulation with TENS of moderate amplitude. Both pain fibers and sympathetic fibers are of small diameter, making them relatively unexcitable to TENS. High-amplitude, painful stimulation would be necessary to activate such fibers, and failure to do so may explain the lack of response to conventional TENS over dorsal roots.

The axon reflex has classically been described in skin and may be one mechanism of the cutaneous response to distally applied acupuncturelike TENS. Lewis[53] described the result of the axon reflex as the transient cutaneous "flare," in the triple response to noxious stimulation, the flare being the result of vasodilation. The triple response consists of a red line followed by the red flare, and finally a wheal (extrusion of fluid into tissue to cause a raised area). The afferent fibers responsible for the axon reflex are also thought to be type III (A delta) and type IV (C) pain fibers.[22,23] *Electroacupuncture* with low-rate, high-amplitude TENS presumably stimulates type III and IV (pain) fibers, and as mentioned above, this type of TENS has been associated with enhanced blood flow.

Because electroacupuncture is thought to have its effects on pain by the release of endorphins and enkephalins (opioids),[54,55] it is tempting to speculate that the vascular responses also result from *humoral mediators*. This temptation to speculate is especially true because cutaneous vasodilation with low-frequency acupuncturelike TENS is delayed in onset and prolonged in duration,[39,48,49] a fact that suggests mediation by a humoral agent or a metabolite rather than by a reflex arc. The mediator has been postulated to act through sympathetic dilator nerves.[39] The results of an elegant set of experiments designed to identify possible mediators of TENS-induced vasodilation enabled Kaada and associates[39,56] to cast doubt on the role of several mechanisms including beta adrenergic, cholinergic, histaminergic, dopaminergic, and purinergic systems, as well as prostaglandins, plasma kinins, angiotensin II, potassium ions (K^+), and certain peptides.

Serotonin may be one humoral mediator of TENS-induced vasodilation. In patients with Raynaud's disease or diabetic polyneuropathy, acupuncturelike stimulation was found to elevate skin temperature to normal levels. Cyproheptadine, a serotonin receptor blocker, blocked this vasodilatory response, thereby implicating serotonin involvement.[49] Unlike the analgesic response to acupuncturelike stimulation, however, naloxone, an opioid receptor blocker, did not block the vasodilatory response.[48] Kaada and Eielson[49] reasoned that the analgesic effects and the vascular effects of acupuncturelike TENS were mediated by different central humoral pathways involving opioids and serotonin, respectively. As those authors noted, this conclusion must be qualified by the assumption that the in vivo doses of the receptor blockers were sufficient for complete receptor blockade.

Other humoral mediators may also play a role in TENS-induced vasodilation. There are several other known vasoactive substances whose roles in this phenomenon await further clarification. *Vasoactive intestinal polypeptide* (VIP) is one substance that may play a role. Plasma VIP levels were found to elevate with acupuncturelike TENS, but a causal relation between VIP and cutaneous vasodilation could not be established.[50]

Thus, cutaneous vasodilation with acupuncturelike TENS is probably due to at least two mechanisms: (1) the *axon reflex*, a local phenomenon involving antidromic conduction down side branches of type III and IV fibers, and (2) *central release of serotonin and other humoral mediators*.

The effects of other forms of TENS on cutaneous blood flow have not been studied as well as those of low-frequency acupuncturelike TENS. The available studies on the systemic autonomic effects and cutaneous blood flow with so-called conventional TENS[40,57,58] have had conflicting results, so whether and how conventional TENS affects skin circulation is unknown. If conventional mode or other modes of TENS do increase cutaneous blood flow, it is conceivable that the mechanisms are quite different from acupuncturelike TENS. At least some applications of ES do increase cutaneous blood flow, which provides support for designing treatment protocols.

The Effects of Electrical Stimulation on Microcirculatory Exchange (Edema)

Of all the forms of ES, the advent of *high-voltage pulsed current* (HVPC) as a treatment modality has been associated with claims that such stimulation is remarkable in its ability to reduce soft tissue edema. Several authors have advocated the use of HVPC for clinical edema reduction, based on empirical evidence.[46,59–65]

The results of some investigations support the contention that HVPC can reduce or minimize edema, whereas others do not. Crisler[66] used HVPC to induce muscle pumping in sprains and strains, and this was associated with edema reduction. Alon[67] and Quillen (Quillen, WS: unpublished data, 1983) described successful use of HVPC in reducing ankle edema after sprains without employing muscle pumping (sensory stimulation only). Delp and Newton (Delp, H and Newton, R: unpublished data,

1980) could not demonstrate reduction of volumetric measurements with HVPC in chronic hand edema, but associated HVPC with improvement in measured hand joint range of motion and patients' subjective reports of improved joint mobility. In a carefully controlled study, Bettany and associates[68] found that serial HVPC treatments significantly reduced edema in acutely injured frog hindlimbs, although edema increased between treatments so that by 24 hours postinjury no difference was found between treated and untreated limbs.

In contrast to these positive findings, Michlovitz and co-workers[69] found that the addition of HVPC to treatment with ice and elevation of the affected limb did not accelerate edema reduction in the treatment of acute ankle sprains. Similarly, Mohr and colleagues[70] did not demonstrate an acceleration of edema reduction with HVPC in a controlled study on rats.

Mechanisms that have been postulated to account for the purported edema reductions with HVPC include reduced leakage of serum proteins as a result of charge repulsion of the proteins[61] or by reduced microvascular permeability to the proteins;[71] accelerated lymphatic uptake of leaked proteins;[62] and enhanced venous and lymphatic fluid reabsorption as result of muscle pumping.[62]

Of these mechanisms, *fluid reabsorption with muscle pumping* is inherently the most plausible. When electrically stimulated muscle pumping is employed in subacute conditions, bulk flow of fluid from the interstitium into the vascular system occurs because of enhanced pressure gradients. The interstitial hydrostatic pressure (P_i) is increased, causing net reabsorption of fluid; capillary hydrostatic pressure (P_c) is consequently increased, creating a greater pressure gradient from the periphery to the right atrium. These events should assist local edema reduction. In some reports of HVPC-induced edema reduction, however, only sensory level (not motor level) stimulation was used.[67,68] This fact suggests that microcirculatory exchange was directly affected by HVPC.

Reed[71] investigated the hypothesis that HVPC reduced microvessel leakage of plasma proteins under conditions of simulated acute inflammation. This was done by quantifying the extravascular appearance of plasma macromolecules with and without HVPC in the histamine-superfused hamster cheek pouch. Fluorescein-labeled dextran was used intravenously as a tracer of protein leaks. Because the molecular size of the dextran was similar to that of plasma proteins, its escape into the interstitium was indicative of a protein leak(s) (Fig. 6–5). At or above a threshold amplitude of HVPC, protein leakage was indeed reduced (Fig. 6–6). Reed maintained that charge repulsion could not have been responsible for his results because the fluorescein-dextran tracer was electrically neutral, and that reduced permeability to plasma proteins might therefore have been involved.[71]

The effect of HVPC on *lymphatic uptake of protein and fluid* remains to be determined, as does the direct effect of HVPC on microvessel hemodynamics in vivo. In vitro ES causes constriction of resistance vessels, probably due to neural mechanisms and, possibly, to direct activation of vascular smooth muscle.[72] The reduced protein leakage with HVPC demonstrated by Reed[71] may have resulted from hemodynamic changes such as reduced microvascular blood flow because of upstream constriction of arterioles. In this case, the reduced leakage might have resulted more from decreased blood flow than from reduced permeability of the microvessels.

There is no reason to assume a priori that there is anything unique about the HVPC waveform with respect to edema reduction. Other waveforms, such as sine

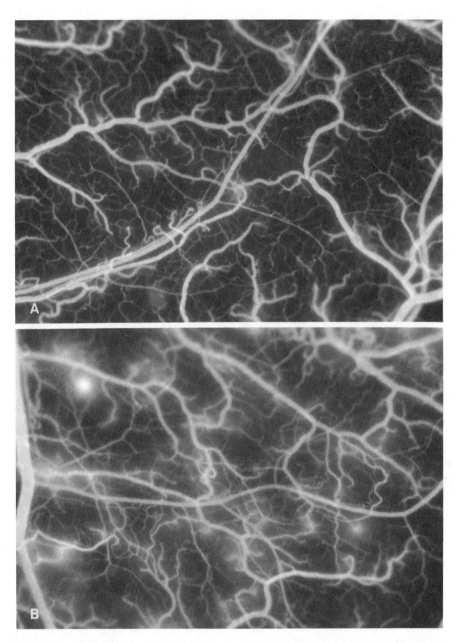

FIGURE 6–5. Microvascular bed outlined by fluorescein-dextran *(A)* before and *(B)* during perfusion with 10^{-5} histamine. Note beginning protein leaks indicated by fluorescent (opaque) spots in illustration B (magnification $\times 25$). (From Reed,[71] pp. 491–495. Reprinted from PHYSICAL THERAPY with the permission of the American Physical Therapy Association.)

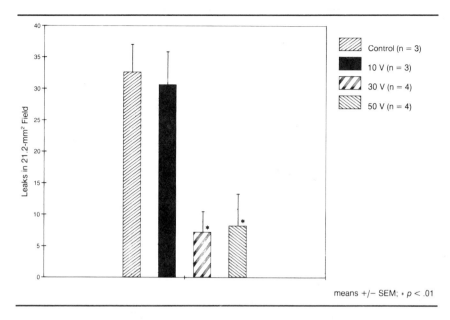

FIGURE 6–6. Posthistamine protein leaks shown by treatment group (means +/− SEM; asterisk indicates $p < .01$). (From Reed,[71] pp. 491–495. Reprinted from PHYSICAL THERAPY with the permission of the American Physical Therapy Association.)

waves of 2500 Hz, may have the same effect as the HVPC if applied at appropriate amplitudes or burst frequencies.

In summary, *the efficacy of HVPC in treating soft tissue edema is still not firmly established*. The fact that findings have been equivocal supports the need for additional clinical and basic research. Under some circumstances, HVPC may limit the edema formation associated with acute injury, but the optimal clinical applications, stimulus variables, and physiologic mechanisms remain to be defined.

The Effects of Electrical Stimulation on Venous Blood Flow

ES-induced muscle contractions of the extremities have been known for some time to increase *venous return*. This phenomenon was observed by Gaskell[73] in 1877 and confirmed by later investigators. In 1948, Wakim used occlusion plethysmography to demonstrate increased venous return with ES in spastic paraplegic and healthy subjects, but the phenomenon did not occur in flaccid paraplegics who had no motor response to ES. This experiment provided evidence that the increased venous flow resulted from skeletal muscle contractions that compressed the leg veins, thus squeezing blood towards the heart.[74] Also in 1948, Apperly and Cary[75] demonstrated that intermittent ES to the legs could counteract orthostatic hypotension effectively.

At about the same time, researchers became interested in the possibility that ES might be effective in reducing the incidence of postoperative *deep vein thrombosis* (DVT) and the associated risk of pulmonary embolism. They reasoned that venous stasis precipitated thrombus formation; if ES reduced venous stasis, it might also prevent DVT. This use of ES was perceived as an important application because of the commonness of the problem and the morbidity and mortality associated with it.

Anecdotal reports indicated reduced incidences of venous thrombi and pulmonary emboli with postoperative rhythmic ES.[75-78] In the 1960s, Doran and associates conducted controlled, single-blind studies of venous return and the incidence of postoperative thrombi using radioactive tracers.[4,79] They found that venous return was decreased significantly during general anesthesia, especially when muscle relaxants were used, and that this venous stasis could be effectively counteracted with ES of the calf muscles during surgery.[79] Furthermore, the risk of deep vein thrombosis was shown to be significantly reduced in legs that received ES during surgery compared with those that did not.[4] These findings were later confirmed by studies in which sensitive testing with fibrinogen labeled with iodine 125 was used to detect thrombi.[80-83] The reduction in incidence of thrombosis from 20.9 to 8.2 percent observed by Browse and Negus[79] was a typical result. Others also reported good results in large clinical trials.[84]

Nicolaides and co-workers[81] suggested that the decreased incidence of deep vein thrombosis with ES might be the result of enhanced venous fibrinolysis as well as of reduced venous stasis, but this suggestion was not supported by later assays.[85]

Other studies did not demonstrate a reduction of DVT incidence with ES. Dejode and associates[86] failed to find a significant difference in DVT-stimulated legs and unstimulated legs. The sample size in this study was relatively small (n = 64), and the stimulation frequency was relatively fast (30 pps), and these factors may have accounted for the negative result.

Prior to 1982, investigators had used a wide variety of stimulus characteristics for enhancing venous return, and stimulation amplitudes often were not specified. Lindstrom and colleagues[85] studied the effects of a variety of ES stimuli to determine the optimal stimulation characteristics. They reported that for patients under general anesthesia each monophasic pulse needed a minimum duration of 25 milliseconds, and was best given as a train at a frequency of about eight 1-second bursts per minute and with 6 to 8 pulses contained within each burst. Adequate current amplitude was determined to be about 40 to 50 mA.[85]

Studies to date on *stimulation of muscles* of the legs for the purpose of *enhancing venous return* have used either monophasic square waves or relatively low-frequency alternating currents. Studies with newer generation waveforms such as HVPC, 2500-Hz AC, or IFC waveforms ought to be undertaken to determine their effectiveness for improving venous return, because they do produce strong skeletal muscle contractions with transcutaneous stimulation.

All of the studies on intraoperative or postoperative ES have reported no serious risks associated with the treatment. Problems were limited to isolated incidents of minor burns when electrodes were applied improperly, and minor patient discomfort with some postoperative treatments. In addition, strict precautions for minimizing the risk of explosion of anesthetic gases were necessary in the operating room. The problems of burns and discomfort probably could be minimized with some of the newer electrical waveforms having zero net charge or short pulse duration, or both.

Venous thrombosis remains a serious problem. Depending on the type of surgery and the age of the patients, the incidence of postoperative DVT in patients who are not treated prophylactically can be in excess of 40 percent. Elderly orthopedic patients, especially those undergoing hip surgery, are at risk.[87] Although the incidence of pulmonary embolism is much lower than that of DVT, morbidity from DVT in the form of varicosities, pain, and chronic venous insufficiency is common.

There is much literature on the application of ES for prevention of DVT, and it seems clear that the treatment is simple, cost-effective, and entails minimal risks. Strangely enough, however, neither intraoperative nor postoperative ES is widely used for DVT prevention or treatment in the United States at this time.[3] The most common prophylactic treatments for DVT in the United States are pharmacologic (involving anticoagulants); intermittent compression of the lower extremities;[87] and repeated voluntary contractions of the calf muscles. Further research is necessary to determine the efficacy of ES relative to the other therapies, and of combined ES and pharmacologic therapy.

Other Clinical Effects: Wound Healing

Enhanced *wound healing* has been associated with subthreshold motor or sensory level ES for some time. This phenomenon is certainly not a result of the vascular effects of ES alone, but, depending on the type of lesion, vascular responses probably do play some role. This section will briefly survey the evidence for enhanced wound healing with ES and consider proposed mechanisms for the effect.

The idea of using electrical current to enhance wound healing dates back as far as 1688, when Digby advocated the use of gold leaf to prevent smallpox scars.[88] Gold leaf holds an electrostatic charge; thus it can be considered a form of electrotherapy. Gold leaf was used as recently as the 1960s[89,90] for treatment of cutaneous lesions including chronic ischemic ulcers.[90]

CONTINUOUS DIRECT (MICRO) CURRENT STIMULATION

Since the 1960s, several studies have reported enhanced wound healing with continuous direct current ES. In studies on humans, direct current at amplitudes of up to 1 mA and for treatment periods of 4 to 6 hours daily was applied with good results.[91-93] In animal studies, continuous direct current was associated with accelerated wound closure and increased wound tensile strength.[94,95]

The relative benefits of anodal (+) versus cathodal (−) stimulation is a topic of controversy. With animal models there have been mixed findings. Assimacopoulis[94] used negative polarity stimulation, whereas Alvarez and associates[95] used positive polarity stimulation; these investigators observed enhanced wound healing and wound tensile strength. Other investigators,[96,97] however, have been unable to demonstrate an advantage of one polarity over the other with microamperage levels of direct current. Studies on humans have typically alternated the polarity of the treatment electrode, and this type of protocol has yielded consistently good results. The protocols began with the cathode as the treatment electrode for about 3 days, or until a plateau in the rate of healing was observed, and then switched to the anode.[91-93] In at least one case, direct current (DC) polarity was reversed daily after a second healing plateau was reached.[91]

The studies on continuous DC promoted the use of an empirical guideline (still used today) for determining the amplitude of current to be used. If copious serous exudate from the wound being treated was observed, the amplitude was considered too low; if an excessively bloody exudate was observed, the current was too high. The optimal amplitude was deemed to be somewhere between these two extremes.[91-93]

HIGH-VOLTAGE PULSED CURRENT STIMULATION

Despite the evidence for enhanced wound healing with low-voltage DC, most clinics presently use pulsed ES waveforms, especially *high-voltage pulsed current* (HVPC), because of the greater comfort and reduced risk of burns afforded. Only very recently, however, has a body of literature begun to support the clinical efficacy of HVPC, and treatment protocols remain poorly defined.

There have been several studies of the effects of HVPC on wound healing in animals. Young[98] reported that HVPC prevented gangrene and promoted full recovery in dogs that had had their hindlimb circulation compromised for 12 hours by means of a tourniquet.[98] In a series of studies in which healing tissues were analyzed after 4 and 7 days of HVPC treatment, Brown and Gogia investigated the effects of HVPC on wound healing and tensile strength in rabbits. They found that cathodal stimulation enhanced healing after 4 days of treatment but delayed healing relative to controls after 7 days.[99] Anodal stimulation, however was associated with delayed wound closure after 4 days and accelerated closure thereafter, to the point where there was no difference between treated and control animals after 7 days.[100] A third study was conducted, in which the polarity of the active electrode was alternated.[101] The protocol consisted of ($-$) stimulation for the first 3 days and ($+$) stimulation for the last 4 days. This polarity arrangement resulted in a significant increase in the degree of wound closure between treated animals and controls. Histologic analysis suggested that this resulted from increased epithelialization in the HVPC-treated animals.

Curiously enough, although collagen production was also increased in the treated animals, the tensile strength of the wounds was not increased. This collagen/tensile strength condition may have been because of the early stage of healing, when collagen fiber orientation was still fairly random.[101] In any case, these data indicated that wound healing could be accelerated by changing HVPC polarity during the course of treatment, even if the effect with 1 week of treatment was primarily epidermal and not dermal. The fact that HVPC can increase *collagen synthesis* is reinforced by the work of Bourguinon and Bourguinon,[102] who demonstrated that phenomenon in vitro. If applied for periods longer than 1 week, the alternating-polarity HVPC treatment might have resulted in increased tensile strength as well as accelerated closure.[101] Confirmation of this possibility awaits further research.

With respect to humans, there have been some clinical case reports on HVPC in wound healing. These cases concerned a decubitus ulcer,[46] a purulent abscess,[43] and wound healing after podiatric surgery.[44] Treatment was deemed to be beneficial in each of these reports.

The most convincing evidence for the clinical value of HVPC for wound healing comes from a controlled clinical study by Kloth and Feedar[47] involving patients with stage IV dermal ulcers. The protocol was dissimilar to Brown and associate's[101] in that the polarity sequence was opposite. As in previous studies with continuous direct current, the positive electrode was initially placed over the wound (Fig. 6–7), and this orientation was maintained until a plateau in healing was observed. At that point, the treatment electrode was made negative. If a second plateau was reached, polarity was alternated daily. The HVPC-treated patients healed at a mean rate of 44.8 percent over a mean period of 7.3 weeks, with complete closure in all cases (Fig. 6–8). By contrast, the ulcers of control patients increased in area an average of 28.9 percent over a mean period of 7.4 weeks.

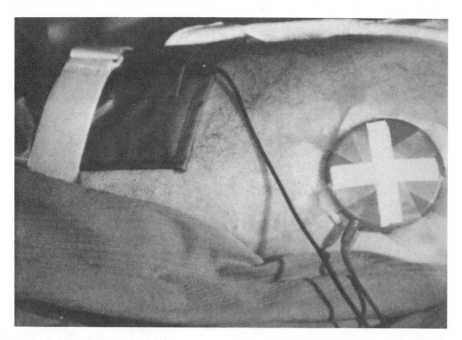

FIGURE 6–7. Electrode placement on wound site, showing the relation of the anode and the cathode to the neuraxis. (From Kloth and Feedar,[48] pp. 503–508. Reprinted from PHYSICAL THERAPY with the permission of the American Physical Therapy Association.)

POSSIBLE MECHANISMS

There is a rationale for alternating the polarity of the treatment electrode. Humans, as well as other species of animals, have measureable tissue potentials.[103–106] *Skin surface potentials* are oriented with positive polarity over the neuraxis and increasing negativity towards the periphery.[105] Furthermore, when tissue is injured, tissue potentials change, becoming strongly positive for 3 or 4 days, then negative.[103–105] Presumably, the wound potential provides an error signal to the central nervous system (CNS), and this in turn amplifies growth and repair responses. Electrical stimulation has been hypothesized to accelerate healing by augmenting these naturally occurring wound potentials.[104–106] This phenomenon has, in fact, been demonstrated in salamanders,[104] and it may be one mechanism by which wound healing was enhanced with continuous direct current[91–93] or pulsed current[43,46,47] in humans.

Predictably, there are contradictions in the literature. The usual scheme for alternating polarity has been to start with positive, then switch to negative polarity, and to alternate as needed thereafter. In their series of studies on rabbits, Brown and associates[99–101] found that with HVPC this polarity sequence actually hampered wound healing, and that the opposite scheme (negative, then positive stimulation) was superior. Perhaps species differences can account for these findings; this is another area that awaits clarification.

Another mechanism of enhanced wound healing may be a *bactericidal effect* of ES. Continuous direct current was reported to have bactericidal effects in vitro and in vivo when cathodal[91–93,105,107] or anodal[107] stimulation was used. Most investigators have used cathodal stimulation for bactericidal effects in humans,[47] so this may be another reason to begin the treatment of infected wounds with that polarity.

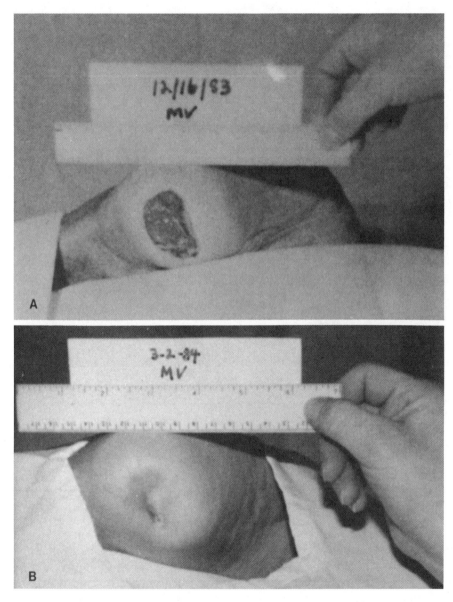

FIGURE 6–8. Decubitus ulcer, *(A)* prior to and *(B)* after 10 weeks of high voltage stimulation. (From Kloth and Feedar,[48] pp. 503–508. Reprinted from PHYSICAL THERAPY with the permission of the American Physical Therapy Association.)

Whether *increased local blood flow* is a mechanism by which ES promotes healing is unknown. In areas where the active electrode overlaps intact skin, ES probably induces an axon reflex, at the least. When acupuncturelike TENS is used, there may also be humorally mediated increases in blood flow as well.[39,48–50,56] The increase in cutaneous blood flow may accelerate inflammation and repair, bolster the immune response to antigens, and thus accelerate closure from the periphery of the wound. In open areas of a wound, however, these reflex effects cannot occur because they are cutaneous in nature. Kaada[45] studied the effect of acupuncturelike TENS on wound

TABLE 6–1 Chart of Treatment Rationales for Various Clinical Conditions

Rationale	RSD*	Localized Edema	DVT (Prevention)† & Venous Stasis	Wounds
		Clinical Condition		
Muscle contraction		X subacute	X	
Humoral vasodilation	X			X
Axon reflex	X			
Reduction of Π_i‡		X acute injury		
Augment wound potentials				X

*RSD: Reflex sympathetic dystrophy.
†DVT: Deep venous thrombosis.
‡Π_i: Interstitial oncotic pressure.

healing in patients with chronic leg and sacral ulcers of various etiologies. He reported enhanced wound healing associated with prolonged increases in cutaneous blood flow as indicated by increased skin temperature. The cathode was placed on the web space between the first and second metacarpal bones, and the anode was placed on the ulnar border of the same hand. Because of this remote electrode placement, the results seem more likely due to reflex vascular events than to augmentation of wound potentials. Thus, with some forms of ES, increased blood flow may be a mechanism by which wound healing can be enhanced. Much, however, remains to be determined regarding optimal waveforms and protocols for promoting wound healing.

In summary, there is good evidence that *some forms of ES can enhance wound healing by accelerating epithelialization and collagen production, and by killing infectious organisms.* Some of these effects may be mediated through *enhanced blood flow*, yet much remains to be determined with respect to optimal waveforms and treatment protocols for promoting wound healing.

TREATMENT RATIONALES AND PROTOCOLS

Electrotherapy for the purpose of affecting the vascular system should be applied according to the physiologic principles described. Table 6–1 displays treatment rationales for the various vascular diseases that can be treated with electrotherapy. These rationales and applications are based on an interpretation of the literature to date. One notable omission from the applications is arterial occlusive disease, because effective electrotherapeutic treatment of arterial occlusive disease has not been demonstrated. In fact, if ES-induced muscle contractions are used in arterial occlusive disease, there is a risk that metabolic demand will exceed the available blood supply.

Protocols

The following protocols assume familiarity with the principles of electrical stimulation. The listings of waveforms do not necessarily include all possible waveforms. Polarity refers to the treatment electrode.

Muscle Contraction

Polarity	$(-)$
Pulse frequency	>25 pulses, bursts, or beats/second[108]
On/off ratio	1:5 on/off[108]; for maximal venous return, induce about 12 contractions per minute
Amplitude	To tolerance; goal is rhythmic, tetanic contractions; may be ramped for graded contractions
Electrode placement	Cathode over muscle motor point; anode distal to muscle belly
Possible waveforms	Pulsed current including HVPC and compensated waveforms; AC including IFC

*Humoral Vasodilation**

Polarity	$(-)$
Pulse frequency	2 to 4 pulses or bursts per second, continuous
Amplitude	To level of tolerable discomfort; local muscle contraction
Electrode placement	Cathode at appropriate acupuncture points; anode at some distant location
Treatment duration	30 to 45 minutes; up to three sessions daily

---

*Kaada and associates observed good results with stimulation only at the Baxie 28 point (web between the first and second metacarpal bones).[39,45,48-50,56]

Axon reflex

Polarity	$(-)$
Pulse frequency†	70 to 100 pulses or bursts per second, continuous
Amplitude†	Perceptible sensory stimulation but not uncomfortable
Electrode placement†	For neurovascular syndromes such as reflex sympathetic dystrophy (RSD) or Raynaud's, electrodes should span the involved area. Alon and DeDomenico[3] have suggested using bifurcated electrodes for this purpose.
Possible waveforms	Pulsed currents including compensated waveforms; monophasic; AC such as 2500-Hz burst 50 times per second; low-amplitude DC
Treatment duration	20 to 30 minutes daily

---

†These treatment variables are similar to those of "conventional" TENS. This may be useful for the treatment of patients with neurovascular problems who exhibit hypersensitivity and therefore cannot tolerate acupuncturelike TENS.

Reduction of Π_i‡

Polarity	$(+)$ or $(-)$
Pulse frequency	120 pps
Amplitude	Subthreshold to motor response; comfortable
Electrode placement	Treatment electrode over edematous area; dispersive electrode some distant location; immersion technique may be used.

Possible waveforms   HVPC
Treatment duration   >30 minutes, at least twice daily

---

‡This protocol is based on animal research[65,68] and has not been proven clinically. Data suggest that for carry-over effect, multiple treatments (e.g., out-of-clinic) may be indicated.

Augmentation of Wound Potentials

Polarity   (+) for first 3 to 4 days, then (−) until a plateau in the rate of healing is reached; continue to switch polarity when plateaus are reached.
Pulse frequency   100 pps for pulsed currents; does not apply for continuous DC
Amplitude   Two guidelines:
                                 1. HVPC: subthreshold to motor responses, comfortable.
                                 2. HVPC or continuous DC; stronger than the amplitude that produces a copious serous exudate, but not so strong that an excessively bloody exudate results.§
Electrode placement   Treatment electrode over wound, anode always cephalad and closer to neuraxis than cathode
Possible waveforms   HVPC; continuous DC
Treatment duration   45 minutes, daily

---

§HVPC offers greater comfort and reduced risk of electrical burns compared with continuous DC.

SUMMARY

Physiologic regulation of the arterial resistance vessels is mediated through both intrinsic and extrinsic controllers. The extrinsic controllers are generally neural and humoral in nature, whereas the local controllers are such things as metabolites, prostaglandins, and the inherent myogenicity of the arterioles. Regional blood flow at any given time reflects the degree of balance between the intrinsic and extrinsic control systems.

Electrical stimulation (ES) can affect arterial blood flow through central (humoral vasodilation) or local (axon reflex) reflexes, or by the production of local metabolites via muscle contraction. In skeletal muscle, there may be an additional somatosympathetic reflex in which ergoreceptors induce increased blood flow through reduced sympathetic outflow to the arterioles. At present there is no clear evidence that electrically induced contraction will increase local blood flow beyond what is required to meet metabolic demand.

Physiologic regulation of microvascular fluid flux is due to the relative balance of Starling forces. The Starling forces are the hydrostatic and oncotic gradients between the exchange vessels and the interstitium. Lymphatic vessels help to prevent excessive fluid accumulation in the interstitium (edema) by removing leaked plasma proteins and fluid.

Although controlled clinical studies are lacking, there is a good possibility that ES can affect edema. Some evidence exists that certain types of ES can minimize acute edema formation when applied at sensory-level amplitudes. Researchers have hypothesized that this effect is due to reduced microvascular permeability to plasma proteins or enhanced lymphatic uptake of proteins and fluid in the interstitium. Prolonged application of ES may be necessary for optimal results. In addition, electrically induced rhythmic contractions in skeletal muscles (motor-level stimulation) presumably helps to reduce subacute edema by pumping plasma from the microvessels to the right side of the heart through the veins.

Physiologic regulation of venous blood flow is accomplished through sympathetically mediated venous tone and by the pumping effect of contracting skeletal muscles. Properly applied ES can create an involuntary muscle pumping effect, which increases venous return. This pumping effect is an especially important application during and following surgery, in that it reduces the risk of deep vein thrombosis. In the United States, ES is not commonly used for the prevention of deep vein thrombosis.

Physiologic wound healing is complex, but recent theory suggests that one of the broad control mechanisms involves changes in electrical potentials in tissues as well as larger electrical "currents of injury" from the periphery to the neuraxis. There now is good evidence that ES can promote wound healing. Two types of current seem to be useful. Continuous low-amplitude direct current can be an effective bacteriocide in infected wounds. Monophasic pulsed currents of short pulse duration promote wound closure, presumably by augmenting injury currents. The augmented injury currents cause unknown central responses that enhance healing. It is also possible that increased blood flow, perhaps from humoral vasodilation or axon reflexes, might further promote wound healing.

The physiologic regulation of the peripheral vascular system has been reviewed along with the general vascular responses to ES. The ES affects on the arterial blood flow, on microcirculatory exchange, on venous blood flow, and on wound healing are discussed. The treatment rationale and clinical protocols for using ES to affect the vascular system follow the above discussions. Information presented on vascular activity should help the clinician gain insight into ES treatments for problems arising from pathology of the vascular system.

REFERENCES

1. Vander, AJ, Sherman, JH, and Luciano, DS: Human Physiology, ed 3. McGraw-Hill, New York, NY, 1980, pp 285–289.
2. Tallis, RC, Illis, LS, Sedgwick, EM, et al: Spinal cord stimulation in peripheral vascular disease. J Neurosurg Psychiatry 46:478–484, 1983.
3. Alon, G and De Domenico, G: Peripheral blood circulation. In High Voltage Stimulation: An Integrated Approach to Clinical Electrotherapy. Chattanooga Corp, Chattanooga, TN, 1987, pp 147–167.
4. Doran, FSA and White, HM: A demonstration that the risk of postoperative deep vein thrombosis is reduced by stimulating the calf muscles electrically during the operation. Br J Surg 54:686–689, 1967.
5. Duckles, SP: Transmural electrical stimulation: Distinguishing between activation of nerves and smooth muscle. In Bevan, JA, et al (eds): Vascular Neuroeffector Mechanisms. Raven Press, New York, NY, 1980, pp 33–35.
6. Mohr, T, Akers, TK, and Wessman, HC: Effect of high voltage stimulation on blood flow in the rat hind limb. Phys Ther 67:526–533, 1987.
7. Currier, DP, Petrilli, CR, and Threlkeld, AJ: Effect of graded electrical stimulation on blood flow to healthy muscle. Phys Ther 66:937–943, 1986.
8. Folkow, B and Halicka, H: A comparison between "red" and "white" muscle with respect to blood supply, capillary surface area and oxygen uptake during rest and exercise. Microvasc Res 1:1–14, 1968.

9. Wakim, KG: Influence of frequency of muscle stimulation on circulation in the stimulated extremity. Arch Phys Med Rehabil 34:291–295, 1953.

10. Crayton, SC, Aung-Din, R, Fixler, DE, et al: Distribution of cardiac output during induced isometric exercise in dogs. Am J Physiol 236:H218–H224, 1979.

11. Randall, BF, Imig, CJ, and Hines, HM: Effect of electrical stimulation upon blood flow and temperature of skeletal muscle. Am J Phys Med Rehabil 32:22–26, 1953.

12. Folkow, B, Gaskell, P, and Waaler, BA: Blood flow through limb muscles during heavy rhythmic exercise. Acta Physiol Scand 80:61–72, 1970.

13. Clement, DL and Shepherd, JT: Influence of muscle afferents on cutaneous and muscle vessels of the dog. Circ Res 35:177–183, 1974.

14. Tracy, JE, Currier, DP, and Threlkeld, AJ: Comparison of selected pulse frequencies from two different electrical stimulators on blood flow in healthy subjects. Phys Ther 68:1526–1532, 1988.

15. Kjellmer, I: On the competition between metabolic vasodilation and neurogenic vasoconstriction in skeletal muscle. Acta Physiol Scand 63:450–459, 1965.

16. Berne, RM and Levy, MN: Cardiovascular Physiology, ed 3. CV Mosby, Saint Louis, MO, 1977, pp 130–154.

17. Gray, SD and Staub, NC: Resistance to blood flow in leg muscles of dog during tetanic isometric contraction. Am J Physiol 213:677–682, 1967.

18. Petrofsky, JS, Phillips, CA, Sawka, MN, et al: Blood flow and metabolism during isometric contractions in cat skeletal muscle. J Appl Physiol 50:493–502, 1981.

19. Kniffki, KD, Mense, S, and Schmidt, RF: Muscle receptors with fine afferent fibers which may evoke circulatory reflexes. Circ Res (Suppl 1)48:25–31, 1981.

20. Kalia, M, Mei, SS, and Kao, FK: Central projections from ergoreceptors (c- fibers) in muscle involved in cardiopulmonary response to static exercise. Circ Res (Suppl 1)48:48–62, 1981.

21. Bayliss, WM: On the origin from the spinal cord of the vaso-dilator fibres of the hindlimb and on the nature of these fibres. J Physiol (Lond) 26:173–209, 1901.

22. Celander, O and Folkow, B: The nature and the distribution of afferent fibers provided with the axon reflex arrangement. Acta Physiol Scand 29:359–370, 1953.

23. Hilton, SM and Marshall, JM: Dorsal root vasodilation in cat skeletal muscle. J Physiol (London) 299:277–288, 1980.

24. Cook, AW, Oygar, A, Baggenstos, P, et al: Vascular disease of the extremities: Electric stimulation of spinal cord and posterior roots. New York State Journal of Medicine 76:366–368, 1976.

25. Dooley, DM and Kasprak, M: Modification of blood flow to the extremities by electrical stimulation of the nervous system. South Med J 69:1309–1311, 1976.

26. Meglio, M, Cioni, B, Dal Lago, A, et al: Pain control and improvement of peripheral blood flow following epidural spinal cord stimulation: Case report. J Neurosurg 54:821–823, 1981.

27. Hinsey, JC and Gasser, HS: The component of the dorsal root mediating vasodilation and the Sherrington contracture. Am J Physiol 92:679–689, 1930.

28. Currier, DP: Electrical stimulation for improving muscular strength and blood flow. In Nelson, RM and Currier, DP (eds): Clinical Electrotherapy. Appleton & Lange, Norwalk, CT, 1987, pp 141–164.

29. Alon, G, Bainbridge, J, Croson, G, et al: High voltage pulsed direct current effects on peripheral blood flow (abstract). Phys Ther 61:734, 1981.

30. Hecker, B, Carron, H, and Schwartz, DP: Pulsed galvanic stimulation: Effects of current frequency and polarity on blood flow in healthy subjects. Arch Phys Med Rehabil 66:369–371, 1985.

31. Walker, DC, Currier, DP, and Threlkeld, AJ: Effects of high voltage pulsed electrical stimulation on blood flow. Phys Ther 68:481–485, 1988.

32. Foerster, O: The dermatomes in man. Brain 56:1–39, 1933.

33. Beck, L, et al: Sustained dilation elicited by sympathetic nerve stimulation. Federation Proceedings 25:1596–1610, 1966.

34. Zimmerman, BG: Sympathetic vasodilation in the dog's paw. J Pharmacol Exp Ther 152:81–87, 1966.

35. Zimmerman, BG: Influence of sympathetic stimulation on segmental vascular resistance before and after neuronal blockade. Arch Int Pharmacodyn Ther 160:66–82, 1966.

36. Brody, M and Schaffer, RA: Distribution of vasodilator nerves in the canine hindlimb. Am J Physiol 218:470–474, 1970.

37. Rolewicz, TF and Zimmerman, BG: Peripheral distribution of cutaneous sympathetic vasodilator system. Am J Physiol 223:939–944, 1972.

38. Rolewicz, TF and Zimmerman, BG: Activation of sustained sympathetic vasodilation in the dog by spinal cord stimulation. Experientia 32:1447–1449, 1976.

39. Kaada, B and Eielsen, O: In search of mediators of skin vasodilation induced by transcutaneous nerve stimulation: I. Failure to block the response by antagonists of endogenous vasodilators. Gen Pharmacol 14:623–633, 1983.

40. Owens, S, Atkinson, ER, and Lees, DE: Thermographic evidence of reduced sympathetic tone with transcutaneous nerve stimulation. Anesthesiology 50:62–65, 1979.
41. Augustinsson, LE, Carlsson, CA, Holm, J, et al: Epidural stimulation in severe limb ischemia: Pain relief, increased blood flow and a possible limb saving effect. Ann Surg 202:103–110, 1985.
42. Augustinsson, LE, Carlsson, CA, and Fall, M: Autonomic effects of electrostimulation. Appl Neurophysiol 45:185–189, 1982.
43. Thurman, BF and Christian, EL: Response of a serious circulatory lesion to electrical stimulation. Phys Ther 51:1107–1110, 1971.
44. Ross, CR and Segal, D: High voltage galvanic stimulation: An aid to postoperative healing. Current Podiatry 30:19–25, 1981.
45. Kaada, B: Promoted healing of chronic ulceration by transcutaneous nerve stimulation. VASA Journal for Vascular Disorders 12:262–269, 1983.
46. Akers, T and Gabrielson, A: The effect of high voltage galvanic stimulation on the rate of healing of decubitus ulcers. Biomed Sci Instrum 20:99–100, 1984.
47. Kloth, LC and Feedar, JA: Acceleration of wound healing with high voltage, monophasic, pulsed current. Phys Ther 68:503–508, 1988.
48. Kaada, B: Vasodilation induced by transcutaneous nerve stimulation in peripheral ischemia (Raynaud's phenomenon and diabetic polyneuropathy). Eur Heart J 3:303–314, 1982.
49. Kaada, B and Eielsen, O: In search of mediators of skin vasodilation induced by transcutaneous nerve stimulation: II. Seratonin implicated. Gen Pharmacol 14:635–641, 1983.
50. Kaada, B, Olsen, E, and Eielsen, O: In search of mediators of skin vasodilation induced by transcutaneous nerve stimulation: III. Increase in plasma VIP in normal subjects and in Raynaud's disease. Gen Pharmacol 15:107–113, 1984.
51. Richlin, DM, Carron, H, Rowlingson, JC, et al: Reflex sympathetic dystrophy: Successful treatment by transcutaneous nerve stimulation. J Pediatr 93:84–86, 1978.
52. Bodenheim, R and Bennett, JH: Reversal of a Sudeck's atrophy by the adjunctive use of trancutaneous electrical nerve stimulation: A case report. Phys Ther 63:1287–1288, 1983.
53. Lewis, T: The Blood Vessels of the Human Skin and Their Responses. Shaw & Sons Ltd, London, 1927.
54. Sjolund, B and Erikson, M: The influence of naloxone on analgesia produced by peripheral conditioning stimulation. Brain Res 173:295–301, 1979.
55. Editorial: How does acupuncture work? BMJ 283:746–748, 1981.
56. Kaada, B and Helle, KB: In search of mediators of skin vasodilation induced by transcutaneous nerve stimulation: IV. In vitro bioassay of the vasoinhibitory activity of sera from patients suffering from peripheral ischemia. Gen Pharmacol 15:115–122, 1984.
57. Ebersold, MJ, Laws, ER, and Albers, JW: Measurements of autonomic function before, during and after transcutaneous stimulation in patients with chronic pain and in control subjects. Mayo Clin Proc 52:228–232, 1977.
58. Wong, RA and Jette, DV: Changes in sympathetic tone associated with different forms of transcutaneous electrical nerve stimulation in healthy subjects. Phys Ther 64:478–482, 1984.
59. Newton, RA: Electrotherapeutic Treatment: Selecting Appropriate Waveform Characteristics. JA Preston Corp, Clifton, NJ, 1984.
60. Mannheimer, JS and Lampe, GN: Clinical Transcutaneous Electrical Nerve Stimulation. FA Davis, Philadelphia, 1984, p 335.
61. Newton, RA: High voltage pulsed galvanic stimulation: Theoretical bases and clinical application. In Nelson, RM and Currier, DP (eds): Clinical Electrotherapy. Appleton & Lange, East Norwalk, CT, 1987, p 176.
62. Alon, G and De Domenco, G: Joint effusion and interstitial edema. In High Voltage Stimulation: An Integrated Approach to Clinical Electrotherapy. Chattanooga Corp, Chattanooga, TN, 1987, pp 129–146.
63. Smith, W: High volt galvanic therapy in the symptomatic management of acute tibial fracture. Athletic Training 16:59, 1981.
64. Lamboni, P and Harris, B: The use of ice airsplints and high voltage galvanic stimulation in effusion reduction. Athletic Training 18:23, 1983.
65. Voight, ML: Reduction of posttraumatic ankle edema with high voltage pulsed galvanic stimulation. Athletic Training 19:278–279, 1984.
66. Crisler, GR: Sprains and strains treated with the Ultrafaradic M-4 impulse generator. J Fla Med Assoc 40:32–34, 1953.
67. Alon, G: High Voltage Stimulation. Chattanooga Corp, Chattanooga, TN, 1984.
68. Bettany, JA, Fish, DR, and Mendel, FC: Influence of high voltage pulsed galvanic stimulation on edema formation following impact injury (abstr). Phys Ther 69:164, 1989.

69. Michlovitz, S, Smith, W, and Watkins, M: Ice and high voltage pulsed stimulation in treatment of acute lateral ankle sprains. Journal of Orthopaedic and Sports Physical Therapy 9:301–304, 1988.

70. Mohr, TM, Akers, TK, and Landry, RG: Effect of high voltage stimulation on edema reduction in the rat hind limb. Phys Ther 67:1703–1707, 1987.

71. Reed, BV: Effect of high voltage pulsed electrical stimulation on microvascular permeability to plasma proteins: A possible mechanism in minimizing edema. Phys Ther 68:491–495, 1988.

72. Duckles, SP and Silverman, RW: Transmural nerve stimulation of blood vessels in vitro: A critical examination. Blood Vessels 17:53–57, 1980.

73. Gaskell, WH: On the changes of the blood-stream in muscles through stimulation of their nerves. J Anat 11:360–402, 1877.

74. Wakim, KG, Terrier, JC, Elkins, EC, et al: Effects of percutaneous stimulation on the circulation in normal and in paralyzed lower extremities. Am J Physiol 153:183–189, 1948.

75. Apperly, FL and Cary, M: The control of circulatory stasis by the electrical stimulation of large muscle groups. Am J Med Sci 216:403–406, 1948.

76. Tichy, VL and Zankel, HT: Prevention of venous thrombosis and embolism by electrical stimulation of calf muscles. Arch Phys Med Rehabil 30:711–715, 1948.

77. Tichy, VL: Prevention of venous thrombosis on pulmonary embolism by electrical stimulation of leg muscles. Surgery 26:109–116, 1949.

78. Martella, J, Cincotti, JJ, and Springer, WP: Prevention of thromboembolic disease by electrical stimulation of the leg muscles. Arch Phys Med Rehabil 35:24–29, 1954.

79. Doran, FS, Drury, M, and Sivyer, A: A simple way to combat the venous stasis which occurs in the limbs during surgical operations. Br J Surg 51:486–492, 1964.

80. Browse, NL and Negus, D: Prevention of leg vein thrombosis by electrical muscle stimulation: An evaluation with ^{125}I-labelled fibrinogen. BMJ 3:615–618, 1970.

81. Nicolaides, AN, Kakkar, VV, Field, ES, et al: Optimal electrical stimulus for prevention of deep vein thrombosis. BMJ 3:756–758, 1972.

82. Becker, J and Schampi, B: The incidence of postoperative venous thrombosis of the legs. Acta Chir Scand 139:357–367, 1973.

83. Rosenberg, IL, Evans, M, and Pollock, AV: Prophylaxis of postoperative leg vein thrombosis by low dose subcutaneous heparin or peroperative calf muscle stimulation: A controlled clinical trial. BMJ 1:649–651, 1975.

84. Powley, JM and Doran, FSA: Galvanic stimulation to prevent deep-vein thrombosis. Lancet 1:406–407, 1973.

85. Lindstrom, B, Korsan, K, Jonsson, BO, et al: Electrically induced short-lasting tetanus of the calf muscles for prevention of deep vein thrombosis. Br J Surg 69:203–206, 1982.

86. Dejode, LR, Kurshid, M, and Walther, WW: The influence of electrical stimulation of the leg during surgical operations on the subsequent development of deep-vein thrombosis. Br J Surg 60:31, 1973.

87. Goldhaber, SZ: Prevention of venous thromboembolism. In Goldhaber, SZ (ed): Pulmonary Embolism and Deep Venous Thrombosis. WB Saunders, Philadelphia, PA 1985, pp 135–158.

88. Robertson, WGA: Digby's receipts. Annals of Medical History 7:219, 1925.

89. Kanof, N: Gold leaf in the treatment of cutaneous ulcers. J Invest Dermatol 43:441–442, 1964.

90. Wolf, M, Wheeler, PC, and Wolcott, LE: Gold-leaf treatment of ischemic skin ulcers. JAMA 196:693–696, 1966.

91. Wolcott, LE, Wheeler, PC, Hardwicke, HM, et al: Accelerated healing of skin ulcers by electrotherapy. South Med J 62:795–801, 1969.

92. Gault, WR and Gatens, PF: Use of low intensity direct current in management of ischemic skin ulcers. Phys Ther 56:265–269, 1976.

93. Carley, PJ and Wainapel, SF: Electrotherapy for acceleration of wound healing: Low intensity direct current. Arch Phys Med Rehabil 66:443–446, 1985.

94. Assimacopoulos, DA: Wound helaing promotion by the use of negative electric current. Am Surg 34:423–431, 1968.

95. Alvarez, OM, Merta, PM, Smerbeck, RV, et al: The healing of superficial skin wounds is stimulated by external electrical current. J Invest Dermatol 81:144–148, 1983.

96. Carey, LC and Lepley, D: Effects of continuous direct electric current on healing wounds. Surgical Forum 13:33–35, 1962.

97. Wu, KT, Go, N, Dennis, C, et al: Effects of electrical currents and interfacial potentials on wound healing. J Surg Res 7:122–128, 1967.

98. Young, GH: Electric impulse therapy aids wound healing. Modern Verterinary Practice 47:60–62, 1966.

99. Brown, M and Gogia, PP: Effects of high voltage stimulation on cutaneous wound healing in rabbits. Phys Ther 67:662–667, 1987.

100. Brown, M, McDonnell, MK, and Menton, DN: Electrical stimulation effects on cutaneous wound healing in rabbits: A follow-up study. Phys Ther 68:955–960, 1988.
101. Brown, M, McDonnell, MK, and Menton, DN: Polarity effects on wound healing using electric stimulation in rabbits. Arch Phys Med Rehabil 70:624–627, 1989.
102. Bourguignon, GJ and Bourguignon, LYW: Electric stimulation of protein and DNA synthesis in human fibroblasts. FASEB J 1:398–402, 1987.
103. Burr, HS, Harvey, SC, and Taffel, M: Bio-electric correlates of wound healing. Yale J Biol Med 11:103–107, 1938–1939.
104. Becker, RO: The bioelectric factors in amphibian-limb regeneration. J Bone Joint Surg [Am] 43:643–656, 1961.
105. Becker, RO, Bachman, CH, and Friedman, H: The direct current control system: A link between environment and organism. New York State Journal of Medicine 62:1169–1176, 1962.
106. Foulds, IS and Barker, AT: Human skin battery potentials and their possible role in wound healing. Br J Dermatol 109:515–522, 1983.
107. Rowley, BA, McKenna, JM, Chase, GR, et al: The influence of electrical current on an infecting microorganism in wounds. Ann NY Acad Sci 238:543–551, 1974.
108. Benton, LA, Baker, LL, Bowman, BR, et al: Functional Electrical Stimulation: A Practical Clinical Guide, ed 2. Professional Staff Association Rancho Los Amigos Medical Center, Downey, CA, 1981.

CHAPTER 7

Human Skeletal Muscle Fatigue

Carl G. Kukulka, Ph.D., P.T.

Human motor performance, whether on the athletic field, in activities of daily life, or in the physical therapy clinic, is influenced by fatigue. Efforts to obtain or maintain peak performance frequently seek to abate or delay the onset of fatigue. An understanding of the processes underlying fatigue should therefore be a prerequisite for anyone responsible for establishing a training or prescribing a clinical treatment.

Fatigue is not a single process, and the evaluation of these processes is complicated by a myriad of accompanying sensations. Eight hours spent in the preparation of a written document, such as a review article on fatigue, produces feelings best described as mental exhaustion. An hour's concentrated workout at a local gym will lead to the feeling of being physically spent. For most daily activities, the feelings of fatigue will include the mental and the physical, and on any given day may be further influenced by encroaching psychologic factors that may add to, or detract from, the final outcome of a given performance. The interaction of these physical, mental, and psychologic variables therefore poses difficulties in attempts to define fatigue.

Several possible definitions for fatigue have been proposed.[1] The definition used here is that given by Simonson and Weiser[2] as cited by Bigland-Ritchie and colleagues[3]: "Fatigue is defined as a transient loss of performance capacity resulting from preceding performance regardless of whether the current performance is affected." This definition best reflects our current interpretations of experimental results obtained over the past 30 to 40 years. It recognizes that fatigue processes may be operative from the onset of activity and that these processes act along a continuum. In addition, the definition is not task specific insofar as it relates to any type of motor performance and the measurement of that performance.

The purpose of this chapter is to provide a review of the basic physiologic processes underlying fatigue and how these processes may affect performance. Experiments are designed to reveal underlying processes and incorporate strict controls for minimizing or accounting for concomitant changes in a subject's perception of effort

163

and motivation to perform. These confounding variables are most certainly important in performance outside the laboratory, but failure to control, or at least account for, such changes can lead to false interpretation of results and erroneous conclusions regarding mechanisms. In turn, the exercising of strict controls, a prerequisite to good scientific methodology, might lead to criticism of the relevance of such experiments to "real world" conditions. This chapter will attempt to describe this relevance as well as to point out the restrictions and limitations in interpretations and the need for continued research efforts.

SITES OF FATIGUE

In a discussion of fatigue, it is informative to review the events associated with the generation of a muscle contraction. In so doing, both the possible anatomic sites of fatigue and the associated contributing physiologic processes can be identified. Two general categories of fatigue (Table 7–1) have been described, based on anatomic sites. The first, central fatigue, is associated with sites that reside within the central nervous system (CNS) and the second, peripheral fatigue, with sites residing outside the CNS. Historically, investigators have attempted to differentiate between central and peripheral sites of failure. Until the early 1950s, fatigue was thought to be primarily a centrally mediated event, the function of which was to act as a protective mechanism for restricting muscle overexertion.[4,5] It was believed that the CNS was not capable of fully activating muscle, and that this ability worsened with fatigue.[5] These two suppositions were not seriously challenged until Merton[6] set the stage for a modern assault on the problem.

Table 7–1 also depicts an alternative classification of fatigue based on two general sets of processes associated with the chain of events that lead to a muscle contraction. The first set of processes involves the delivery of electrical excitation to the muscle. The second deals with the metabolic and enzymatic processes involved in providing the energy for contraction. With the advent of modern electrophysiologic measurement techniques, this classification scheme has proved quite useful in discerning between failure of electrical excitation versus failure within the contractile apparatus. Parallel declines in both force and electrical activity are interpreted as excitation failure, whereas a loss of force without electrical decrements is suggestive of contractile system failure. This logic has been used extensively over the past 40 years and has provided us with much of our current insight into fatigue processes.

CENTRAL VERSUS PERIPHERAL FATIGUE

Since the late 1800s, two fundamental problems of fatigue have been the focus of much research. The first was concerned with differentiating between central and peripheral fatigue; the second dealt with whether the CNS was capable of fully activating a muscle. Prior to 1954, it was thought that the CNS was not capable of full activation and that this ability worsened with fatigue, implying a central failure in force generation. The experiments of Merton[6] and others in the 1970s and 1980s changed much of our thinking.

The basic premise underlying experiments designed to test CNS involvement in

TABLE 7–1 Chain of Events Leading to a Muscle Contraction

Chain of Events Leading to a Muscle Contraction (Anatomic Sites of Fatigue)		Mechanisms Involved in Processing Information through the Chain of Events (Physiologic Processes Responsible for Fatigue)
Central fatigue	Limbic, premotor, and association cortices →	Insufficient motivation or incentive
	Sensorimotor cortex →	Insufficient cortical motoneuron activation
	Spinal cord →	Depressed alpha motoneuron excitability
		Processes involved in delivery of sufficient electrical excitation from CNS to muscle
Peripheral fatigue	Peripheral motoneurons →	Failure in neural transmission
	Neuromuscular junction →	Failure in neuromuscular transmission
	Sarcolemma →	Depressed muscle membrane excitability
	Transverse tubules →	Failure of muscle action potential propagation
	Sacroplasmic reticulum →	Insufficient release and/or reuptake of Ca^{2+}
	Formation of actin-myosin cross-bridges →	Failure in excitation-contraction coupling, insufficient energy supplies, inadequate energy supply replenishment, metabolite accumulation
		Metabolic and enzymatic processes involved in providing sufficient energy for contraction
	Muscle contraction	

fatigue is to compare the force of a maximum voluntary contraction with that of a maximum electrically stimulated contraction. Trains of electrical stimuli are delivered to a muscle's nerve at a rate (50 pps to 100 pps depending on the muscle studied) sufficient to produce a complete tetanic fusion of the muscle response. The electrically stimulated contractions effectively eliminate the CNS from participation in force generation. When the two forces match, central fatigue is ruled out. If the electrically generated force rises above the voluntary force, central fatigue is inferred.

Figure 7–1 demonstrates this experimental procedure for sustained maximum isometric contractions of adductor pollicis and quadriceps femoris muscles. The max-

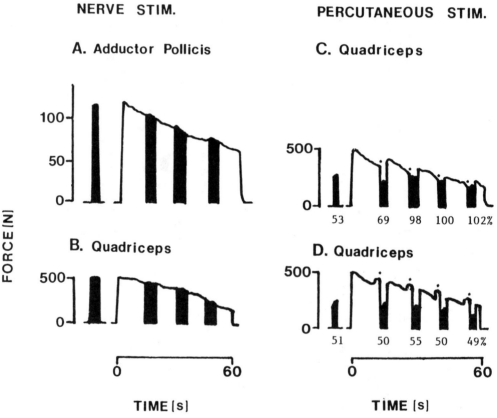

FIGURE 7–1. Force records for sustained voluntary isometric contractions of adductor pollicis and quadriceps femoris muscles. (*A* and *B*) 50/second tetanic stimulation was delivered to the ulnar, *A*, and femoral, *B*, nerves prior to and during the sustained efforts *(shaded regions)*. The tetanic stimulated contractions matched those at the onset of voluntary contraction indicating maximal voluntary activation of the CNS. The stimulated contractions also matched those of the voluntary effort throughout the 60-second contraction, indicating a lack of central fatigue. (*C*) Percutaneous stimulation of the quadriceps femoris muscle produced a 53 percent maximum contraction prior to the sustained effort. When the stimulated contractions were compared to the voluntary efforts just prior to delivery of the stimuli (asterisks), the percentage of stimulated contractions gradually increased to 102 percent of the voluntary effort after 60 seconds. The enhanced contraction produced with electrical stimulation is taken as evidence for central fatigue. (*D*) Same experimental paradigm as in C. Immediately prior to delivery of stimuli, the subject was instructed to produce an extra effort. When the stimulated contractions were compared to these extra efforts (asterisks), the ratio of stimulated to voluntary efforts remained relatively stable, indicating the subject's ability to overcome the central failure. (Adapted from Bigland-Ritchie,[65,66] pp. 95 and 137.)

imal force of tetanic stimulation (shaded area) matched that of the initial voluntary effort (Fig. 7–1A and B), confirming the ability of the subject to maximally activate the CNS. Interpolated 5-second tetanic stimulations at 15, 30, and 45 seconds into a sustained voluntary effort revealed a matching of voluntary to stimulated force production, indicating a lack of central failure.

Evidence for central failure has been reported in the quadriceps femoris muscle when percutaneous stimulation of a fraction of the muscle was used (Fig. 7–1C and D) rather than femoral nerve stimulation. In these experiments, it was assumed that if the stimulated contraction remained the same percentage of the voluntary effort, central fatigue could be ruled out. Comparison of tetanic force to voluntary effort was made for the voluntary force just prior to stimulation (as shown by asterisks in figure). As seen in Figure 7–1C, the stimulated contraction went from an initial 53 percent of the maximum voluntary effort to 102 percent of the effort after 60 seconds of sustained effort, indicating a letup in central activation. This central fatigue could be overcome by asking the subject to make an extra effort just prior to stimulation (indicated by the brief rise in force prior to stimulus delivery in Fig. 7–1D).

The general conclusion drawn from these experiments is that motivated, healthy subjects can fully activate the CNS to produce maximal isometric contractions of the adductor pollicis and quadriceps femoris muscles. Although central fatigue can be demonstrated in the quadriceps femoris muscle, this fatigue can be overcome by an enhanced concentrated effort by the subject. The question remains as to the generalization of this conclusion for different muscle groups, for different types of contraction, and for different populations of subjects. Recent investigations, using a variation of the tetanic stimulation technique, have been directed at these issues.

Supramaximal tetanic stimulation of a peripheral nerve, as used in the previously described experiment, is an effective means for fully activating a muscle, but moderate pain and discomfort is associated with it. An alternative, less painful method, first described by Denny-Brown,[7] consists of delivering single shocks to a peripheral nerve during a voluntary contraction rather than a train of tetanizing pulses. If the muscle were not fully activated, the electrical shocks would add a detectable twitch response to the voluntary force record. At rest or at low levels of voluntary contraction, twitch responses are clearly discernible (Figure 7–2A). At higher voluntary forces, the interpolated twitch becomes smaller, until at maximum no added force is observed. This method has been used to test the ability of healthy subjects to maximally activate isometrically the adductor pollicis,[6,8] soleus,[8–12] tibialis anterior,[11–13] biceps brachii,[8,14] quadriceps femoris,[14] and diaphragm muscles.[15] In all instances, a percentage of the subjects were capable of fully activating the CNS with little evidence for central fatigue. Most studies also reported that a percentage of the individuals tested were either incapable of fully activating the CNS or else could fully activate only after additional concentrated efforts.

The conclusion that the CNS may be fully activated and therefore has little role in fatigue deserves at least two qualifying remarks. First, full CNS activation and lack of central fatigue require cooperative, highly motivated individuals who have practiced producing maximum contractions and who receive appropriate feedback of their performance. Implementation of this method in a patient population would therefore require familiarization of the patient with the method of producing maximum contractions. Second, certain muscle groups such as the ankle plantarflexors, quadriceps femoris, and biceps brachii are more difficult to fully activate than others. A conclusion of central failure in these muscles (or in muscles not yet investigated) should therefore

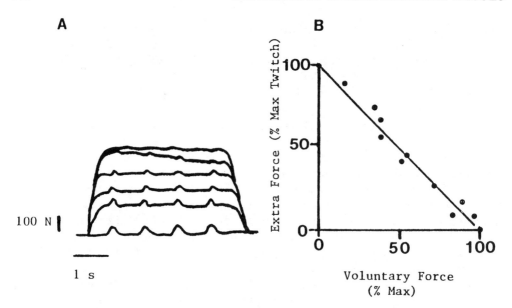

FIGURE 7–2. Demonstration of the interpolated twitch method in quadriceps femoris muscle. *(A)* Single, constant voltage shocks delivered to the femoral nerve at rest and at five levels of voluntary effort. The interpolated twitch is seen to decrease in amplitude as the level of background force is increased. *(B)* Quantification of interpolated twitch data. The background level of voluntary force is plotted on the *x* axis versus the extra force added by the interpolated twitch. (Adapted from Chapman, et al.,[17] p. 3P.)

be approached with some hesitancy and should be carefully validated by supplementary tests.

The clinical implications for using the interpolated twitch have only recently begun to be recognized. Tests for maximum effort have been made on individuals with musculoskeletal disorders[14] and psychiatric problems,[12] and for comparison of strength training regimes in patients with neuromuscular disorders.[16] Such investigations show promise for distinguishing among sites of neuromuscular impairment. For example, three patient groups have recently been distinguished from among 13 patients presenting with a mixture of musculoskeletal disorders: patients experiencing pain and inability to completely activate the CNS, patients without pain and inability to fully activate, and patients without pain but with the ability to fully activate.[14] The last group most likely represented patients who used all of their contractile capabilities to perform functional activities. The other two groups demonstrated untapped potential that would require special consideration in first determining the cause for decreased activation such as pain, lack of motivation, and reflex inhibition. Once the cause for the decreased activation has been determined, the appropriate adjustments to treatment can be made.

Results from these clinical trials are promising yet will require further attention to the verification and establishment of standardized testing protocols. One advantage of the technique is that access to a peripheral nerve for stimulation is not a prerequisite. Percutaneous stimulation of the quadriceps femoris muscle that activates a substantial fraction of that muscle produced results comparable with nerve stimulation.[14,17] The interpolated twitch on any of the large proximal muscles of the body should therefore be possible. On a more cautionary note, the evidence presented on clinical trials to date has been largely descriptive. A recent attempt at using a modified interpolated twitch method to assess training effects in the triceps brachii muscle produced equivocal results as to the repeatability of the technique.[18] More rigorous tests of the validity and reliability of this technique for larger patient populations and for different muscle groups will therefore be necessary.

A final question regarding central versus peripheral fatigue concerns the generalization of findings from maximal isometric contractions to other types of contractions. For fatigue of intermittent submaximal isometric contractions, lack of central fatigue could be demonstrated in quadriceps femoris and adductor pollicis muscles but not in soleus muscle.[19] Likewise, central failure was not evident in quadriceps femoris muscle for fatigue of sustained submaximal isometric contractions.[3] To my knowledge, similar experiments have yet to be done with nonisometric contractions.

ELECTROMYOGRAPHIC CHANGES ASSOCIATED WITH FATIGUE

A rudimentary appreciation of fatigue processes may be gained from examination of gross muscle force and surface electromyographic (EMG) records. Figure 7–3 depicts two examples of how the EMG may change under two different experimental conditions. For a sustained maximum isometric contraction (Fig. 7–3A), the force and EMG are seen to decline in parallel. Mechanisms underlying these changes will be discussed later. For a sustained constant submaximal contraction, the EMG is seen to increase over the period of contraction (Fig. 7–3B). This EMG finding has been consistently verified in independent laboratories and under a variety of experimental conditions.[3,19–23]

The classical interpretation of the finding is that to maintain a constant force level, additional motor units must be recruited,[20] or the firing rate of units already active must increase, or both.[3,22] Other evidence indicates that these may not be the only factors responsible for the EMG changes. First, power spectral shifts in the EMG signal to lower frequencies have been consistently reported[24–26] and are believed to be a result of peripheral changes such as the slowing of muscle action potential conduction velocity.[24,27,28] This low-frequency shift in EMG, together with the low pass filtering characteristics of muscle, effectively augments the EMG signal recorded[29,30] and may account in part for the EMG increase observed with submaximal contractions. Correction for this artifactual enhancement in EMG has been recommended.[30] Second, recent findings suggest that the increase in EMG may be task or muscle specific. Evidence for a task specificity effect comes from experiments in which few surface EMG changes were observed in wrist flexor and extensor muscles taken to their limits of endurance in a hand grasp task.[31] Finally, evidence for muscle specificity effects comes from preliminary EMG measurements of erector spinae muscle, which show inconsistent EMG increases with various levels of submaximal isometric contractions of the low back.[32] A reassessment of the accepted interpretation for the EMG increases during submaximal efforts therefore seems timely. Future experiments will need to address the EMG power spectrum changes as well as possible task or muscle dependent effects on the EMG, and the increased synchronization of muscle discharge.

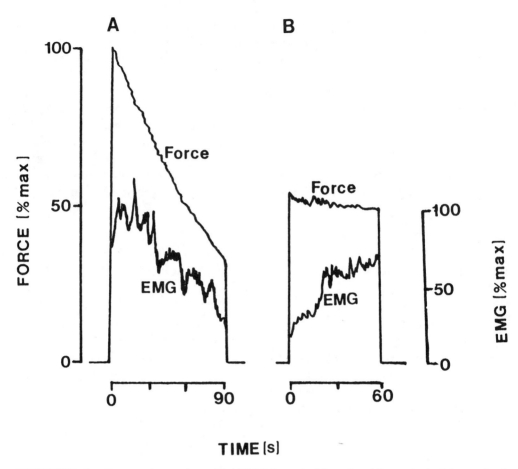

FIGURE 7–3. Force and smooth rectified EMG from the biceps brachii muscle during sustained, isometric contractions during *(A)* a maximal sustained contraction, and *(B)* a 50 percent maximal contraction. (Adapted from Bigland-Ritchie,[65] p. 88.)

NEUROMUSCULAR TRANSMISSION

With the demonstration that central activation can be fully maintained under a variety of experimental conditions and in different muscles, the question remains as to where fatigue may occur. The first peripheral site of failure (Table 7–1) is at the neuromuscular junction. Neuromuscular transmission may be tested by measuring the size of the muscle's compound action potential (M wave) evoked by single, supra-maximal shocks to its nerve.[6,33,34] During a fatiguing contraction, the lack of a decline in the M wave, assuring full central activation, is taken as evidence indicating unimpaired neuromuscular transmission, and that fatigue must be within the muscle itself.

Evidence for lack of neuromuscular transmission failure was first given by Merton,[6] disputed briefly in the early 1970s,[33] but later reconfirmed by Bigland-Ritchie and colleagues.[35] Evidence for the lack of neuromuscular transmission failure (Fig. 7–4) has been reported in a number of muscles for sustained maximal and submaximal isometric contractions[3,35] and for intermittent submaximal isometric contractions.[19] The most convincing evidence comes from experiments designed to circumvent neu-

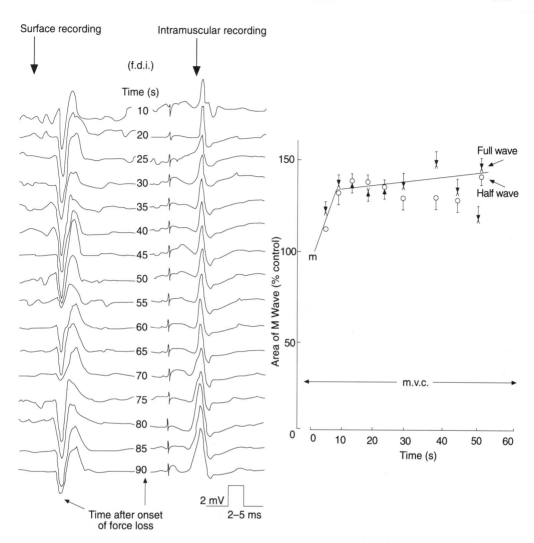

FIGURE 7–4. Evidence for preservation of neuromuscular transmission during fatigue of voluntary sustained isometric contractions. *(A)* Surface and intramuscular evoked M-wave responses from the first dorsal interosseus muscle during a sustained maximal isometric contraction. *(B)* Quantification of M-wave responses from two experiments each, in four subjects. Areas of the M-waves were calculated for both full-wave and half-wave analyses. Mean values are plotted together with their standard deviations. The lack of a decrease in the M-wave is indicative of preservation of the neuromuscular junction. (From Bigland-Ritchie, et al.,[35] pp. 269 and 271, with permission.)

romuscular junction involvement in fatiguing contractions. Jones and co-workers[36] very eloquently demonstrated that tetanic stimulation of curarized mouse muscle could be made to mimic the force loss of voluntary fatigue. The blocking of neuromuscular transmission by curare leaves little doubt that the artificially induced force loss of this experiment was the result of processes outside the muscle. Second, direct stimulation of human muscle following electrically induced, fatiguing contractions has been shown to produce a 12-fold reduction in twitch contractile properties.[37] These contractile changes, independent of neuromuscular transmission, are similar to those seen with fatigue of voluntary effort and lend strong support to fatigue occurring distal to the neuromuscular junction.

Although considerable evidence indicates that neuromuscular transmission failure plays a small role in the fatigue of voluntary contractions, conflicting opinions continue to be expressed. Recently, Marsden and colleagues[38] challenged the concept of a total lack of neuromuscular transmission failure. They reported that the M wave stability is maintained primarily within the first 60 seconds of a contraction (the period most frequently assessed by most investigators). After 60 seconds, they reported that neuromuscular failure becomes more evident.[38]

A complete and final resolution to this problem may not be tenable in human studies, given a number of the complicating findings. Repetitive stimulation of single muscle fibers is known to produce a diminution of the intracellularly recorded action potential.[39] The frequencies of such stimulation are substantially higher than those seen with voluntary activation of motoneurons, but if the total number of action potentials delivered to a muscle is a determining factor in force maintenance,[38] then muscle action potential failure may be a contributing factor in the latter portion of a fatiguing task. Separation of this factor from neuromuscular block is presently technically not feasible in humans. Second, investigations of human[40] and cat motor units[41] indicate that the site of fatigue may depend on the properties of type of motor unit. These cautionary notes prompt serious reflection on the interpretation of surface EMG and whole muscle force measurements.

SLOWING OF MOTONEURON FIRING AND MUSCLE MECHANICAL CHANGES

A persistent observation in fatigue of voluntary contractions is a progressive slowing of motoneuron firing frequencies.[9,10,38,42–44] Although the time course of the slowing appears related to the muscle investigated, taking longer in a postural muscle, the soleus,[9,10] than in a hand muscle, the adductor pollicis,[45] the pattern is stereotypical and consists of two distinct phases: A rapid initial decline in firing followed by a secondary, gradual decline. A similar pattern of slowing can be electrically induced.[34,38] A consequence of this induced slowing is that a force pattern is produced (Fig. 7–5E) that very closely mimics the force decline seen with a voluntary effort (Fig. 7–5A, F). Indeed, if the excitation frequencies are maintained at constant levels (Fig. 7–5B,C,D), the rate of force loss is substantially greater than with voluntary efforts or with the progressive reduction in neuromuscular electrical stimulation frequency. In addition, neuromuscular transmission, as measured by action potential generation (bottom traces of Fig. 7–5), is severely impaired with constant frequency stimulation (Fig. 7–5B,C,D), and essentially preserved for voluntary efforts (Fig. 7–5A,F) or with progressive decreases from electrical stimulation (Fig. 7–5E).

Several function consequences regarding the maintenance of optimal motor performance have been postulated, based on these findings.[34,38,45,46] First, high-frequency fatigue, as demonstrated by the failure of neuromuscular transmission and exaggerated force declines with 100- and 50-pps frequency stimulation (Fig. 7–5B,C) and does not appear to play a significant role in fatigue of voluntary contractions (Figs. 7–4 and 7–5A,F). The maintenance of neuromuscular transmission with voluntary efforts may be attributed to the slowing of motoneuron firing frequencies. Without the slowing, ensuing neuromuscular block would result, with a consequent hastening of

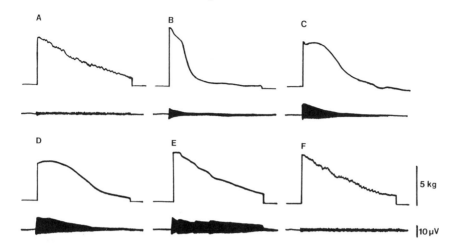

FIGURE 7–5. Surface EMG *(bottom traces)* and force records *(top traces)* for approximately 95-second voluntary isometric contractions *(A and F)* and tetanically stimulated contractions *(B–E)* of the adductor pollicis muscle. In records B, C, and D, a constant train of tetanic stimuli were delivered at 100, 50, and 35 pps, respectively. In E, stimuli were progressively decreased (8 seconds at 60 per second, 17 seconds at 45 per second, 15 seconds at 30 per second, and 55 seconds at 20 per second). (Adapted from Marsden, et al.,[38] p. 177.)

force loss. At least three factors may contribute to motoneuron slowing: the natural adaptation of the motoneurons to prolonged activation,[47] facilitation of the recurrent inhibitory pathway,[10,48] and reflex modulation of motoneurons resulting from fatigue-induced changes within the muscle.[13,44] The difficult challenge ahead will be the separation of their relative contributions to the total firing pattern. Whatever future results reveal, the unmistakable slowing of motoneuron firing frequencies undoubtedly assists in maintaining appropriate neuromuscular transmission during fatiguing voluntary efforts.

The slowing of motoneuron frequencies is accompanied by a prolongation of the muscle's twitch response.[45] A consequence of these concomitant changes may be to optimize the force-generating capabilities of the muscle. It is well established that the firing frequency of a motoneuron for producing tetanic fusion of its muscle fibers is closely matched to the muscle's twitch duration.[49,50] Twitches of short duration require a higher stimulation frequency for tetanic fusion than do twitches of long duration.[51–53] Bigland-Ritchie and colleagues[19] postulated, based on fatigue-induced enhancement of 7-pps frequency twitch summation (Fig. 7–6), that fatigue may induce a shift in the force-frequency relation of muscle (Fig. 7–7). A stimulation frequency for generating a 100 percent maximum effort in the unfatigued state (80 per second; right arrow in Fig. 7–7) could be halved in the fatigued state (left arrow in Fig. 7–7) yet still generate a 100 percent effort. A substantial saving in neural energy would therefore be accompanied by an optimization of muscle force output.

This shift in the force-frequency curve could also act to help preserve frequency modulation of muscle force under conditions of changing neural drive and muscle contractile alterations. The natural firing frequencies of human motor units are in the range of 6 to 30 pps.[8,50,54,55] These frequencies are subtantially lower than those needed to tetanize muscle (Fig. 7–7), and are most likely because of the improvement in fusion capabilities associated with the natural asynchronous discharge of motoneurons versus synchronous stimulation.[56] A decrease in motoneuron firing frequencies,

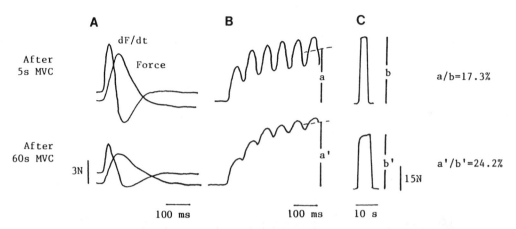

FIGURE 7–6. Mechanical changes in twitch response in adductor pollicis muscle to ulnar nerve stimulation. *(A)* Twitch force and its derivative (dF/dt), 5 seconds into a maximum contraction *(top)* and immediately after a 60-second maximum contraction *(bottom)*. Slight slowing of the contraction time (CT) is evident by the depressed positive deflection in dF/dt after the 60-second contraction. The most dramatic change following fatigue was the pronounced slowing of the relaxation phase of the twitch as exemplified by the severe depression of the negative phase of dF/dt. *(B)* Twitch summation at 7 pps demonstrates an enhancement in the fusion frequency following fatigue *(bottom trace)*. *(C)* Stimulation at 50 pps demonstrates a decrease in maximum tetanic force (b'<b) but an enhancement in the 7 pps tetanus/50 pps tetanus ratio (a/b<a'/b'). The results in both B and C indicate an enhancement in 7 pps frequency summation following fatiguing contractions. (Adapted from Bigland-Ritchie, et al.,[45] p. 318.)

as seen during fatigue, would therefore more closely match the contractile slowly, as demonstrated by the predicted leftward shift of the force-frequency curve. The final result of this matching would be the preserving of frequency modulation of a wide range of forces over a reduced range of firing frequencies.

In summary, the slowing of motoneuron firing rates during fatigue would act to preserve neuromuscular transmission throughout a contraction. This motoneuron slowing, together with the prolongation of the muscle's twitch duration, would ensure that both the full range of force modulation through frequency coding and the optimization of force output would be maintained. What at first glance appear to be detrimental changes in neural activity and muscle mechanical responses, are what in actuality helps to preserve and maintain optimum performance under adverse conditions.

A perplexing problem associated with the matching of contractile properties and motoneuron frequencies is the precise mechanism underlying such changes. The major change in twitch duration is caused by a slowing in relaxation rate.[9,10,45,46] The relation between tetanic fusion frequency and twitch duration predicts that complete fusion of a motor unit would occur when the stimulus intervals are slightly longer than half the time to peak twitch.[52] How a slowing in relaxation time could account for the improvement in twitch summation is therefore difficult to envision. Possibly, this paradox is the result of attempts to draw conclusions on whole muscle investigations using results from single unit experiments. If differences in fatigue sites among motor units holds true,[41,42] then whole muscle results may be misleading. Resolution of this problem will likely require concomitant experimentation at both levels of analyses.

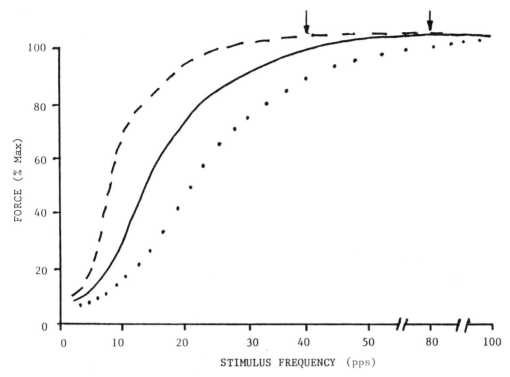

FIGURE 7–7. Demonstration of the force-frequency relationship for whole muscle in the un-fatigued state *(solid line)*, and the displacements of the curve as predicted with contractile slowing *(dashed line)* and with an impairment in low-frequency fusion capabilities *(dotted line)* (i.e., low-frequency fatigue). (Adapted from Bigland-Ritchie, et al.,[45] p. 323, and from Gibson and Edwards,[64] p. 123.)

HIGH-FREQUENCY FATIGUE VERSUS LOW-FREQUENCY FATIGUE

A most fascinating finding in research on fatigue concerns the differential response of fatigued muscle to high-frequency versus low-frequency stimulation. High-frequency fatigue, as demonstrated with sustained (35 to 100 pps) stimulation (see Fig. 7–5B,C,D), has been shown to be of minor consequence in fatigue of voluntary contraction, due in part to the natural slowing of motoneuron firing. Of more functional interest may be what Edwards[57] has referred to as low-frequency (1 to 20 pps) fatigue.[57] This type of fatigue has been demonstrated under anaerobic isometric conditions[57] as well as with eccentric quadriceps femoris muscle contractions.[58] The characteristic finding (Fig. 7–8) is a selective compromising of low-frequency fusion capabilities of muscle that may last from several hours to several days. This impairment in low-frequency force-generating capabilities effectively shifts the force-frequency curve to the right and suggests that generation of any desired prefatigue force level must be accompanied by compensatory changes in firing frequency or recruitment of additional motor units. Whereas high-frequency (35 to 100 pps) fatigue results from failure of excitation, failure in low-frequency fatigue is postulated to occur at the level of excitation-contraction coupling,[57] possibly secondary to sarcomere destruction.[59]

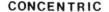

CONCENTRIC

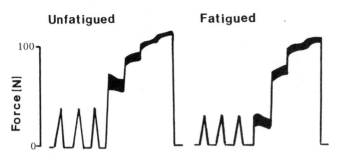

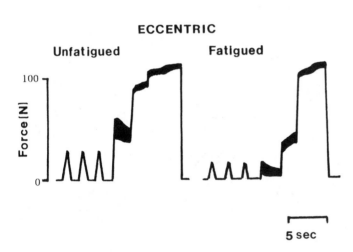

FIGURE 7–8. Mechanical response of quadriceps femoris muscle to stimulation frequencies of 1, 10, 20, 50 and 100 per second before fatigue and following fatigue induced by concentric *(top)* and eccentric *(bottom)* exercises. The response to 50- and 100-per-second frequency stimulation is minimally impaired for both types of exercise. The response to low-frequency stimulation (1, 10, and 20 per second) is mildly impaired for concentric exercise and severely impaired for the eccentric exercise. (Adapted from Newham, et al.,[58] p. 58.)

MUSCULAR EVENTS ASSOCIATED WITH FATIGUE

The most dramatic demonstration of fatigue being the result of muscular events was made more than 30 years ago.[6] Figure 7–9 is taken from this work and depicts the force of voluntary contraction (top traces) and evoked M wave responses (bottom traces). The traces to the right were obtained when ischemia was induced in the subject by inflation of sphygmomanometer cuff. It is readily apparent that (1) force is less and fatigue occurs at a greater rate under ischemic conditions, (2) the recovery of the twitch responses occurs only when the ischemia is relieved, and (3) evidence for neuromuscular block is lacking (as shown by persistent M waves) even under ischemic conditions. Such evidence strongly implicates muscular processes involved in fatigue.

Two recent review articles have succinctly provided excellent overviews of research concerned with muscular events associated with fatigue.[60,61] Two major hypotheses for muscular fatigue have been proposed, and a synopsis of these ideas is presented here.[61] The first hypothesis states that an accumulation of metabolites such as hydrogen ions, ammonia and the ammonium ion, or inorganic phosphate occurs during prolonged or strenuous muscle activity. The accumulation of these products leads to alterations in the extracellular milieu and complex metabolic changes. The most thor-

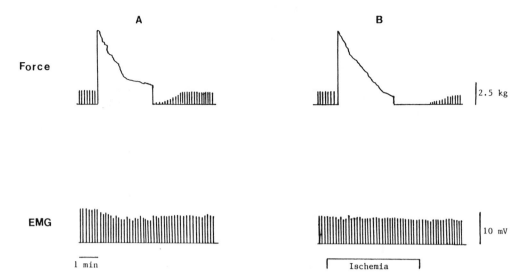

FIGURE 7–9. Force *(top)* and M-wave *(bottom)* changes in adductor pollicis during sustained maximum isometric contractions. Twitch responses of the muscle precede and follow the voluntary efforts. Under ischemic conditions *(B)*, the twitch response does not recover until the blood supply is restored, indicating that fatigue sites must reside within the muscle. (Adapted from Merton,[6] p. 556.)

oughly studied metabolite change is the elevation of extracellular hydrogen ion concentration and consequent depressions of glycolysis and the contractile process (Table 7–2). Less is known about the detrimental effects of ammonia and inorganic phosphate accumulation, yet both have been implicated in the decrement in performance associated with fatigue.

The second hypothesis, the exhaustion hypothesis, states that fatigue occurs as a result of the depletion of key energy substrates such as adenosine triphosphate (ATP), glycogen, and phosphocreatine. Although considerable evidence has been accumulated in support of such a hypothesis, the precise role of any of these substrate depletions has yet to be formulated. Difficulties in so doing are most likely the result of the complex biochemical interactions among the substrates as well as their interactions with the accumulation of metabolites, as described above. Nonetheless, it is an unequivocal fact that fatigue processes within muscle play key roles in the deterioration of performance associated with fatigue.

Considerable insight into muscular events responsible for fatigue has been gained from the study of abnormalities associated with inborn errors in metabolism. The specific problems with such disorders have been thoroughly reviewed by Edwards and Jones,[62] and the implication of these enzymatic deficiencies for fatigue processes has been presented elsewhere.[61] The findings from such studies have aroused serious questioning of several long-held beliefs concerning muscular fatigue. For example, the accumulation of lactic acid had long been thought to be a major contributing factor to the development of fatigue and ensuing muscle cramps. In McArdle's disease, characterized by a lack of lactic acid buildup following ischemic exercise, muscle cramps and fatigue were nonetheless quite evident .[63,64] Continued research into such disorders, together with the application of advanced measurement technologies such as magnetic resonance spectroscopy, should greatly aid in our unraveling of the

TABLE 7–2 Possible Effects of Elevated Hydrogen Ion Concentration Produced during Fatigue on Various Enzymatic and Metabolic Processes

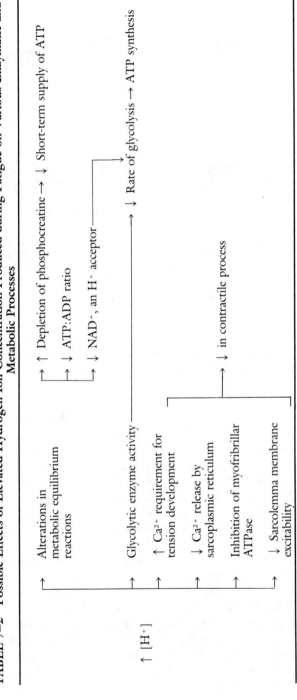

Adapted from MacLaren et al.,[61] pp. 34–35.

association between muscular metabolic events and excitation events associated with fatigue.

SUMMARY

The basic physiologic processes of fatigue and their effects on human performance were reviewed. Sites of fatigue were categorized according to general anatomic site of involvement (central versus peripheral) or according to general physiologic processes (electrical excitation versus metabolic/enzymatic processes). Differentiation of central versus peripheral fatigue could be established through comparisons of voluntary contraction efforts to tetanic stimulation of a muscle or its nerve supply. For sustained or intermittent isometric contractions in a variety of upper extremity and lower extremity muscles, most healthy subjects are capable of full activation of the CNS with little evidence of central fatigue. The ability to fully activate the CNS is dependent, however, on the muscle group studied, with some groups being easier to activate than others, and on the individuals tested. In most studies, a percentage of individuals were either incapable of fully activating the CNS or else could fully activate only after additional concentrated efforts. Neuromuscular transmission failure does not appear to be a major cause of fatigue for voluntary efforts, and may be due largely to the slowing of motoneuron firing during fatigue. The slowing of motoneuron firing is also accompanied by a concomitant prolongation of a muscle's twitch response; the functional consequence of these neuromuscular changes may be to maintain a full range of motoneuron firing rate modulation for optimizing force output during fatigue.

ACKNOWLEDGMENTS

The author was supported by NIH grant NS24991 during the writing of this chapter. Stimulating discussions with Major John S. Halle, P.T., Ph.D. greatly assisted in the clarification of several concepts within this chapter.

REFERENCES

1. Edwards, RHT: Human muscle function and fatigue. Ciba Found Symp 82:1–18, 1981.
2. Simonson, E and Weiser, P: Physiological Aspects and Physiological Correlates of Work Capacity and Fatigue. Charles C Thomas, Springfield, IL, 1976.
3. Bigland-Ritchie, B, Cafarelli, and Vollested, NK: Fatigue of submaximal static contractions. Acta Physiol Scand 128(Suppl)556:137–148, 1986.
4. Waller, AD: The sense of effort: An objective study. Brain 14:179–249, 1891.
5. Reid, C: The mechanism of voluntary muscular fatigue. Quarterly Journal of Experimental Physiology 19:17–42, 1928.
6. Merton, PA: Voluntary strength and fatigue. J Physiol (Lond) 128:553–564, 1954.
7. Denny-Brown, D: On inhibition as a reflex accompaniment of the tendon jerk and of other forms of active muscular response. Proc R Soc Lond [Biol] 103:321–336, 1928.
8. Bellemare, F, Woods, JJ, Johansson, R, et al: Motor unit discharge rates in maximal voluntary contractions of three human muscles. J Neurophysiol 50:1380–1392, 1983.
9. Kukulka, CG, Russell, AG, and Moore, MA: Electrical and mechanical changes in human soleus muscle during sustained maximum isometric contractions. Brain Res 362:47–54, 1986.
10. Kukulka, CG, Moore, MA, and Russell, AG: Changes in human alpha motoneuron excitability during sustained maximum isometric contractions. Neurosci Lett 68:327–333, 1986.

11. Belanger, AY and McComas, AJ: Extent of motor unit activation during effort. J Appl Physiol 51:1131–1135, 1981.
12. McComas, AJ, Kereshi, S, and Quinlan, J: A method for detecting functional weakness. J Neurol Neurosurg Psychiatry 46:280–282, 1983.
13. Garland, SJ, Garner, SH, and McComas, AJ: Reduced voluntary electromyographic activity after fatiguing stimulation of human muscle. J Physiol (Lond) 401:547–556, 1988.
14. Rutherford, OM, Jones, DA, and Newham, DJ: Clinical and experimental application of the percutaneous twitch superimposition technique for the study of human muscle activation. J Neurol Neurosurg Psychiatry 49:1288–1291, 1986.
15. Bellemare, F and Bigland-Ritchie, B: Assessment of human diaphragm strength and activation using phrenic nerve stimulation. Respir Physiol 58:263–277, 1984.
16. McCartney, N, Moroz, D, Garner, SH, et al: The effects of strength training in patients with selected neuromuscular disorders. Med Sci Sport Exerc 20:362–368, 1988.
17. Chapman, SJ, Edwards, RHT, Creig, C, et al: Practical application of the twitch interpolation technique for the study of voluntary contraction of the quadriceps muscle in man. J Physiol (Lond) 353:3P, 1984.
18. Barr, JO: Neural versus Muscular Responses to Isometric Strength Training of the Triceps Brachii. Graduate Program in Physical Therapy, University of Iowa, Iowa City, 1989. Doctoral dissertation.
19. Bigland-Ritchie, B. Furbush, F, and Woods, JJ: Fatigue of intermittent submaximal voluntary contractions: Central and peripheral factors. J Appl Physiol 61:421–429, 1986.
20. Edwards, RG and Lippold, OCJ: The relation between force and integrated electrical activity in fatigued muscle. J Physiol (Lond) 132:677–681, 1956.
21. Viitasalo, J and Komi, PV: Signal characteristics of EMG during fatigue. Eur J Appl Physiol 37:111–211, 1977.
22. Lind, AR and Petrofsky, JS: Amplitude of the surface electromyogram during fatiguing isometric contractions. Muscle Nerve 2:257–264, 1979.
23. Hakkinen, K and Komi, PV: Effects of fatigue and recovery on electromyographic and isometric force- and relaxation-time characteristics of human skeletal muscle. Eur J Appl Physiol 55:588–596, 1986.
24. Lindstrom, LH and Magnusson, RI: Interpretation of myoelectric power spectra: A model and its application. Proc IEEE 65:653–662, 1977.
25. Lindstrom, LH, Kadefors, R, and Petersen, I: An electromyographic index for localized muscle fatigue. J Appl Physiol 43:750–754, 1977.
26. Stulen, FB and DeLuca, CJ: Frequency parameters of the myoelectric signal as a measure of muscle conduction velocity. IEEE Trans Biomed Eng 28:515–523, 1981.
27. Lynn, PA: Direct on-line estimation of muscle fibre conduction velocity by surface electromyogram. IEEE Trans Biomed Eng 26:564–571, 1979.
28. Kranz, H, Williams, AM, Cassell, J, et al: Factors determining the frequency content of the electromyogram. J Appl Physiol 55:392–399, 1983.
29. DeLuca, CJ: Physiology and mathematics of myoelectric signals. IEEE Trans Biomed Eng 26:313–325, 1979.
30. Kranz, H, Cassell, JF and Inbar, GF: Relation between electromyogram and force in fatigue. J Appl Physiol 59:821–825, 1985.
31. Davenport, ME: The Effects of Varying Work-rest Cycles on the Performance of a Repetitive Handgripping Task. Graduate Program in Physical Therapy, The University of Iowa, Iowa City, 1989. Master's thesis.
32. Halle, JS and Smidt, GL: Unpublished results from pilot experiments into EMG changes associated with low back fatigue. Physical Therapy Research Laboratories, University of Iowa, Iowa City, 1989.
33. Stephens, JA and Taylor, A: Fatigue of maintained voluntary muscle contraction in man. J Physiol (Lond) 220:1–18, 1972.
34. Bigland-Ritchie, B, Jones, DA, and Woods, JJ: Excitation frequency and muscle fatigue: electrical responses during human voluntary and stimulated contractions. Exp Neurol 64:414–427, 1979.
35. Bigland-Ritchie, B, Kukulka, CG, and Lippold, OCJ, et al: The absence of neuromuscular transmission failure in sustained maximal voluntary contractions. J Physiol (Lond) 330:256–278, 1982.
36. Jones, DA, Bigland-Ritchie, B, and Edwards, RHT: Excitation frequency and muscle fatigue: Mechanical responses during voluntary and stimulated contractions. Exp Neurol 64:401–413, 1979.
37. Merton, PA, Hill, DK, and Morton, HB: Indirect and direct stimulation of fatigued human muscle. Ciba Found Symp 82:120–129, 1981.
38. Marsden, CD, Meadows, JC, and Merton, PA: "Muscular wisdom" that minimizes fatigue during prolonged effort in man: Peak rates of motoneuron discharge and slowing of discharge during fatigue. Adv Neurol 39:169–211, 1983.
39. Luttgau, HC: The effect of metabolic inhibitors on the fatigue of the action potential in single muscle fibers. J Physiol (Lond) 178:45–67, 1965.
40. Borg, J, Grimby, L, and Hannerz, J: The fatigue of voluntary contraction and the peripheral electrical propagation of single motor units in man. J Physiol (Lond) 340:435–444, 1983.
41. Clamann, HP and Robinson, AJ: A comparison of electromyographic and mechanical fatigue properties in motor units of the cat hindlimb. Brain Res 327:203–219, 1985.

42. Grimby, L, Hannerz, J, and Hedman, B: The fatigue and voluntary discharge properties of single motor units in man. J Physiol (Lond) 316:545–554, 1981.
43. Bigland-Ritchie, B, Johansson, R, Lippold, OCJ, et al: Changes in motoneuron firing rates during sustained maximal voluntary contractions. J Physiol (Lond) 340:335–346, 1983.
44. Bigland-Ritchie, B, Dawson, NJ, Johansson, RS, et al: Reflex origin for the slowing of motoneuron firing rates in fatigue of human voluntary contractions. J Physiol (Lond) 379:451–459, 1986.
45. Bigland-Ritchie, B, Johansson, R, Lippold, OCJ, et al: Contractile speed and EMG changes during fatigue of sustained maximal voluntary contractions. J Neurophysiol 50:313–324, 1983.
46. Jones, DA: Muscle fatigue due to changes beyond the neuromuscular junction. In Potter, R and Whelan, J (eds): Physiological Mechanisms. Ciba Found Symp 82:178–196, 1981.
47. Kernell, D, Monster, AW: Motoneurone properties and motor fatigue. Exp Brain Res 46:197–204, 1982.
48. McNabb, N, Frank, JS, and Green, HJ: Recurrent inhibition during sustained submaximal contractions in humans. Neuroscience Abstracts 14:948, 1988.
49. Eccles, JC, Eccles, RM, and Lundberg, A: Action potentials of alpha motoneurons supplying fast and slow muscles. J Physiol (Lond) 193:45–55, 1958.
50. Grimby, L, Hannerz, J, and Hedman, B: Contraction time and voluntary discharge properties of individual short toe extensor motor units in man. J Physiol (Lond) 289:191–201, 1979.
51. Wuerker, RB, McPhedram, AM, and Hernneman, E: Properties of motor units in a heterogeneous pale muscle (m. gastrocnemius) of the cat. J Neurophysiol 28:85–99, 1965.
52. Burke, RE: Motor unit types of cat triceps surae muscle. J Physiol (Lond) 193:141–160, 1967.
53. Binder-Macleod, SA: Force-frequency Relationship in Skeletal Muscle. In Currier, DP and Nelson, RM: Excitable and Connective Tissue: Current Issue. FA Davis, Philadelphia, 1990.
54. Milner-Brown, HS, Stein, RB, and Yemm, R: Changes in firing rate of human motor units during voluntary isometric contractions. J Physiol (Lond) 230:359–370, 1973.
55. Kukulka, CG and Clamann, HP: Comparison of the recruitment and discharge properties of motor units in human brachial biceps and adductor pollicis during isometric contractions. Brain Res 219:45–55, 1981.
56. Rack, PMH and Westbury, DR: The effects of length and stimulus rate on tension in the isometric cat soleus muscle. J Physiol (Lond) 204:443–460, 1969.
57. Edwards, RHT, Hill, DK, Jones, DA, et al: Fatigue of long duration in human skeletal muscle after exercise. J Physiol (Lond) 272:769–778, 1977.
58. Newham, DJ, Mills, KR, Quigley, BM, et al: Pain and fatigue following concentric and eccentric muscle contractions. Clin Sci 64:55–62, 1983.
59. Newham, DJ, McPhail, G, Mills, KR, et al: Ultrastructural changes after concentric and eccentric contractions. J Neurol Sci 61:109–122, 1983.
60. Fitts, RH and Metzger, JM: Mechanisms of muscular fatigue. In Poortmans, JR (ed): Principles of Exercise Biochemistry. Vol 27, Medical Sports Science. Karger, Basel, 1988, pp 212–229.
61. MacLaren, DPM, Gibson, H, Parry-Billings, M, et al: A review of metabolic and physiological factors in fatigue. Exerc Sport Sci Rev 17:29–66, 1989.
62. Edwards, RHT and Jones, DA: Diseases of skeletal muscles. In Peachey, LD (ed): Handbook of Physiology. Section 10: Skeletal Muscle. The American Physiology Society, Baltimore, MD, Williams & Wilkins, 1983, pp 633–672.
63. McArdle, B: Myopathy due to a defect in glycogen breakdown. Clin Sci 10:13–35, 1951.
64. Gibson, H and Edwards, RHT: Muscular exercise and fatigue. Sports Med 2:120–132, 1985.
65. Bigland-Ritchie, B: EMG/force relations and fatigue of human voluntary contractions. In Hutton, RS and Miller, DI (ed): Exercise and Sport Science Reviews, Vol 9. 1981, pp 75–117.
66. Bigland-Ritchie, B: EMG and fatigue of human voluntary and stimulated contractions. Ciba Found Symp 82:130–156, 1981.

CHAPTER **8**

Functional Electrical Stimulation of Paralytic Muscle*

Elizabeth R. Gardner, M.S., P.T.
Lucinda L. Baker, Ph.D., P.T.

Although electrical stimulation for therapeutic purposes has been in existence for centuries, functional applications were not reported until the 1960s.[1,2] With increasingly sophisticated technology, functional stimulation systems have become more elaborate and can now be used for complex tasks.

Functional electrical stimulation (FES) is defined as the application of electrical stimuli to an intact peripheral nerve in an effort to replace lost upper motor neuron control and generate functional, goal-oriented movement. FES is a component of neuromuscular electrical stimulation (NMES), which encompasses the application of electrical stimuli to obtain a neuromuscular response for therapeutic as well as functional purposes. Strengthening, range of motion, and facilitation are examples of therapeutic applications. Walking represents a functional application. Appropriate candidates for FES systems are those with central nervous system impairment as a result of neurologic insults such as spinal cord injury (SCI), cerebrovascular accident (CVA), traumatic brain injury (TBI), cerebral palsy (CP), and other disease processes. Because sensory and motor portions of an intact peripheral nerve can respond to an adequate electrical stimulus, it is possible for movement to be altered or enhanced via afferent and efferent pathways.

The rationale for developing electrical stimulation systems for functional use is, in part, a consequence of the limitations of orthoses and assistive devices, which can restrict mobility or are unable to substitute adequately for lost function. One advantage of FES systems is the use of the existing neuromuscular mechanism that is intact but

---

*This material was submitted for publication in January 1990.

lacks central control. In some cases, facilitation of the recovery of volitional control has resulted from activation of this intact pathway, which demonstrates the potential for therapeutic as well as functional benefit.[3-13] In addition, electrical stimulation systems may be more cosmetically acceptable than alternative devices.

The purposes of this chapter are to describe FES systems that are being developed or are currently in use with some neurologically involved populations; to review methods for evaluating functional ability provided by the systems; and to discuss practical considerations related to system use such as training, control devices, electrodes, and orthotics. Although the availability of complex systems is limited, application of simple FES systems with neurologically involved individuals in the clinical setting will be discussed briefly.

FUNCTIONAL APPLICATIONS

Lower Extremity: Standing

DESCRIPTION OF STANDING SYSTEMS

The use of FES to achieve standing has primarily involved the adult[14-28] and, more recently, the pediatric spinal cord–injured populations. This is because the majority of patients who recover from a CVA, TBI, or central nervous system pathology such as multiple sclerosis, usually regain the ability to stand with conventional intervention, whereas individuals with complete SCI at the thoracic and lumbar levels rarely regain this ability. Orthoses can assist some individuals with SCI to stand, but the effort involved in rising from a seated position, as well as donning and removing the devices, often makes them impractical.

Standing with a minimal FES system is achieved by continuous stimulation of the quadriceps femoris muscles.[15-17,26-28] Depending on the sophistication of the system, the gluteus maximus, gluteus medius, hamstring, adductor magnus, gastrocnemius, and soleus muscles are included to enhance the duration and quality of standing.[14,19-22,25,27] Although upper extremity support as a balance assist is necessary, one extremity is often free to perform functional tasks once the standing position has been attained.[15,20,25-27] Systems using continuous stimulation to achieve standing would be classified as "open loop" systems because the stimulator receives no feedback regarding the standing state (i.e., from goniometers or force sensors) and therefore cannot alter its output in response to postural demands. In the case of the able-bodied individual, sensory feedback allows postural muscles to be active only when necessary to maintain a stable upright position in a highly efficient manner.

The obvious drawback to standing with continuous stimulation is limitation of standing time because of muscular fatigue. Stimulus frequency is usually between 18 and 25 pps in order to minimize fatigue,[16,17,20-22,25,26,28] however, synchronous contraction of muscle fibers in response to stimulation remains a problem. Attempts to resolve this problem have included intramuscular sequential stimulation,[29] sequential neural stimulation,[19] posture switching,[18,24] and the use of "closed loop" controllers.[23,30-32]

Intramuscular sequential stimulation simulates normal recruitment and allows muscle fibers to be stimulated noncontinuously by systematically rotating between multiple electrodes located in the same muscle. In addition, a subtetanic response of individual portions of muscle can result in a fused response of the whole muscle, further promoting fatigue resistance. Although this idea seems attractive and has resulted in fatigue reduction with upper extremity applications,[29] it has not, as yet, been demonstrated in the lower extremity. Sequential stimulation of the nerve is conceptually similar, except a cuff electrode is used to provide submaximal stimulation to several sites located around the circumference of the nerve. Portions of the nerve supplying a particular muscle can be activated asynchronously allowing a prolonged muscle response to stimulation. Although this technique has resulted in functional endurance with stimulation of the phrenic nerve for diaphragmatic paced breathing, improvement in quadriceps femoris muscle endurance that exceeds endurance pro-duced by continuous stimulation is not apparent.[19] Complexity of the hardware and corrosion of the implanted anode contribute to implementation problems.

Posture switching involves the shifting of body weight to allow certain muscles to rest for brief periods. For example, alignment of body weight in front of the knee joint allows the quadriceps femoris muscle to rest while the ankle plantarflexors, hip extensors, and upper extremities prevent the person from falling forward. A backward shift in weight would allow hip extensors and plantarflexors to rest while the quad-riceps femoris muscles are activated. Standing times ranging from 10 to 60 minutes as a result of continuous stimulation have more than doubled by incorporating posture switching, with exceptional subjects standing for up to 5 hours.[18,24] It is not known, however, if the shift in posture interferes with the performance of functional tasks. The open loop nature of this system limits the user to a preestablished on-off pattern of muscle activation, and therefore of postural shifts, which may or may not be task appropriate.

Of greater potential usefulness than the open loop system is the development of closed loop controllers that simulate normal postural control by providing feedback of the postural state to the stimulator, which can then regulate muscle activity in response to postural demand.[23,30–32] Jaeger describes computer simulations of postural control that demonstrate the feasibility of using intermittent stimulated muscle activity to maintain upright posture under restricted circumstances.[23] Clinical trails of closed loop controllers have taken place with paraplegic individuals using a hybrid orthosis developed in Glasgow, Scotland.[30–32] This device uses the combination of a floor reaction orthosis, electrogoniometers to detect knee joint position, and force-sensing resistors (FSR) to detect loading or unloading of the suprapatellar strap of the device. Goniometric and FSR information is fed back to the stimulator so as to turn the quadriceps femoris muscles on or off as the body sways forward and backward, thereby simulating normal postural control for standing. Preliminary trials of this device indicate that the standing time of an individual can be increased well in excess of that achieved by the same person using continuous stimulation, while allowing a posture that is adequate for functional use of the upper extremities.

Although all people with spinal cord injuries will not benefit from this technology, results from 10 years of research using FES systems with adults who have complete thoracic level SCI in Ljubljana, Yugoslavia suggest that a substantial percentage of individuals are able to regain the ability to stand. Of 500 adults representing the entire SCI population seen at the University Rehabilitation Institute at Ljubljana, 54 were selected to participate in the FES program, and 50 achieved the ability to stand using an FES system. Of the 50 participants able to stand, 29 continued to use the system to stand at home following 3 months of initial home use.[27] Yarkony and associates[26] describe the ability of 18 paraplegic adults to stand successfully in the laboratory setting. However, only four of the participants demonstrated the ability to stand at home.[26]

EVALUATION OF STANDING FUNCTION

Standing function is usually quantified by the length of time the individual is able to stand with bilateral upper extremity support, the amount of upper extremity support needed to stand, the standing posture as documented on film, the ability to withstand an induced perturbation, and, more recently, by application of a standardized test of upper extremity function performed in the standing position. Standing ability varies substantially among subjects and is dependent on a variety of factors including subject characteristics such as stimulated and/or voluntary strength and endurance, joint range of motion, cardiovascular condition, status of the peripheral nerves, level of spinal cord injury, motivation, and system characteristics such as electrodes, number of channels, orthoses, and stimulator output. Because of these multiple factors, wide ranges exist for quantified standing ability as reported in the literature. Standing times of trained individuals range from only a few minutes to several hours.[15,17,18,20–22,24,28] The amount of support necessary to maintain standing, reported as the percentage of body weight borne by the upper extremities, ranges from 5 to 60 percent.[20,21,26,28] Standing posture typically includes either relatively normal posture, lordotic "C" posture to maintain mechanical stability as with the use of knee-ankle-foot orthoses (KAFOs), or a flexed posture at the trunk and hips to bear weight on assistive devices.[14–17,19–21,26–28,30,31] Induced perturbations are used to test standing stability and the function of closed loop controllers, which correct for postural disturbances in stance.[33] The use of closed loop control at the hip and trunk appears to reduce the need for upper extremity support in response to perturbation while standing. This hip and trunk control may provide users with an increased opportunity for hand use.[33]

Although standing for therapeutic purposes may be of benefit to some neurologically impaired individuals who are otherwise unable to stand, the primary reason for developing FES standing systems has been to promote function. Such functions as gaining access to otherwise unreachable places are more easily accomplished in standing than in the sitting position. To assess the ability of individuals to use their arms while standing with an FES system, a standardized test was developed.[34] This test was modified from an upper extremity function test that had hitherto been performed in the sitting position.[35] Normal values for performing the standing test have been reported for the adolescent age group and these values have been used for comparison with adolescents who stand with FES and the support of one upper extremity.[34] Although other methods may provide quantitative information about standing performance with an FES system, the advantage of this type of test is that it provides some information about the ability of the FES system user to function in the standing position and can therefore be used to compare FES with more traditional orthotic systems or to compare one stimulation system with another. Ultimately, the practicality of FES standing systems will be decided by the level of function they allow when compared to conventional systems, and by the ease with which they can be donned, used, and maintained.

Lower Extremity: Walking

DESCRIPTION OF WALKING SYSTEMS

Adults, adolescents, and children with neurologic impairments including CVA, CP, complete thoracic or lumbar level SCI, and incomplete SCI at any level, have participated in the development of FES walking systems, both simple and complex. Goals vary between programs, but generally include restoration of walking ability to nonambulatory individuals, improvement of walking ability among ambulatory individuals who use stimulation in place of an orthosis, and improvement of walking ability among ambulatory individuals who use stimulation to augment the function of a conventional orthosis.

The simplest walking system, and the first to be developed, was the peroneal stimulator, which delivered electrical stimulation to the peroneal nerve in order to correct footdrop during the swing phase and initial double limb support phase of walking. The device included a small portable stimulator, a single channel of stimulation to the peroneal nerve, and a heel-switch trigger to start and stop the stimulation.[1,2] Many variations of this system have been made available and continue to be used. They range in complexity from a totally implanted device that uses a nerve cuff electrode and signal transmission via radio frequency, to a completely external system that provides stimulation via a surface electrode garment.[3,4,6-8,10,11,36-42] Although these devices demonstrate the feasibility of using electrical stimulation as a long-term orthotic substitute for a variety of patient populations, they do not meet the needs of the majority of neurologically impaired individuals who demonstrate inadequate volitional control of many muscle groups and therefore require multiple channels of stimulation to enhance function.

An interim step between the development of simple and complex walking systems was the development of a hybrid system combining conventional orthoses—such as the Reciprocating Gait Orthosis (RGO) or Hip Guidance Orthosis (HGO)—with stimulation so as to improve the quality and efficiency of walking with the orthotic device.[43-47] These systems are typically intended for use by individuals with complete thoracic level SCI. Surface electrodes, embedded in an easily donned garment or attached with adhesives, are used to stimulate the quadriceps femoris, gluteus maximus, and hamstring muscles. The quadriceps femoris muscles are used to achieve the standing position. Sensors mounted onto the orthosis allow the mechanical knee joint to be automatically locked once the standing position has been achieved. The typical walking pattern of an individual using a conventional RGO is facilitated by stimulation of the gluteus maximus and hamstring muscles of one leg, which assists the opposite leg with forward progression. The user controls the onset of stimulation with crutch-mounted switches. Without the assistance of stimulation, this motion would be generated from the upper trunk. The major advantage of this system compared with bracing alone is improved efficiency as measured by decreased energy cost, increased velocity, decreased upper extremity support, and increased walking endurance.[43-47] Advantages of this system compared with walking systems using stimulation alone include increased safety in the event of a stimulation system failure, prevention of undesirable motions such as excessive rotation or hyperextension of joints, and availability. A major drawback of this system is the extent of bracing required. It takes time to don and remove, may not be cosmetically appealing to some individuals, and does not approximate a normal walking pattern. Whereas the energy cost of using this system may be superior to that of bracing alone, it is not clear whether other stimulation systems may offer walking that is energy consuming.

Of those systems using electrical stimulation as the primary mode of forward progression, a moderately complex system would include four to eight channels of stimulation, activating two to four muscles per lower extremity.[15,20,21,27,48-57] For the SCI population, the major hip and knee extensors (quadriceps femoris, gluteals, hamstring muscles) are activated for support phases of gait, and a cutaneous flexion reflex is typically elicited for limb clearance. The success of a four-channel FES system, which allows some individuals with thoracic level SCI to walk, has been demonstrated.[51,54,56] Of 50 subjects with complete thoracic level SCI using the four-channel system, 25 were able to walk at home with the use of crutches or walkers. At the 3-month follow-up, only 16 continued to walk at home because of the inconvenience of donning and removing the device and difficulty adapting the system for home use.[56] Of 26 subjects with incomplete SCI, all were able to walk with the assistance of one or more channels of stimulation, with the majority requiring stimulation to elicit a flexion reflex for limb clearance during swing.[54] The user of this system has control over the timing of gait events (swing, stance) such that walking can be adapted to the demands of the environment. For the SCI population, drawbacks of these systems compared with more complex walking systems might include slowness of walking, inefficiency of walking, inadequate approximation of a normal walking pattern, reflex habituation, and the possibility of joint damage because of the reliance on ligaments and soft tissue structures for mechanical stability. The possibility for home use, and availability on at least a limited basis, contribute to the desirability of these systems.

For hemiparetic adults, moderately complex FES walking systems offer as many as eight channels of stimulation, which can be combined in any configuration depending on the needs of the individual.[58-68] Short-term stimulation can provide facilitation of voluntary movement in the paretic lower extremity, which has been shown to enhance walking ability[61,65-68]; but some patients do not demonstrate long-term carry-over of improved walking ability.[67] For these individuals, the continuation of stimulation on a chronic basis as a permanent orthotic substitute to either permit or enhance walking ability is a logical progression of intervention. Unfortunately, this has been prevented by inconsistency of patient response to stimulation and difficulty with daily set-up[61,65,68] except under special conditions.[62,63]

At this time, complex walking systems are typically used with nonambulatory individuals, such as those with complete thoracic level SCI to restore their ability to walk within the laboratory setting for research and development purposes.[69-74] These systems can include up to 48 channels of stimulation, the majority of which are intramuscular. Nearly all muscles typically active during normal walking can be controlled by stimulation including some lower trunk muscles.[70,72,73] Ankle-foot orthoses (AFO) are frequently employed with these systems to assist in controlling ankle and foot motion.[71] As in the case of the peroneal stimulator, foot-switches are often used as a simple form of closed loop control to start and stop stimulation for swing and stance phases of each limb.[73,74] Steps can also be triggered manually by the investigator or the subject. Assistive devices such as rolling walkers or Lofstrand crutches are necessary for balance and for some support of the upper extremity and trunk. Subjects may have control over the choice of functions they are able to perform (e.g., standing, walking, sitting, or exercising) via thumb or crutch switches that allow pattern selection and activation.

For multichannel systems, stimulation patterns (parameters and timing) for walking are determined individually, case by case. Each channel of stimulation, and therefore the muscle it activates, can be controlled independently. The stimulation pattern that will allow a particular subject to walk is typically determined by a repetitive process of trial programming, followed by subjective and objective gait assessment and reprogramming to optimize the speed, stability, and quality of walking.[25,73,75] This labor intensive process can be complicated by inconsistent neuromuscular response to stimulation from trial to trial and day to day as a result of fatigue, variable stimulation threshold or response gain (or both), interfering muscle spasms, and other factors that are not well understood. Some systems allow the stimulus pattern to be transferred to a portable stimulator after an adequate walking pattern is established during programming, and thus provide the user some freedom to walk outside the confines of the laboratory with supervision.[25,74]

There appear to be advantages to the independent control of multiple channels of stimulation afforded by complex systems that require the use of an implantable electrode, such as intramuscular, epimyseal, or nerve cuff electrodes. Advantages may include walking velocities that approach normal speed, less reliance on the upper extremities and assistive devices for support, decreased energy cost, and a closer approximation of normal movement.[73,74] Use of the flexion reflex, which can be slow and unreliable, is not necessary because multiple muscles can be stimulated to achieve limb clearance. A major disadvantage lies in the complexity and maintenance of these systems. Because the current generation of systems uses implanted electrodes that exit the skin, leads and connectors are subject to frequent breakage. These systems represent an interim step and research platform for the development of totally implantable systems. For this reason, multichannel system use is at present largely limited to the laboratory. Although it is unlikely that a system of this complexity will be available for home use soon, development continues because the feasibility of restoring walking ability to individuals with substantial paralysis has been demonstrated.

EVALUATION OF WALKING FUNCTION

Stimulated walking has been described and quantified by numerous methods including measurement of gait timing and distance parameters, gait symmetry, upper extremity support, joint motion, and energy cost, in addition to clinical observation. Quantification of locomotor ability has generally involved limited numbers of subjects of differing diagnoses using a variety of functional stimulation systems. Although studies of limited numbers of subjects makes it difficult to describe stimulated walking or compare the merits of various systems with each other or to normal walking, some general statements can be made.

Electrically stimulated walking is slower than normal walking, and subjects are able to cover only limited distances. Walking speed is typically measured over short distances, such as a 6-meter laboratory walkway. For individuals with complete thoracic level SCI, speeds range from 2 to 54 m/minute depending on the subject and the sophistication of the walking system.[25,27,49,53,56,73,74,76–78] By contrast, normal walking speed is about 90 m/minute.[79] When walking velocities approach normal values, the distance that an individual is capable of traversing is usually limited. Combined RGO or HGO/FES systems provide walking speeds which range from 7 to 33 m/minute.[43,47] Speed has been shown to be greater, energy cost reduced, and upper extremity support lessened with the stimulation/orthosis system than with the orthosis alone.[43–47] Maximal walking distances that can be traversed by subjects using FES walking systems are rarely reported. For paraplegic individuals with complete spinal cord injuries, distances range from 100 to 400 meters.[25,56,74]

For those individuals with minimal or no ability to walk because of varying degrees of impairment as a result of CVA, TBI, or incomplete SCI, FES-assisted walking velocities from 1 to 31 m/minute have been reported.[66,67,80] For ambulatory individuals post-CVA, single channel peroneal stimulation has been shown to increase walking velocity from 35 m/minute, using an AFO prior to electrode implantation, to 47 m/minute. A direct comparison of free walking velocity with and without stimulation following surgery indicated a 4-m/minute increase from 43 to 47 m/minute.[37]

The gait pattern afforded by stimulation allows some nonambulatory individuals to walk and improves the existing walking pattern of others. Nonetheless, there is impairment of joint motion and timing of interlimb and intralimb movement compared with normal walking. When peroneal stimulators are used by hemiparetic adults and children with cerebral palsy, reductions in gait deviations include increased limb clearance during swing phase with an associated decrease in compensatory movements such as hip hiking, and improved floor contact patterns during initial and midstance, as exemplified by initial heel instead of toe contact.[6,13,40,42] Some hemiparetic adults using more complex three- or six-channel stimulation systems have demonstrated improvements in gait, which include (1) decreased equinovarus during swing and stance; (2) increased hip and knee flexion during initial and midswing with decreased compensatory motion; (3) increased knee extension in terminal swing; (4) increased step length; (5) improved knee stability in stance, as indicated by a decrease in knee hyperextension or in excessive knee flexion; (6) improved heel rise in terminal stance; and (7) improved interlimb symmetry.[59,61,63]

For complete thoracic level SCI subjects, walking ability measured within and between days is variable. Substantial differences in walking ability exist between subjects using the same system, as well as between subjects using different systems, making it difficult to describe a typical walking pattern. In general, subjects spend excessive time in the double limb support phase of gait and less than the normal amount of time in the swing or single limb support phases.[25,49,53] The double limb support phases tend to be static rather then transitional phases, as indicated by the fully extended position of both knees during loading response and preswing.[25,49,53,73] Often the subject uses this time to advance the walker or walking device in preparation for the next swing phase. Maximal upper extremity support occurs during single limb support and loading response, as would be expected, and has been reported to be between 30 and 60 percent of body weight.[25,70,73] Rapid transition of body weight and forward progression during double limb support phases are critical to efficient walking. Achieving this ability is hampered, however, by difficulty in generating sufficient muscular forces at certain joints, difficulty in precisely controlling the timing and extent of movement, and difficulty in coordinating stimulated movement with the subject's voluntary effort. Substantial progress has been made toward improving the quality of stimulated gait by inclusion of nearly all of the muscles active during normal walking and by the addition of simple closed loop control.[70,72,74,76,77] Some current examples of stimulated walking that approach normal walking in terms of speed and quality are encouraging.[73] More sophisticated closed loop control, such as multijoint goniometric feedback, is expected to help minimize the remaining gait deficits.

Finally, the energy cost of walking with an FES system is greater than that of normal walking, as would be expected. For the paraplegic population, stimulated walking at a speed of 30 m/minute has been reported to require 2.2 times the metabolic energy of normal walking at comparable speeds.[77] Nonetheless, stimulated walking may be more efficient than walking with conventional braces when both systems are compared at comparable fast walking speeds.[74,78] In light of evidence that walking with orthoses alone is often rejected by the SCI population for its high energy consumption, among other reasons, it will be important to optimize the efficiency of stimulated walking and demonstrate its superiority to walking with orthoses if FES systems are to be accepted as practical orthotic substitutes.

Upper Extremity: Hand Function

DESCRIPTION OF SYSTEMS

Appropriate candidates for FES hand systems usually have significantly impaired or absent voluntary hand function but have sufficient proximal arm and trunk control to be able to manipulate objects if grasp and release were available to them.[81] Individuals with a cervical level SCI at the C-6 level or higher and some individuals with central nervous system involvement as a result of TBI, CVA, or cerebral palsy fall into this category. Although orthoses, such as tenodesis splints, can be of assistance in the performance of functional tasks for this population, they are usually limited in the variety of functions they can afford and are unusable by some patients. Also, adaptation of everyday objects is often necessary to permit functional independence. Surgical intervention, such as tendon transfers, is an option for select patients who retain sufficient voluntary control over certain muscles to allow successful transfer. However, the needs of a large number of more severely impaired individuals remain unaddressed by orthoses and surgery alone. The introduction of FES hand systems into the array of available technology may allow a much greater segment of this population to obtain functional hand use and, therefore, greater independence than is now possible.

Simple FES hand systems use two to four channels of stimulation and some form of controller.[39,60,82–84] For those individuals with quadriplegia, one hand is chosen for stimulation and will become the dominant hand. For hemiparetic individuals, the paretic arm is stimulated. Usually the opposite arm, via shoulder motion, is used to activate and control contralateral hand motion. Whereas cyclical, predictable movement is an inherent characteristic of walking, this is not true of hand function. It would not be appropriate for a user to initiate stimulation and have it continue in a preprogrammed manner, as is the case with walking systems. For this reason, the command input, that is, the way in which the user operates the FES device, is critical to acceptable function of the FES system. As discussed by Peckham, "the input must have a rapid and accurate response, with proportional gradation of the output . . . it should supply the user with information on its magnitude, be easily learned and operatable, and be simply applied and cosmetically acceptable."[81] Many controllers have been proposed and tested, including simple on-off switches, myoelectric (EMG) controllers, voice-activated controllers, and joint position controllers.[39,82–90]

The muscles chosen for stimulation depend on the ability and needs of the user. Hemiparetic adults often have preserved grasp with absent voluntary finger and wrist extension for release.[39,82,83,90] Stimulation of the radial and ulnar wrist extensors combined with stimulation of the finger extensors allows hand opening and, therefore, significantly improved function with minimal training for some hemiparetic adults.[84,90] Other hemiparetic and quadriparetic adults require stimulation of both finger and wrist flexors and extensors to obtain grasp and release. Although this can be achieved with multiple channels of surface stimulation,[87,89] greater fine control of movement, more forceful movement, and more consistent movement can often be obtained using a more sophisticated multichannel intramuscular or epimyseal stimulation system.[81,88,90,91]

Substantial progress has been made on a multichannel hand system using intramuscular electrodes, which has been in development over the past 20 years.[81,86,91–93] The system is intended for use by individuals with C-5–C-6 level SCI. Activation of the device is achieved by depressing a chest-mounted switch. The same switch allows the user to choose between lateral and palmar grasp patterns. Once the desired grasp pattern has been selected, a transducer attached to the shoulder and sternum controls the stimulation by detecting the extent and speed of shoulder elevation/depression and protraction/retraction. As the shoulder is moved through the range of motion that controls stimulation, the muscles responsible for opening and closing the hand are activated. This device also allows the user to "lock" the grasp or control the position and force of the grasp. The primary flexors and extensors of the fingers and thumb are stimulated; these can include the abductor pollicis brevis, opponens pollicis, adductor pollicis, flexor pollicis longus/brevis, extensor pollicis longus, flexor digitorum superficialis and profundus, and the extensor digitorum communis muscles. Stimulation is often combined with surgery, such as joint arthrodesis or tendon transfer, to optimize the quality of the grasp and release that can be achieved.[81,93] Although the intrinsic muscles of the hand are not under stimulated control with the current system, there is some indication that hand position and function could be further improved with inclusion of these muscles into the palmar grasp pattern.[94]

Advantages of the FES system over orthoses and surgery alone include the amount of force that can be achieved; the choice of more than one grasp pattern, thus affording a wider variety of function; the ability to use objects at work or home without modification; and the ability to manipulate objects in space.[81] The drawbacks of this system are primarily related to maintaining the intramuscular electrodes and cables. The release of this technology to several other clinical centers for distribution to selected outpatients for use at home, school, and work is indicative of progress toward a practical FES system.

EVALUATION OF FUNCTION

The hand function possible with the FES system has been quantified by a battery of timed tests in which the user must grasp, move, and release a variety of standard and common objects.[95] The ability to pick up an object, such as a cup, represents a simple task. The ability to perform integrated tasks that involve an increased level of difficulty in terms of object manipulation, such as handling a floppy disk or brushing one's teeth, are also assessed.[81,88,90,92] Function has been evaluated on a more pragmatic level by requiring system users to report their daily use of the system at home, work, or school by task and frequency of use. As modification of objects in the environment is often necessary to make them usable for individuals with quadriplegia, the ability to use unmodified objects is considered to be an indication of improved function with the FES system. The outcome of these evaluations has not yet been reported. Stimulation systems cannot be considered practical unless they are durable and reliable, so the user is required to keep a record of all failures and problems with system use.

Upper Extremity: Shoulder Subluxation

DESCRIPTION OF SYSTEMS

Shoulder subluxation is a problem requiring intervention for many adults who are hemiparetic as a result of stroke or head injury.[96] Pain, swelling, and limited use of the involved upper extremity may result from unmanaged glenohumeral subluxation.[96-99] To date, only surface stimulation systems have been used to reduce or correct the subluxation. Surface electrical stimulation appears to be superior to conventional interventions, such as slings and lap boards, in terms of the degree of correction of the deformity.[100] Because one channel of stimulation is sufficient for this system, the potential exists for widespread clinical application.

With surface stimulation, the cathode is usually placed over the posterior head of the deltoid muscle and the anode over the muscle mass covering the supraspinous fossa. The polarity of the leads can be reversed; however, this often results in excessive shoulder elevation from stimulation of the superficially located trapezius muscle.[100,101] Because it is undesirable to have the humerus slipping in and out of the glenoid fossa with the stimulus on-off cycle, extensive training is necessary in order for this system to act as an orthotic substitute. A 12:1 on-off ratio that can be maintained for several hours per day during the course of a 4 to 6–week training period can often be achieved.[100]

Although some individuals regain proper glenohumeral positioning with stimulation and are able to maintain it without stimulation because of recovery, others require the stimulation system as a permanent orthotic substitute. For this reason, an implanted system is currently being developed. Implantation of electrodes would allow repeatable electrode placement and eliminate much of the variability of response from surface stimulation. The implanted electrodes would substantially reduce the time and effort required by the user to don and remove the system. The issue of skin irritation would be avoided. An added benefit would be the reduction of power consumption, which results from the proximity of the electrode to the nerve it stimulates. This reduction of power consumption would mean increased wear time with less maintenance for the user.

EVALUATION OF FUNCTION

Because these systems maintain proper joint position, evaluation of the ability of the system to perform that function takes the form of clinical and radiographic measurement of the subluxation. These measurements are compared with those taken with the use of conventional intervention, which includes various types of upper extremity slings and supports. Studies have indicated that whereas conventional intervention rarely achieves or maintains proper joint alignment, stimulation can provide nearly normal alignment and maintain that alignment for many appropriate candidates.[100] Additional benefits that have not been measured objectively to date may include improved cosmesis, body image, and use of the involved extremity.

PRACTICAL CONSIDERATIONS

Training Issues

INTENT OF TRAINING

The training issues to be discussed will be limited to those having to do with muscular exercise for neurologically impaired individuals via electrical stimulation in preparation for using an FES system. This information may therefore differ substantially from that found in the literature on electrically stimulated exercise with able-bodied or orthopedically involved individuals.

The goal of training via electrical stimulation is to increase the stimulated strength and endurance of the muscles intended for functional use to a level sufficient for the individual to use the system reliably for an adequate length of time to accomplish the desired task. A clear definition of muscular strength that has meaning for a variety of functions and situations is difficult to provide. Muscular strength can broadly be defined as the force that a muscle or group of synergistic muscles is capable of producing in order to achieve a particular joint position and maintain that position if necessary. Depending on the function, the forces required are often a combination of those produced isotonically (concentrically and eccentrically) and isometrically. Endurance could then be defined as the ability to continue to produce sufficient force, either cyclically or continuously over time, to move a joint or maintain it in a position so as to allow the activity to continue until completion.

Determining the force that a muscle or group of muscles must produce and for how long the muscle is required to produce that force so as to enable function is a complicated matter. For example, consider the forces required of the quadriceps femoris muscles for an individual to stand from a chair, take an object from an overhead shelf, and return to sitting. The quadriceps are required to extend the knees enough to lift the body against gravity. Once the standing position is attained, the quadriceps are required to maintain an extended knee joint position in the presence of postural perturbations when the object is being moved. The quadriceps are then required to allow the knees to flex in a controlled, gradual manner so that the individual returns to the seated position. Forces generated from soft tissues, other joints, and upper extremity support could add to or lessen force requirements for the quadriceps femoris muscles.

How to measure stimulated strength and endurance in a way that relates to function, and the degree to which muscles need to be conditioned for functional use, are questions that remain largely unanswered. However, the fact that training has an effect on paretic muscular performance, and that this training does in some way affect the individual's ability to use an FES system, has been demonstrated by numerous investigators.

TRAINING REGIMENS AND EFFECTS OF TRAINING

For those individuals with complete paralysis as a result of SCI, both stimulated strength and endurance for a variety of muscle groups have been shown to increase with exercise.[19,27,102–109] Measurements that reflect stimulated strength changes have included increase in the amount of weight the individual is able to lift against gravity, increase in the isometric moment produced at various ranges about a particular joint, increase in the isokinetic moment produced at various speeds and through various ranges for a particular joint, and increase in the amount of resistance through which an individual is able to pedal a bicycle ergometer. Endurance is usually characterized by the time required for the isometric moment to drop to 50 percent of its initial value, or as the ratio of the initial isometric moment to the moment after some arbitrary time of continuous or cyclic stimulation.

Because testing and training methods vary greatly between and within studies, the stimulus and exercise conditions necessary for inducing changes in strength and endurance cannot be determined. Also, the time course during which these changes occur is difficult to determine. For able-bodied individuals, it is generally accepted that a strength training regimen would involve exercise against maximal resistance for a low number of repetitions per session, repeated 3 to 5 days per week. Endurance training would involve exercise against a low percentage of maximal resistance for a high number of repetitions per session, repeated 5 to 7 days per week. There is some indication that these general statements may be true for electrically induced exercise with the complete SCI population. Gardner and Triolo[110] have reported increases in the isometric knee extension moment of paraplegic children following only three test sessions over a 3-week period involving approximately 60 maximal contractions per test session. Others who have reported increases in stimulated strength allowed subjects to exercise isometrically at high levels of stimulated force,[102,106] or isotonically against gravity, resistance from weights, or bicycle ergometry.[19,27,103–105,107–109] Whereas no changes in endurance were demonstrated from an exercise regimen involving a minimal number of repetitions performed once per week,[110] daily exercise for 30 minutes or more per day appears to induce increases in stimulated endurance.[27,102–104,106–109]

For individuals who have paresis, such as those with an incomplete SCI, stroke, head injury, or cerebral palsy, the influence of stimulated exercise on muscular performance is less clear because of the presence of some degree of volitional movement. Also, differences in testing and training methods between and within studies add to the difficulty in making statements regarding the effects of exercise. Endurance is often not measured or reported in studies involving these patient populations. Subjects seem to fall into three general categories in terms of the effect that an electrical stimulation exercise program has on their muscular performance. There are those who gain voluntary and stimulated strength, those who gain stimulated strength with no change in voluntary strength, and those whose stimulated and voluntary strength do not appear to change.* Some of those who gain voluntary strength can maintain the increase without additional stimulation, whereas others cannot. Also, gains in volitional movement in a test situation do not always result in improvement during the desired functional activity. For neurologically involved patient populations with some volitional control, frequent reassessment is necessary once a stimulation exercise program has been initiated, in order to determine whether the individual has gained sufficient volitional control to perform the desired function without stimulation. Some degree of stimulation may be required to maintain the volitional gains, or the stimulation may be needed as a permanent orthotic substitute when no volitional gains have been made. Reassessment is also necessary to determine whether the muscular force produced by the stimulation is sufficient for functional use.

---

*References 1, 3, 5, 7, 8–11, 13, 40, 63, 66, 67, 106, 107, 111–118.

RELATIONSHIP OF TRAINING TO FUNCTION

To think that conditions for inducing electrically stimulated strength and endurance changes in the neurologically involved population are not substantially different from those used to induce volitional strength and endurance changes in the able-bodied population is intuitively appealing. Such a premise, however, is overly simplistic. There are several weaknesses in the literature regarding electrically induced exercise as related to function with neurologically involved patients. For instance, for lower extremity applications, training effects have most often been reported for the quadriceps femoris muscles, probably because of the importance of the quadriceps femoris muscles to standing and walking ability and the ease of measuring the force generated by this muscle group. However, the effects of quadriceps femoris muscle training is probably not generalizable to other muscle groups. Although several investigators claim to have conducted exercise of the hip extensors with their subjects[19,66,67,74,103,119] or claim to have stimulated hip extensors during standing or walking,* few have reported stimulated hip extension strength or the effects of exercise on the force the hip extensors are capable of generating.[66,67,119] When they are reported, methods for testing and training the hip extensors are different from quadriceps femoris muscle training and testing. The author's experience and that of other researchers indicate that stimulation of the hip extensors, and the production of measurable forces from this muscle group with electrical stimulation, is difficult.[27,58,61,103] The difficulty in stimulating hip extensors is the likely reason why it is rarely reported by other investigators. Unfortunately, this situation creates the illusion that the generation of forces about the hip joint is not critical to stimulated standing and walking, when in fact it is one of the more difficult issues to be addressed.

The lack of apparent relationship between training and function is a substantial weakness in the literature and in our collective knowledge regarding the amount and type of training necessary to prepare an individual for continued use of an FES system. The amount of muscular force sufficient to achieve a particular function and the ability to maintain that force over time are obviously task specific. Therefore, the training required to obtain and maintain strength and endurance sufficient for FES system use is also task and system specific. Most training programs, however, are prescribed for an arbitrary length of time that is not necessarily related to the task, after which the system user is permitted to perform the functional activity. Whether all subjects need to complete training prior to system use is not known because, for most applications, the degree of muscular strength and endurance required is not known. Peckham and associates[102] reported that approximately 1 kg of grip strength is necessary to grasp common objects. It is this sort of knowledge, which relates measured strength to functional requirements, that is needed if training is to be purposeful and specific. Some FES systems, such as that used to control shoulder subluxation, measure training effects by observing the function being performed. In this way, training is directly related to function. Stimulus on-off ratio and duration of the stimulation period are intensified according to the ability of the user to tolerate stimulation without losing glenohumeral alignment, which is both palpable and visible and therefore clinically measureable. For training to be appropriate, it must be based directly on the user's ability to perform the task. Strength and endurance values must be determined by additional research, which would allow traditional means of measurement such as dynamometry to be meaningfully related to the functional task.

---

*References 20, 21, 24, 25, 43–49, 53, 61, 70, 72, 76.

USER INTERFACE

The method by which the user controls the FES system is critical to the successful operation of the system. Depending on the system, the user may have control over turning the system on and off, choosing the mode of operation and the function to be performed, grading the muscular force produced by the stimulus, and altering the speed of movement. There are numerous ways by which the user can provide such commands to the stimulator. The choice of command input has to do with the ability of the user to operate various controls; the type of stimulation system to be controlled; and the reliability, cosmesis, and ease of operation that the controls afford. For example, for individuals with quadriplegia, the command input must be voice activated or operated by a body part under volitional control. The command input would have to be placed in such a way as not to interfere with use of either upper extremity, and it should be easily and reliably donned and operated. The entire system would not, however, necessarily need to be miniaturized to the size of a walking system, because most of the device could be attached to the wheelchair.

Examples of user interfaces include transducers that are activated by movement of some body part under volitional control. These transducers may be myoelectric devices that are activated by the EMG signal from a muscle under volitional control, on-off switches that afford only minimal start-stop control, and voice-activated controls that reduce the amount of equipment required to be attached to the user.[39,81-90] There are instances where it may not be optimal or efficient for the user to have substantial control of the system.[39] For example, the user of a walking system should be able to activate the system and choose to stand or walk, and should be able to choose the speed of walking. However, joint position controllers and foot-contact or force-sensing switches should control individual steps and allow proportional control of movement for walking on rough terrain or unlevel surfaces. A walking system would be limited by excessive user control because the user's attention would be directed to control of the system. One goal for walking-system controllers would be to allow the automaticity that approximates normal walking. Technical advances need to be made before such systems become realized. Continued development should be directed toward the design of controllers that meet the minimal requirements of efficient, reliable, easy, and cosmetically acceptable use.

CHOICE OF ELECTRODES

Electrode choice has to do with specificity of the stimulated response, reliability, and longevity of the electrode; ease of use; connection to the rest of the system; and power consumption. Although electrodes used for surface stimulation are attractive because of their noninvasive and nonpermanent nature, there are numerous drawbacks to choosing surface electrodes for multichannel systems and long-term use. From clinical experience, most therapists would recognize that repeatability of optimal electrode placement is often difficult, and that the system user would have a difficult time donning certain electrodes independently because of their location. Some attempts have been made to commercialize garments that house multiple surface electrodes and could be donned independently by many users.[120] Currently these garments are not customized as to electrode placement and are therefore limited in their capability. The availability of multichannel stimulators to use in conjunction with the garment has been limited, thus far, to bicycle ergometry applications. Moreover, certain muscle groups cannot be adequately stimulated with surface stimulation, and selectivity is often poor. Because of the high impedance of the skin-electrode interface, surface stimulators require substantial power compared with implanted electrode systems. This means either that the system is heavy with batteries or that it requires frequent recharging. Problems with skin integrity after prolonged use of surface electrodes is an additional drawback.

Epimyseal, percutaneous fine wire, and nerve cuff electodes solve many of the problems associated with surface stimulation, but these have their own unique problems. Epimyseal electrodes require a surgical incision for implantation. Each electrode is sewn onto the connective tissue surface near the motor point of the muscle to be stimulated. These electrodes require more power than fine wire and nerve cuff electrodes but less than surface electrodes. Because of the extent of the implantation procedure, however, these electrodes tend to be stable once implanted. For this reason, they represent a good electrode choice for multiple channel stimulation systems. They are currently in use as part of a totally implanted upper extremity system in development,[93,121] and are also in use with multiple channel walking systems.[66,67]

Percutaneous fine wire electrodes have the advantage of requiring only a minimal surgical procedure, which is similar to insertion of EMG recording electrodes.[122,123] Traditionally, these fine wire electrodes have been used as temporary devices for research purposes, testing and validating of concepts important to the development of totally implantable systems. Unfortunately, these electrodes are susceptible to movement from the motor point because they are not sutured into the body, and to breakage because of their delicate nature. Although the implantation procedure is time consuming, removal and replacement of broken or nonfunctioning electrodes is minimally invasive. Thus far, this electrode has exited the skin in order to be connected to the stimulator. However, continued development allowing total implantation of such electrodes will solve some maintenance problems currently encountered. Improvements in their design is ongoing, and continued development may one day make them a good choice for multiple channel systems.

Considerable time and effort has been spent investigating the feasibility of using nerve cuff electrodes for multiple channel systems. These electrodes have been used successfully in humans with the totally implanted one-channel peroneal stimulator system. However, concerns regarding nerve damage and the extent of surgery necessary for implantation have prevented their acceptance as a viable electrode for multiple channel systems in the near future.[124] Advantages of this type of electrode include proximity to the nerve and therefore good specificity of response, low power consumption, and stability and repeatability of the response. Continued research and development may allow this electrode to be a reasonable option for multichannel system use in the future.

ORTHOSES, EFFICIENCY, AND FUNCTIONAL GAIN

If conventional orthoses are to be used in combination with the stimulation system, they must meet the same requirements for ease of application and removal, cosmetic acceptability, and reliable improvement of function. They must be able to be worn all day. One of the goals of developing stimulation systems is to minimize the need for cumbersome orthoses and to exceed the functional ability provided by mechanical means alone. Some orthoses, such as AFOs, however, can augment the stimulation system without further complicating its use. The advantage of combining low-profile orthoses with stimulation can be added stability, simplicity, and improved function that may be difficult to achieve with stimulation alone. The decision to combine conventional orthotic devices with stimulation has to be based on the user's willingness and ability to use the orthosis, as well as on the degree of functional improvement afforded by the orthosis-stimulator combination. If we fail to simplify the combined system such that it is easily usable and acceptable to the patient, then stimulation-orthosis systems will be relegated to the closet, as have many orthotic and prosthetic systems in the past.

The standard by which FES systems must be measured is that of efficiency and the degree of functional improvement. In all likelihood, achieving improved function at the expense of efficiency is not sufficient to warrant system use by the neurologically involved population.[11] At the present time, FES walking systems do not allow walking that is reliable, safe, fast, and low in energy cost.[125] Until this occurs, it is not likely that these systems will meet with widespread acceptance and clinical success.

CLINICAL APPLICATIONS

If one assumes that for a stimulator system to be functional it must be portable, so that it is available to the user throughout the day, then the only functional systems currently available commercially for clinical use are two-channel surface systems. Although these devices are simple and uncomplicated, the potential clinical applications are quite broad. There are numerous functional applications for two-channel surface stimulation systems that could be used with neurologically involved patients. Although the development of multiple channel systems is certainly desirable because of the extent of involvement of a substantial number of neurologically impaired individuals, these units will not be commercially available for some time. In the meantime, there are many patients, particularly hemiparetic individuals, for whom activation of one or two muscle groups of an involved extremity could result in clinically significant functional improvement. Although portable neuromuscular stimulators are used frequently in some rehabilitation centers to promote gain in range of motion or to facilitate movement, therapists often fail to incorporate the devices into a functional program. Too often a functional system is not developed that could be used independently or with set-up assistance on a regular basis at home by the patient. Given the shortcomings of conventional orthotic devices, two-channel functional stimulation systems should regularly by considered as a treatment option by therapists.

For lower extremity applications, two to three muscle groups could be activated in a variety of combinations when the stimulation system is to be used as an orthotic substitute or assist during walking. When one lower extremity is primarily involved, several muscles normally active during stance phase could be stimulated simultaneously, or stance and swing phase muscles could be stimulated reciprocally. Hip extension and abduction can often be obtained simultaneously, with one channel of stimulation allowing one channel for activation of other stance phase muscles, such as the quadriceps femoris. Alternatively, it could be used to assist with limb clearance during swing phase. Although it may be difficult to obtain adequate hip or knee flexion by direct stimulation of these muscle groups using only one or two channels of surface stimulation, mass limb flexion can be obtained in many individuals by eliciting the flexion reflex, which requires only one channel of stimulation.

Most patients with bilateral lower extremity involvement would be likely to require more than two channels of stimulation to assist with gait. There are some individuals in whom stimulation of one muscle group per leg could be of functional benefit, as might be the case with some incomplete SCI patients.

Stimulus timing is critical when the system is to be used as an orthotic substitute or assist. Timing in most commercial stimulators can be controlled by an external trigger switch. This timing must be optimized for each individual by careful placement of the switch that will automatically control the on-off cycle of stimulation. Most stimulators allow the therapist to choose whether the switch will activate stimulation when it is closed, as during weight bearing, or when it is open. Although the switches are often called heel switches, the switch can and should be placed anywhere in the shoe so that it will optimize stimulus timing. Often, placement of the switch in the shoe of the less involved extremity will result in more consistent switch opening or closing, and therefore better stimulus timing.

Upper extremity functional applications for two-channel surface stimulators can include shoulder subluxation reduction, facilitation of hand grasp or release, or assist of tenodesis. Although reducing shoulder subluxation may require substantial training to prepare the user for continuous or nearly continuous stimulation, it does not require the use of switches or special control devices. Using commercially available stimulation systems to allow hand grasp and release requires considerable thought on the part of the therapist about the placement of a trigger that will allow the user to start and stop stimulation, and about the ability of the user to control the stimulation during functional activities. Because the only triggering devices commercially available at the present time are contact closing switches of various types, the user must be able in some way to close or open the switch to initiate stimulation. Controlling the switch with the less involved hand is usually not recommended because it hinders the functional use of that extremity and inhibits bilateral activity. Some individuals with minimal or no cognitive impairment may be able to control the switch if it is placed in a shoe or, if they are wheelchair bound, in some location on the chair. If the system is to provide an actual improvement in functional ability, however, it must be reliable, relatively easy to apply and operate, and must be cosmetically and operationally acceptable to the user. The system would not result in functional improvment if the user is unable or unwilling to don and use the system, as is often the case with cumbersome orthotic and prosthetic devices.

SUMMARY

Functional electrical stimulation systems undoubtedly represent a viable means of restoring or replacing lost function in the neurologically involved population. Although continued technical development is required for multichannel systems to be commercially available, functional application of two-channel surface systems is a powerful clinical tool to which the clinician already has access. Whereas technical development proceeds largely through engineering efforts, it is the clinician who will identify the clinical need, determine the clinical utility, and define the scope of application for FES systems.

REFERENCES

1. Liberson, WT, Holmquest, HJ, Scot, D, et al: Functional electrotherapy: Stimulation of the peroneal nerve synchronized with the swing phase of the gait of hemiplegic patients. Arch Phys Med Rehab 42:101–105, 1961.
2. Vodovnik, L, Dimitrijevic, MR, Prevec, T, et al: Electronic walking aids for patients with peroneal palsy. The European Symposium on Medical Electronics 4:58–61, 1966.
3. Dimitrijevic, MR, Gracanin, F, Prevec, T, et al: Electronic control of paralysed extremities. Bio-Medical Engineering 3:8–19, 1968.
4. Glanville, HJ: Electrical control of paralysis. Proc Roy Soc Med 65:233–235, 1972.
5. Vodovnik, L and Rebersek, S: Improvements in voluntary control of paretic muscles due to electrical stimulation. In Fields, WS (ed): Neural Organization and its Relevance to Prosthetics. Symposia Specialists, Miami, FL, 1973, pp 101–116.
6. Gracanin, F, Vrabic, M, and Vrabic, G: Six years experiences with FES method applied to children. Europa Medicophysica 12:61–68, 1976.
7. Carnstam, B, Larsson, LE, and Prevec, TS: Improvement of gait following functional electrical stimulation. Scand J Rehabil Med 9:7–13, 1977.
8. Merletti, R, Zelaschi, F, Latella, D, et al: A control study of muscle force recovery in hemiparetic patients during treatment with functional electrical stimulation. Scand J Rehabil Med 10:147–154, 1978.
9. Vodovnik, L: Therapeutic effects of functional electrical stimulation of extremities. Med Biol Eng Comput 19:470–478, 1981.
10. Waters, RL, McNeal, DR, and Clifford, B: Correction of footdrop in stroke patients via surgically implanted peroneal nerve stimulator. Acta Orthop Belg 50:285–295, 1984.
11. Waters, RL, McNeal, DR, Faloon, W, et al: Functional electrical stimulation of the peroneal nerve for hemiplegia. J Bone Joint Surg [Am] 67:792–793, 1985.
12. Malezic, M, Kljajic, M, Acimovic-Janezic, R, et al: Therapeutic effects of multisite electric stimulation of gait in motor-disabled patients. Arch Phys Med Rehabil 68:553–560, 1987.
13. Dubowitz, L, Finnie, N, Hyde, SA, et al: Improvement of muscle performance by chronic electrical stimulation in children with cerebral palsy. Lancet 1:587–588, 1988.
14. Kralj, A and Grobelnic, S: Functional electircal stimulatiaon—a new hope for paraplegic patients? Bulletin of Prosthetics Research Fall:75–102, 1973.
15. Kralj, A, Bajd, T, and Turk, R: Electrical stimulation providing functional use of paraplegic patient muscles. Med Prog Technol 7:3–9, 1980.
16. Bajd, T, Kralj, A, Sega, J, et al: Use of a two-channel functional electrical stimulator to stand paraplegic patients. Phys Ther 61:526–527, 1981.
17. Bajd, T, and Kralj, A: Standing-up of a healthy subject and a paraplegic patient. J Biomech 15:1–10, 1982.
18. Kralj, A and Jaeger, RJ: Posture switching enables prolonged standing in paraplegic patients functionally electrically stimulated. Proceedings of the 5th Annual Conference on Rehabilitation Engineering, Houston, TX, 1982, p 60.
19. Holle, J, Frey, M, Gruber, H, et al: Functional electrostimulation of paraplegics. Orthopedics 7:1145–1155, 1984.
20. Braun, Z, Mizrahi, J, Najenson, T, et al: Activation of paraplegic patients by functional electrical stimulation: Training and biomechanical evaluation. Scand J Rehabil Med Suppl 12:93–101, 1985.
21. Isakov, E, Mizrahi, J, and Najenson, T: Biomechanical and physiological evaluation of FES-activated paraplegic patients. J Rehabil Res Dev 23:9–19, 1986.
22. Mizrahi, J, Susak, Z, and Isakov, E: Optimization of stimulus parameters for reduced fatiguability during standing by functional electrical stimulation of paraplegics. Proceedings of the IV Mediterranean Conference on Medical and Biological Engineering, Spain, 1986, pp 353–356.
23. Jaeger, RJ: Design and simulation of closed-loop electrical stimulation orthoses for restoration of quiet standing in paraplegia. J Biomech 19f:825–835, 1986.
24. Krajl, A, Bajd, T, and Turk, R: Posture switching for prolonging functional electrical stimulation standing in paraplegic patients. Paraplegia 24:221–230, 1986.
25. Marsolais, EB and Kobetic, R: Functional electrical stimulation for walking in paraplegia. J Bone Joint Surg [Am] 69:728–733, 1987.
26. Yarkony, G, Jaeger, R, Williamson, T: Standing by functional neuromuscular stimulation in the laboratory and the home: case reports of 18 paraplegic individuals. Proceedings of the 10th Annual Rehabilitation Engineering Society of North America Conference, San Jose, CA, 1987, pp 608–610.
27. Kralj, A and Bajd, T: Functional Electrical Stimulation: Standing and Walking after Spinal Cord Injury. CRC Press, Boca Raton, FL, 1989.
28. Jaeger, RJ, Yarkony, GM, and Smith, RM: Standing the spinal cord injured patient by electrical stimulation: Refinement of a protocol for clinical use. IEEE Transactions on Biomedical Engineering 36:720–728, 1989.
29. Peckham, PH, Van Der Meulen, JP, and Reswick, JB: Electrical activation of skeletal muscle by sequen-

tial stimulation. In Wulfsohn, A and Sances, NL (eds): The Nervous System and Electrical Currents. Plenum Press, New York, 1970, pp 45–49.

30. Andrews, BJ, Baxendale, RH, Barnett, R, et al: A hybrid orthosis for paraplegics incorporating feedback control. Advances in External Control of Human Extremities 9:297–311, 1987.
31. Andrews, BJ, Baxendale, RH, Barnett, R, et al: Hybrid FES orthosis incorporating closed loop control and sensory feedback. J Biomed Eng 10:189–195, 1988.
32. Andrews, BJ, Barnett, RW, and Phillips, GF: Rule-based control of a hybrid FES orthosis for assisting paraplegic locomotion. Automedica 11:175–199, 1989.
33. Chizeck, HJ, Kobetic, R, Marsolais, EB, et al: Control of functional neuromuscular stimulation systems for standing and locomotion in paraplegics. Proceedings of the IEEE 76:1155–1165, 1988.
34. Billau, BW: Proposal for Development of a Functional Standing Evaluation. Department of Biomedical Science, Drexel University, Philadelphia, 1990. (Master's thesis.)
35. Jebsen, RH, Taylor, N, Trieshmann, RB, et al: An objective and standardized test of hand function. Arch Phys Med Rehabil 50:311–319, 1969.
36. Kljajic, M, Bajd, T, and Stanic, U: Quantitative gait evaluation of hemiplegic patients using electrical stimulation orthoses. IEEE Trans Biomed Eng 438–441, 1975.
37. Waters, RL, McNeal, D, and Perry, J: Experimental correction of footdrop by electrical stimulation of the peroneal nerve. J Bone Joint Surg [Am] 57:1047–1054, 1975.
38. Trnkoczy, A, Stanic, U, and Jeglic, T: Electronic peroneal brace with a new sequence of stimulation. Medical and Biological Engineering 570–576, 1975.
39. Vodovnik, L, Krajl, A, and Stanic, U: Recent applications of functional electrical stimulation to stroke patients in Ljubljana. Clin Orthop 131:64–69, 1978.
40. Riso, RR, Crago, PE Sutin, K, et al: An investigation of the carry-over of therapeutic effects of FES in the correction of drop foot in the cerebral palsy child. Proceedings of International Conference on Rehabilitation Engineering, Toronto, Canada, 1980, pp 220–222.
41. Naumann, S, Mifsud, M, Cairns, BJ, et al: Dual-channel electrical stimulators for use by children with diplegic spastic cerebral palsy. Med Biol Eng Comput 23:435–443, 1985.
42. Strojnik, P, Acimovic, R, Vavken, E, et al: Treatment of drop foot using an implantable peroneal underknee stimulator. Scand J Rehabil Med 19:37–43, 1987.
43. Rose, GK: The hybrid parawalker: Rationale and first results. Annual Progress Report No. 11, The Orthotic Research and Locomotor Assessment Unit at the Robert Jones and Agnes Hunt Orthopedic Hospital, Oswestry, Shropshire, England, 1985, pp 35–38.
44. Petrofsky, JS, Phillips, CA, Larson, P, et al: Computer synthesized walking: An application of orthosis and functional electrical stimulation. The Journal of Neurological and Orthopaedic Medicine and Surgery 6:219–230, 1985.
45. Stallard, J, Major, RE, Poiner, R, et al: Engineering design considerations of the ORLAU parawalker and FES hybrid system. Eng Med 15:123–129, 1986.
46. McClelland, M, Andrews, BJ, Patrick, JH, et al: Augmentation of the Oswestry parawalker orthosis by means of surface electrical stimulation: Gait analysis of three patients. Paraplegia 25:32–38, 1987.
47. Hendershot, DM and Phillips, CA: Improvement of efficiency in a quadriplegic individual using an FES-RGO system. IEEE Engineering in Medicine and Biology Society 10th Annual International Conference 1577–1578, 1988.
48. Kralj, A, Bajd, T, Kvesic, Z, et al: Electrical stimulation of incomplete paraplegic patients. 4th Annual Conference on Rehabilitation Engineering, Washington, D.C., 226–228, 1981.
49. Kralj, A, Bajd, T, Turk, R, et al: Gait restoration in paraplegic patients: A feasibility demonstration using multichannel surface electrode FES. J Rehabil Res Dev 20:3–20, 1983.
50. Bajd, T, Kralj, A, Turk, R, et al: The use of a four-channel electrical stimulator as an ambulatory aid for paraplegic patients. Phys Ther 63:1116–1120, 1983.
51. Cybulski, GR, Penn, RD, and Jaeger, RJ: Lower extremity functional neuromuscular stimulation in cases of spinal cord injury. Neurosurgery 15:132–146, 1984.
52. Bajd, T, Andrews, BJ, Kralj, A, et al: Restoration of walking in patients with incomplete spinal cord injuries by use of surface electrical stimulation—Preliminary results. Prosthet Orthot Int 9:109–111, 1985.
53. Mizrahi, J, Braun, Z, Najenson, T, et al: Quantitative weightbearing and gait evaluation of paraplegics using functional electrical stimulation. Med Biol Eng Comput 23:101–107, 1985.
54. Kralj, A, Bajd, T, Turk, R, et al: Results of FES application to 71 SCI patients. Rehabilitation Engineering Society of North America 10th Annual Conference, San Jose, CA, 645–647, 1987.
55. Scroggins, B, Scopp, R, Walker, JB, et al: FES controlled ambulation with surface electrodes and no orthotics. IEEE Engineering in Medicine and Biology Society 10th Annual International Conference, New Orleans, LA, 1575–1576, 1988.
56. Kralj, A, Bajd, T, and Turk, R: Enhancement of gait restoration in spinal injured patients by functional electrical stimulation. Clin Orthop 233:34–43, 1988.
57. Swartz, RS, Weed, HR, Pease, WS, et al: Lower extremity functional electrical stimulation with spinal cord injured subjects at the Ohio State University. IEEE Engineering in Medicine and Biology Society 11th Annual International Conference, Seattle, WA, pp 1693–1694, 1989.

58. Kralj, A, Trnkoczy, A, and Acimovic, R: Hemiplegic gait improvement by means of a three channel functional electrical stimulator. Elektrotehniski Vestnik a12–a15, 1971.
59. Kralj, A, Trnkoczy, A, and Acimovic, R: Improvement of locomotion in hemiplegic patients with multichannel electrical stimulation. In Human Locomotor Engineering. The Institution of Mechanical Engineers, London, 1974, pp 45–50.
60. Kralj, A and Vodovnik, L: Functional electrical stimulation of the extremities: part 2. J Med Eng Technol 1:75–80, 1977.
61. Stanic, U, Acimovic-Janezic, R, Gros, N, et al: Multichannel electrical stimulation for correction of hemiplegic gait. Scand J Rehabil Med 10:75–92, 1978.
62. Marsolais, EB: Engineering applications in orthotic and prosthetic treatment of musculoskeletal defects. Bulletin of Prosthetics Research 10:100–101, 1981.
63. Marsolais, EB and Kobetic, R: Functional walking in paralyzed patients by means of electrical stimulation. Clin Orthop 175:30–36, 1983.
64. Bogataj, U, Kljajic, M, Stanic, U, et al: Gait pattern behaviour of hemiplegic patients under the influence of a six-channel microprocessor stimulator in a real environment. Proceedings of the 2nd International Conference on Rehabilitation Engineering, Ottawa, Canada, 1984, pp 529–530.
65. Malazic, M, Bogataj, U, Gros, N, et al: Evaluation of gait with multichannel electrical stimulation. Orthopedics 10:769–772, 1987.
66. Campbell, J, Nakai, R, and Waters, RL: Epimysial electrical stimulation: Short-term therapeutic applications. RESNA 10th Annual Conference, San Jose, CA, 1987, pp 657–659.
67. Waters, RL, Campbell, JM, and Nakai, R: Therapeutic electrical stimulation of the lower limb by epimysial electrodes. Clin Orthop 233:44–52, 1988.
68. Bogataj, U, Gros, N, Malazic, M, et al: Restoration of gait during two to three weeks of therapy with multichannel electical stimulation. Phys Ther 69:319–327, 1989.
69. Marsolais, EB, Kobetic, R, Cochoff, GF, et al: Reciprocal walking in paraplegic patients using internal functional electrical stimulation. 6th Annual Conference on Rehabilitation Engineering, San Diego, CA, 78–80, 1983.
70. Marsolais, EB, Kobetic, R, Chizeck, H, et al: Improved synthetic walking in the paraplegic patient using implanted electrodes. Proceedings of the 2nd International Conference on Rehabilitation Engineering, Ottawa, Canada, 1984, pp 439–440.
71. Muccio, P and Marsolais, EB: Integration of orthoses with functional neuromuscular stimulation in parplegic subjects. RESNA 9th Annual Conference, Minneapolis, MN, 112–114, 1986.
72. Marsolais, EB: Implementing trunk control in FNS walking systems. RESNA 10th Annual Conference 611–612, 1987.
73. Kobetic, R, Marsolais, EB, and Chizeck, HJ: Control of kinematics in paraplegic gait by functional electrical stimulation. IEEE Engineering in Medicine & Biology Society, 10th Annual International Conference, New Orleans, LA, 1579, 1988.
74. Marsolais, EB and Kobetic, R: Development of a practical electrical stimulation system for restoring gait in the paralyzed patient. Clin Orthop 233:64–74, 1988.
75. McNeal, DR, Meadows, PM, Waters, RL, et al: A system for selection of modulated control sequences for functional electrical stimulation: An overall description. Proceedings of the 2nd International Conference on Rehabilitation Engineering, Ottawa, Canada, 525–526, 1984.
76. Kobetic, R, Pereira, M, and Marsolais, EB: Effect of muscle stimulation on weight shifting in paraplegics. RESNA 8th Annual Conference, Memphis, TN, 234–236, 1985.
77. Marsolais, EB, Kobetic, R, and Chizeck, H: Basic problems in development of FNS-aided crutch walking in the paraplegic individual. IEEE Engineering in Medicine & Biology Society, 10th Annual International Conference, New Orleans, LA, 1569–1570, 1988.
78. Marsolais, EB and Edwards, BG: Energy costs of walking and standing with functional neuromuscular stimulation and long leg braces. Arch Phys Med Rehabil 69:243–249, 1988.
79. Murray, MP, Kory, RC, Clarkson, BH, et al: Comparison of free and fast walking patterns of normal men. Am J Phys Med Rehabil 45:8–24, 1966.
80. Anderson, I, Parkinson, E, Scroggins, B, et al: FES for joint stabilization during stance phase of locomotion in spinal cord injured. IEEE Engineering in Medicine & Biology Society, 10th Annual International Conference, New Orleans, LA, 1571–1572, 1988.
81. Peckham, PH, Keith, MW, and Freehafer, AA: Restoration of functional control by electrical stimulation in the upper extremity of the quadriplegic patient. J Bone Joint Surg [Am] 70:144–148, 1988.
82. Gracanin, F and Dimitrijevic, MR: An electronic brace for externally controlled movement in wrist and fingers of the hemiparetic patient. Proceedings of Symposium on Electronics in Medicine, Ljubljana, 1968, pp 1–6.
83. Gracanin, F: Electrical stimulation as orthotic aid: Experiences and prospects. In Murdoch, G (ed): Prosthetic and Orthotic Practice. Edward Arnold, London, 1970, pp503–511.
84. Merletti, R, Acimovic, R, Grobelnik, S, et al: Electrophysiological orthosis for the upper extremity in hemiplegia: Feasibility study. Arch Phys Med Rehabil 56:507–513, 1975.
85. Vodovnik, L, Long, C, Reswick, JB, et al: Myo-electric control of paralyzed muscles. IEEE Trans Biomed Eng 12:169–172, 1965.

86. Peckham, PH, Marsolais, EB, and Mortimer, JT: Restoration of key grip and release in the C6 tetraplegic patient through functional electrical stimulation. J Hand Surg 5:462–469, 1980.
87. Nathan, RH: Electrostimulation of the upper limb: Programmed hand function. IEEE 8th Annual Conference of the Engineering in Medicine & Biology Society, Dallas, TX, 653–657, 1986.
88. Handa, Y, Handa, T, and Hoshimiya, N: A portable FNS system for the paralyzed extremities. IEEE 8th Annual Conference of the Engineering in Medicine & Biology Society, Dallas, TX, 658–660, 1986.
89. Bohs, L, McElhaney, J, Cooper, E, et al: A voice controlled FES system for restoring hand functions in quadriplegics. IEEE Engineering in Medicine & Biology Society, 10th Annual International Conference, New Orleans, LA, 1566, 1988.
90. Handa, Y, Ohkubo, K, and Hoshimiya, N: A portable multi-channel FES system for restoration of motor function of the paralyzed extremities. Automedica 11:221–231, 1989.
91. Peckham, Ph: Functional neuromuscular stimulation. Phys Technol 12:114–121, 1981.
92. Peckham, PH: Functional electrical stimulation: Current status and future prospects of applications to the neuromuscular system in spinal cord injury. Paraplegia 25:279–288, 1987.
93. Keith, MW, Peckham, PH, Thrope, GB, et al: Functional neuromuscular stimulation neuroprotheses for the tetraplegic hand. Clin Orthop 233:25–33, 1988.
94. Fukamachi, H, Handa, Y, Naito, A, et al: Improvement of finger movement by intrinsic muscles stimulation of the hand. IEEE 9th Annual Conference of the Engineering in Medicine and Biology Society, Boston, MA, 0361, 1987.
95. Stroh, KC, Thrope, GB, Wijman, JC, et al: Functional evaluation of FES hand grasp in C-5 And C-6 quadriplegics. Proceedings of the 4th Annual Applied Neural Control Research Day, Case Western Reserve University, Cleveland, OH, 1989, p 22.
96. Najenson, T and Pikielny, SS: Malignment of the glenohumeral joint following hemiplegia: A review of 500 cases. Annals of Physical Medicine 8:96–101, 1965.
97. Griffin, J, and Redpin, G: Shoulder pain in patients with hemiplegia. Phys Ther 61:1041, 1045, 1981.
98. Teppermann, PS, Greyson, ND, Hilbert, L, et al: Reflex sympathetic dystrophy in hemiplegia. Arch Phys Med Rehabil 65:442–447, 1984.
99. Anderson, LT: Shoulder pain in hemiplegia. Am J Occup Ther 39:11–19, 1985.
100. Baker, LL, and Parker, K: Neuromuscular electrical stimulation of the muscles surrounding the shoulder. Phys Ther 66:1930–1937, 1986.
101. Benton, LA, Baker, LL, Bowman, BR, et al: Functional Electrical Stimulation—A Practical Clinical Guide. Rancho Los Amigos Rehabilitation Engineering Center, Professional Staff Association, Downey, CA, 1981.
102. Peckham, PH, Mortimer, JT, and Marsolais, EB: Alteration in the force and fatigability of skeletal muscle in quadriplegic humans following exercise induced by chronic electrical stimulation. Clin Orthop 114:326–334, 1976.
103. Brindley, GS, Polkey, CE, and Rushton, DN: Electrical splinting of the knee in paraplegia. Paraplegia 16:428–435, 1978.
104. Kralj, A, Bajd, T, and Turk, R: The influence of electrical stimulation on muscle strength and fatigue in paraplegia. Proceedings of International Conference on Rehabilitation Engineering, Toronto, Canada, 1980, pp 223–226.
105. Gruner, JA, Glaser, RM, Feinberg, SD, et al: A system for evaluation and exercise-conditioning of paralyzed leg muscles. J Rehabil Res Dev 20:21–30, 1983.
106. Kiwerski, J, Weiss, M, and Pasniczek, R: Electrostimulation of the median nerve in tetraplegics by means of implanted stimulators. Paraplegia 21:322–326, 1983.
107. Robinson, CJ, Bolam, JM, Chinoy, M, et al: Response to surface electrical stimulation of the quadriceps in individuals with spinal cord injury. RESNA 9th Annual Conference, Minneapolis, MN, 282–284, 1986.
108. Nakai, RJ and McNeal, DR: Tetanic endurance and twitch moment of electically conditioned paralzyed muscle. RESNA 10th Annual Conference, San Jose, CA, 654–656, 1987.
109. Ragnarsson, KT, Pollack, S, O'Daniel, W, et al: Clinical evaluation of computerized functional electrical stimulation after spinal cord injury: A multicenter pilot study. Arch Phys Med Rehabil 69:672–677, 1988.
110. Gardner, ER, Triolo, RJ, and Betz, RR: Repeatability of isometric strength and endurance of the electrically stimulated quadriceps in children with spinal cord injuries. Phys Ther 69:369, 1989.
111. Baker, LL, Yeh, C, Wilson, D, et al: Electrical stimulation of wrist and fingers of hemiplegic patients. Phys Ther 59:1495–1499, 1979.
112. Bowman, BR, Baker, LL, and Waters, RL: Positional feeback and electrical stimulation: An automated treatment for the hemiplegic wrist. Arch Phys Med Rehabil 60:497–502, 1979.
113. Baker, LL, Parker, K, and Sanderson, K: Neuromuscular electrical stimulation for the head-injured patient. Phys Ther 63:1967–1974, 1983.
114. Bajd, T, Kralj, A, Turk, R, et al: FES rehabilitative approach in incomplete SCI patients. RESNA 9th Annual Conference, Minneapolis, MN, 316–318, 1986.
115. Servedio, FJ, Servedio, A, Davis, GM, et al: Voluntary strength gains in paretic muscle after hybrid (FNS-voluntary) exercise training. RESNA 10th Annual Conference, San Jose, CA, 594–596, 1987.

116. Fields, EW: Electromyographically triggered electric muscle stimulation for chronic hemiplegia. Arch Phys Med Rehab 68:407–414, 1987.
117. Milner-Brown, HS and Miller, RG: Muscle strengthening through electric stimulation combined with low-resistance weights in patients with neuromuscular disorders. Arch Phys Med Rehabil 69:20–24, 1988.
118. Murray, JD, Weed, HR, Pease, WS, et al: Lower extremity functional electrical stimulation in a cerebral palsy subject. IEEE Engineering in Medicine & Biology Society, 11th Annual International Conference, Seattle, WA, 1691–1692, 1989.
119. Kobetic, R, Carroll, SG, and Marsolais, EB: Functional electrical stimulation of hip extension and abduction affected by activity of the trunk. RESNA 10th Annual Conference, San Jose, CA, 618–620, 1987.
120. Granek, H and Granek, M: Transcutaneous transducer garments an advanced system of surface electrodes for functional electrical stimulation (FES). IEEE 9th Annual Conference of the Engineering in Medicine & Biology Society, Boston, MA, 0611–0612, 1987.
121. Smith, B, Peckham, PH, Keith, MW, et al: An externally powered, multichannel, implantable stimulator for versatile control of paralyzed muscle. IEEE Trans Biomed Eng 34:499–508, 1987.
122. Peckham, PH, Thrope, GB, and Marsolais, EB: Percutaneous intramuscular excitation of paralyzed skeletal muscle; Electrode reliability. 4th Annual Conference on Rehabilitation Engineering, Washington, DC, 1981, pp 229–231.
123. Marsolais, EB and Kobetic, R: Implantation techniques and experience with percutaneous intramuscular electrodes in the lower extremities. J Rehabil Res Dev 23:1–8, 1986.
124. McNeal, DR, Waters, R, and Reswick, J: Experience with implanted electrodes. Neurosurgery 1:228–229, 1977.
125. Stallard, J, Major, RE, and Patrick, JH: A review of the fundamental design problems of providing ambulation for paraplegic patients. Paraplegia 27:70–75, 1989.

CHAPTER 9

Effects of Acute Pressure on Peripheral Nerve Structure and Function

Arthur J. Nitz, Ph.D., P.T.

This chapter explores the effects of acute compression on peripheral nerves. Following a brief review of nerve structure and function, general features of compressive nerve lesions will be discussed with emphasis on the specific influence of tourniquet application as a model causative agent of such lesions. The impact of neuromuscular dysfunction resulting from nerve compression on clinical decision making and development of treatment regimens will also be discussed.

BASIC SCIENCE REVIEW

Peripheral Nerve Structure

A brief review of the general features of peripheral nerve structure and function is helpful for a better understanding of its response to acute compression. The anatomic and functional unit of the nervous system is the neuron, with its various processes or nerve fibers.[1] Although the term axon strictly applies to a single fiber that conducts neural impulses away from a nerve cell body, it has become common to refer to any long nerve fiber as an axon, regardless of the direction of conduction. Electron microscopy has clearly revealed that the axon has a typical trilaminar plasma membrane, or axolemma, which is intimately applied to the innermost Schwann cell membrane.[2] The axoplasm is replete with longitudinally oriented *neurofilaments* (average diameter 9.5 nm) and *microtubules* (average diameter 25 nm).[3] Less prominent, except near nodes of Ranvier, are *mitochondria*, which provide energy for metabolic activity such as axoplasmic transport (Fig. 9–1).

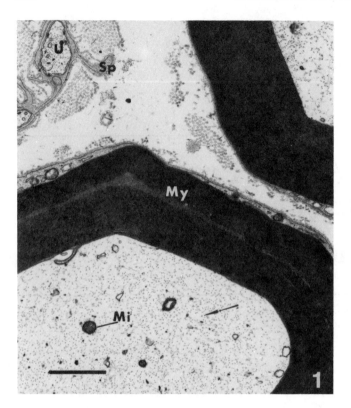

FIGURE 9–1. Electron micrograph cross section of myelinated (My) and unmyelinated (U) axons of a normal rat sciatic nerve. Sp = Schwann cell process; Mi = mitochondria; arrow = microtubules. (Scale bar = 2μm)

Schwann cells bear an intimate relation to axons, whether myelinated or unmyelinated, and subserve a structural and probably a metabolic support role.[4] Myelination of axons results from complex infolding by Schwann cell cytoplasm, the features of which have been delineated by electron microscopy and, at the molecular level, by x-ray diffraction analysis.[5] The consistent repeating lamellar structure of myelin is composed of two Schwann cell membranes (lipoprotein sheets) fused in such a way as to enclose a 2-nm gap that is continuous with the extracellular space.[5] Periodic interruption of myelin occurs where longitudinally sequential Schwann cells meet, forming the *node of Ranvier* (Fig. 9–2). In longitudinal section, this area appears constricted in diameter and is generally characterized by the presence of numerous adjacent mitochondria (Fig. 9–2).[6] The high concentration of sodium channels in this region is consistent with the fact that elevated levels of ionic exchange are known to occur here.[7]

Connective tissue sheaths invest entire nerve fibers (epineurium), fascicles (perineurium), and individual axons (endoneurium) (Fig. 9–3). The tough perineurium provides tensile strength for the nerve fascicles and therefore considerable protection from external trauma. However, nerve stretching has significant deleterious effects on blood delivery flowing through microscopic vessels embedded in the perineurium.[8a,8b] The perineurium also serves a blood-nerve barrier function, providing additional protection from the environment for the nerve.[9,10] Endoneurial fibroblasts are thought to be few but are responsible for producing most of the intraneural connective tissue (Fig. 9–4). Under normal conditions, the fibroblast cell processes are relatively short, and the cell concerns itself with steady-state connective tissue turnover, an essentially maintenance function. This is subject to substantial alteration when the

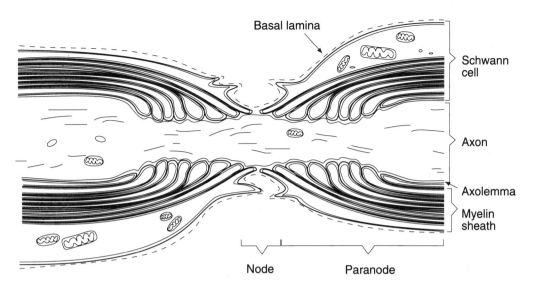

FIGURE 9–2. A node of Ranvier. This diagram represents a typical myelinated axon, which is narrowed at each node of Ranvier. The annular space around the nodal axon is delimited by the basal lamina, the axolemma, and the specialized Schwann cell projections and contains "gap substance," which maintains an ionically active pool of sodium ions for nodal depolarization during saltatory conduction. (From Terzis, JK and Smith, KL: The Peripheral Nerve: Structure, Function, and Reconstruction. Raven Press, New York, 1990, p. 14, with permission.)

nerve is injured. Some investigators contend that the Schwann cells play a role in inducing polymerization of tropocollagen into collagen.[11]

Under normal circumstances, mast cells appear to be quite numerous in *epineural* connective tissue although sparsely distributed *endoneurially*.[12] This differential distribution is altered dramatically when the nerve is injured so that the *endoneurial* mast cell population is markedly increased.[13] The mast cell's normal position, adjacent to blood vessels, along with its numerous biologically active constituent substances (histamine, heparin, serotonin), suggests its possible involvement in postinjury neurogenic edema.[14]

Normal peripheral nerve *function* is largely dependent on sufficient oxygenation from an *extrinsic* vascular system and an *intrinsic* microvascular system. These two vascular systems are integrated but functionally independent, so that complete elimination of the extrinsic system does not necessarily obliterate intraneural nutrition or function,[14,15] because a dynamic vascular plexus in all layers (epineural, perineural, endoneural) can reroute blood through collaterals between layers and between different nerve segments. Periosteal vessels and muscular perforating arteries also contribute to intraneural blood flow when the extrinsic system is embarrassed or eliminated.[14,15] Endoneurial endothelial cells possess tight junctions, rendering the intraneural microvasculature essentially impermeable to proteins.[16] As stated previously, the perineurium also serves as a hindrance to circulating proteins and works jointly with the lining cells of the endoneurial vessels to provide a blood-nerve barrier.[16] Trauma from nerve (limb) compression results in functional deterioration of this barrier and resultant exposure of the nerve to pathologically altered hemodynamics and abnormal intraneural microvascular flow patterns.[14]

The *structural* unit of the nerve (neuron) and muscle (muscle fiber) together form the *functional* unit of the neuromuscular system—*the motor unit*, which is composed

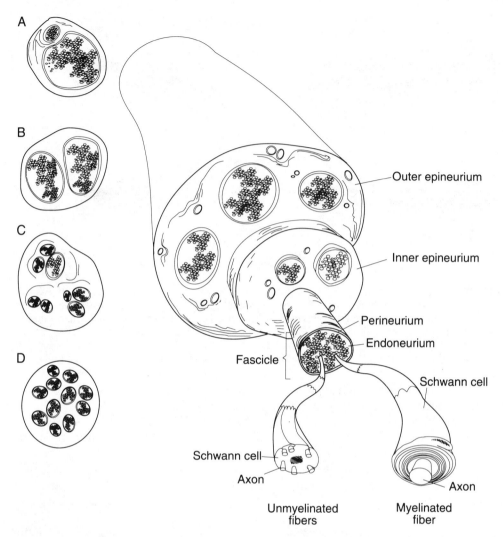

FIGURE 9–3. A peripheral nerve architecture. The connective tissue elements consist of the endoneurium, the perineurium, and the inner and outer epineurium. Individual fascicles contain a heterogeneous mix of myelinated and unmyelinated fibers, but some fascicles demonstrate a preponderance of one type. Basic patterns of intraneural structure are demonstrated. A peripheral nerve is considered monofascicular if it holds one large fascicle *(A)* or oligofascicular for a few large fascicles *(B)*. Polyfascicular nerves consist of many fascicles, which may be grouped *(C)*, or there may be no identifiable group patterns *(D)*. (From Terzis, JK and Smith, KL: The Peripheral Nerve: Structure, Function, and Reconstruction. Raven Press, New York, 1990, p. 16, with permission.)

of the anterior horn cell, its axon, and all muscle fibers innervated by that axon. There is considerable variability in the number of muscle fibers per motor unit (innervation ratio), so that large limb muscles, such as the gastrocnemius, have both far more absolute motor units than do most smaller muscles, and a larger mean number of muscle fibers per motor nerve.[17] Functionally this configuration affords greater precision of movement to small muscles (fewer number of muscle fibers per motor unit), which generally perform more discrete activities than do the larger muscles (greater number of fibers per motor unit) that perform more gross movements. Animal studies

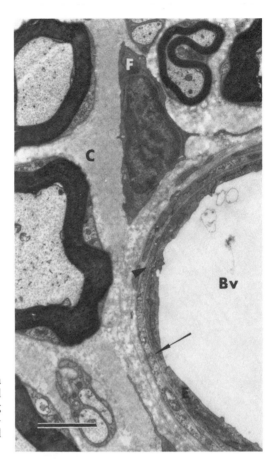

FIGURE 9–4. Electron micrograph from a normal rat sciatic nerve depicting endoneurial fibroblast (F), collagen (C), normal-appearing blood vessel (Bv), endothelial cell (E), and basement membrane (*arrow*). (Scale bar in this and subsequent figures = 3µm.)

have also revealed an interesting motor unit spatial arrangement characterized by extensive intermingling of muscle fibers of different motor units.[18] Because of such overlap, nerve compression must be substantial before evidence of a muscle strength or endurance deficit is clinically recognizable.[19] This fact often makes detection of nerve compression difficult and underscores the need for sophisticated testing of muscle-nerve activity to document otherwise subclinical nerve compression syndromes. Such documentation can be provided, in part, by electrophysiologic testing and possibly by computerized dynamometry.

Peripheral Nerve Function

Nerve tissue has the unique ability to both produce and propagate electrical messages in the form of *action potentials*.[20] Skeletal muscle can conduct electrical signals but is unable to initiate such messages independently. The basis for production and conduction of electrical signals in biologic tissue is the difference in concentration across the cell membrane of the major monovalent ions—potassium (K^+), sodium (Na^+), and chloride (Cl^-). The cell membrane is designed to permit selective permeability of these ions in such a way that unequal distribution of net charge results in a transmembrane potential difference (e.g., the membrane is approximately 50 times more permeable to K^+ than it is to Na^+) (Fig. 9–5). The internal negativity is maintained over time at a steady state (resting membrane potential) by virtue of active transport of Na^+ from inside to outside the cell, and of K^+ from outside to inside (sodium-potassium pump). The active chemical pump expends metabolic energy in the form of high-energy phosphate bonds derived from adenosine triphosphate (ATP).[21] The cell membrane of nerve and muscle fibers therefore serves to separate and insulate the intracellular and extracellular fluids and effectively stores a measurable electrical charge, the resting membrane potential. The membrane potential has been *calculated* to be about −90 mV in giant-squid axons (interior of the cell negative with respect to the extracellular space), and when directly measured by micropipette electrode, to range between −70 mV and −90 mV.[20]

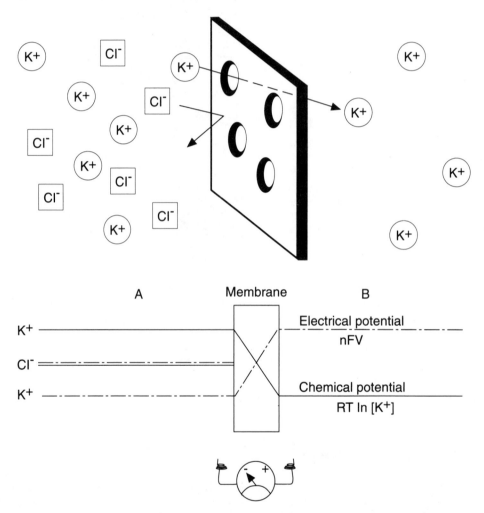

FIGURE 9–5. A semipermeable membrane that allows passage of only positive ions will result in the generation of a transmembrane potential when it is placed between two salt solutions of differing concentrations. The movement of positive ions down their concentration gradient will result in a separation of charges across the membrane, producing a potential gradient that tends to retard movement of the positive ion. At equilibrium, forces due to concentration and potential gradients on the positive ions balance exactly, and no net ion movement occurs. (From Barchi, RL,[20] p. 6, with permission.)

Not only does the nerve (and muscle) cell membrane have the ability to store charge, but it is also excitable. That is, sufficient change in membrane permeability results in local, nonpropagated depolarizing response. If the increase in voltage across the nerve cell membrane exceeds a threshold value of about -55 mV, an "all-or-none," self-perpetrating *action potential* will ensue (Fig. 9–6). This electrical event lasts 1 to 2 milliseconds and is characterized by a rapid reversal of the normal ionic permeability of the membrane to Na^+ and K^+. The spontaneous recovery back to a steady-state resting membrane potential occurs about as quickly as the depolarization itself.

Because action potentials are "propagated," they are continuous. Activation (depolarization) of one portion of the cell membrane leads to a bidirectional, longitudinal spread of current to the adjacent membrane. The net result is a nondecremental, progressive depolarization along the entire length of the axon, followed by spontaneous recovery.

Whereas this brief generic description of depolarization and recovery holds true for unmyelinated axons and muscle fibers, a different mechanism of conduction is at work with myelinated nerve fibers. As mentioned previously, myelin is wrapped radially around axons and is interrupted at the nodes of Ranvier. Nodal regions of the membrane represent a low-resistance pathway to current flow compared with the higher resistance offered by the myelin-wrapped, internodal axon.[20(p33)] Consequently, the locally generated action potential "jumps" from one node to the adjacent inactive node and is referred to as *saltatory conduction*. This form of impulse propagation increases conduction velocity and conserves space while minimizing energy requirements, in that action potentials are only occurring at the nodes of Ranvier.[20(p34–36)]

EFFECTS OF ACUTE COMPRESSION ON NERVE STRUCTURE AND FUNCTION

Pressure on anatomically vulnerable peripheral nerves may result in functional disorders, depending on the precise site of the injury and the severity of the mechanical distortion or ischemia.[22] The extent of functional or structural alteration provides a basis for classification of peripheral nerve injuries as well as information about recovery. Seddon[23,24] proposed the term *neurapraxia* to refer to a local nerve conduction block whose anatomic basis was a discrete demyelination without loss of axonal continuity or Wallerian degeneration. This description was to be distinguished from a *rapidly reversible physiologic block*, which most people have encountered when their arm or leg "goes to sleep" and then recovers immediately following restoration of blood supply to the nerve.[25] Denny-Brown and Brenner[26] were the first to provide experimental evidence that a neurapraxic lesion produced by compressive force is characterized by local demyelination without Wallerian degeneration. Further investigation, using a pneumatic-tourniquet animal model, has revealed that acute pressure of sufficient proportion produces displacement of the node of Ranvier that includes stretching of paranodal myelin on one side of the node and invagination of paranodal myelin on the other.[27]

Examples of neurapraxic lesions include so-called *Saturday night palsy* (radial nerve compression at the spiral groove of the humerus) and *tourniquet palsy*.[22] Clinical features include paralysis or marked reduction in muscle strength in a specific distribution

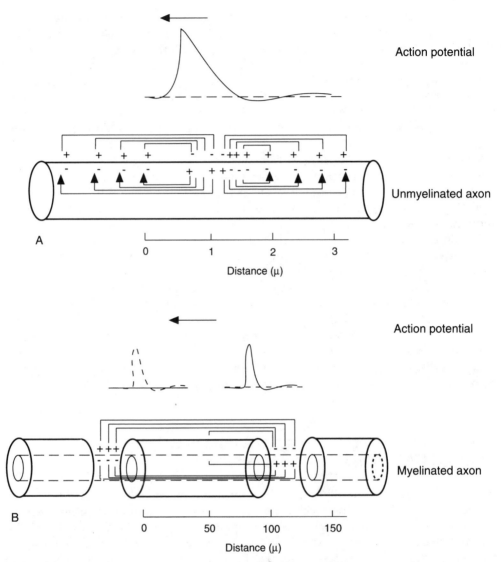

FIGURE 9–6. Propagation of the action potential. *(A)*, In unmyelinated nerve fibers, local currents flowing as the result of depolarization of a small patch of membrane during an action potential produce depolarization and activation of immediately adjacent membrane. Conduction takes place by sequential activation of adjacent membrane regions in a continuous fashion that involves the entire surface membrane. *(B)*, In myelinated fibers, action potential generation is confined to the nodal membrane. Local currents spread along the internode due to the excellent passive properties contributed by the myelin, and exit mainly through the low-resistance pathway provided by the next nodal region. Here depolarization and activation result in another action potential, although the intervening internodal membrane has not been activated. (From Barchi, RL,[20] p. 33, with permission.)

distal to the lesion. Sensation below the level of the lesion may be similarly affected. Nerve *conduction* across the suspected site of lesion is slowed or absent, whereas conduction through nerve segments above and below the lesion is normal. In a similar fashion, *amplitude* of motor and sensory action potentials will be reduced or absent with stimulation at or about the nerve injury, but normal when the nerve is electrically excited below the lesion. Since, classically, no Wallerian degeneration occurs with a neurapraxia, one would not expect to find EMG evidence of denervation (positive sharp waves, fibrillations) in affected muscles, although volitional recruitment of motor units (interference pattern) would be reduced or absent. Consequently, the prognosis for an individual who has sustained such an injury is generally good, in that the anatomic and physiologic abnormality recovers in weeks to months.[22]

The term *axonotmesis* was introduced by Seddon[23,24] to describe a nerve lesion produced by severe compression or stretching that results in "loss of axonal continuity" but leaves the endoneurial connective tissue sheath intact. An alternative classification scheme proposed by Sunderland[28,29] delineates, within this major category, between those injuries in which the endoneurium, perineurium, or epineurium is preserved. At or distal to the site of lesion, axons and myelin sheaths begin to degenerate within 48 hours of a severe injury, resulting in nerve abnormalities described as Wallerian degeneration. Subcellular organelles such as neurofilaments, microtubules, and mitochondria undergo either fragmentation or swelling (Fig. 9–7). This process appears to be under the direction of a calcium-activated enzyme located in the axoplasm.[30] Schwann cells proliferate and are largely responsible for phagocytosis and degradation of both axon and myelin debris, a process nearly completed 2 to 3

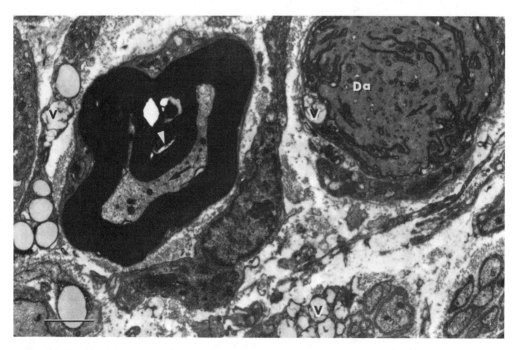

FIGURE 9–7. Sciatic nerve from an animal 1 week after tourniquet compression of 400 mm Hg for 2 hours. Note degenerative state of myelin *(arrowhead)* and axons (Da) and the numerous vacuoles (V). Many neurofilaments *(circled area)* are seen in this axoplasm (compare with the number of neurofilaments in circled areas of Fig. 9–1).

weeks following injury (Fig. 9–8).[31] Nerve compression injury stimulates a progressive increase in collagen content reflected, in part, by an elevated number of intraneural fibroblasts[13] (Fig. 9–9). These fibroblasts appear to be metabolically very active (producing collagen) by virtue of the abundant rough endoplasmic reticulum and the long cell processes (Fig. 9–9).

The effect of the additional intraneural connective tissue is to reduce the endoneurial tubes to as little as 10 to 20 percent of their original diameter during the first 3 months following denervation.[29,32] The abundant collagen and reduced endoneurial tube caliber may present a complication to ensuing attempts by the proximal nerve segment to bridge the nerve injury site with axonal sprouts. In addition to changes distal to the level of the injury, axonal degeneration of a similar nature may proceed up to several centimeters proximal to an axonometic nerve injury.

After axonometic nerve injury, the cell bodies located in either the dorsal root ganglion (sensory) or anterior horn of the spinal cord (motor) undergo a process called *chromatolysis*.[22] The features of this reaction include cell body swelling, proliferation of glial cells, eccentric displacement of nerve cell nucleus and loss of Nissl substance compact arrangement. All these events peak by the seventh postinjury day. Cell body reaction is reflective of metabolic preparation for replacement of the axoplasmic volume lost in the injury. Specifically, a marked increase in protein synthesis directed by RNA-containing material accounts for the elevated cell volume and change in light microscopic staining characteristics.[33]

As the axoplasmic cytoskeleton of the distal nerve segment continues to disintegrate (Wallerian degeneration), axons in the proximal stump produce an excessive number of terminal and collateral sprouts, which grow at an average rate (in humans) of 1 mm per day across the zone of injury toward the distal nerve segment.[22] This growth rate of nerve sprouts conforms, roughly, to the rate of *slow* axoplasmic transport.[34] Some of these sprouts may be misdirected toward intraneural collagen or extraneurally to produce neuromas.[22] However, others, guided by a Schwann cell column, may align themselves with original endoneurial tubes and eventually make contact with the peripheral target organ (muscle fiber or sensory receptor).[22]

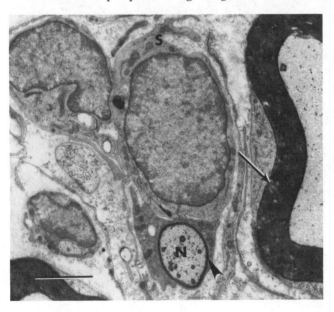

FIGURE 9–8. Electron micrograph of sciatic nerve 3 weeks after epineurectomy showing large Schwann cell (S); small, thinly myelinated nerve fibers (*arrowhead*); and neurofilaments (N). Myelin of large nerve fibers is still disrupted (*arrow*). Small-diameter unmyelinated and thinly myelinated fibers are probably terminal or collateral sprouts.

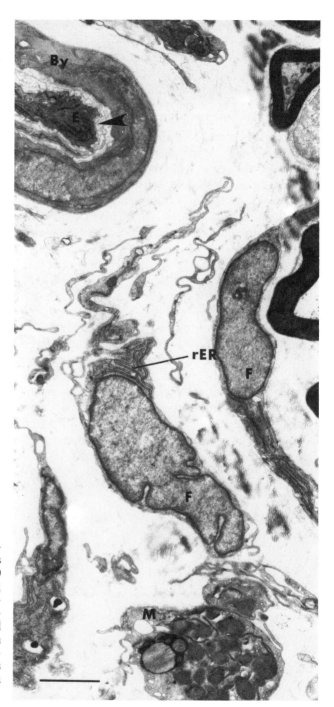

FIGURE 9–9. Electron micrograph of rat sciatic nerve 3 weeks after tourniquet compression of 400 mm Hg for 1 hour. F = fibroblast; rER = rough endoplasmic reticulum; M = mast cell; Bv = abnormal blood vessel; E = endothelial cell; basement membrane region *(arrowhead)*. Note numerous fibroblasts and many long and tortuous cell processes, believed to be a response to nerve injury.

The growth cone at the distal end of each sprout appears to be significantly influenced by the presence of chemotaxic agents such as nerve growth factor (NGF), which seems to exert a regulating effect on the extent and direction of axonal regenration.[35-37] Diffusible substances from Schwann cells or nerve tissue are probably responsible for a tissue specificity such that growing nerve sprouts are preferentially attracted to target tissue of neural origin.[38,39] Also, *contact guidance* appears to be offered to the axonal growth cone by the surfaces of certain cells in the target area.[22]

Clinical examples of axonotmesis include severe peripheral nerve contusions or spinal nerve root compression (SNRC) by the nucleus pulposus of an intervertebral disc, which results in a partially denervated limb. Clinical findings include muscle weakness or paralysis and sensory loss in a specific distribution below the level of the lesion. Conduction of neural impulses *across* the injury site are lost immediately, whereas motor and sensory conduction usually fails below the lesion within several days of the insult.[28] In cases of partial denervation (i.e., SNRC), conduction velocity is often normal, but the amplitude of evoked motor or sensory response is reduced, suggesting a functional or structural loss of excitable axons. Electromyographic examination of involved muscles between 14 and 21 days postinjury reveals electrical evidence of membrane instability resulting from denervation; that is, fibrillations and positive sharp waves (Fig. 9–10). Volitional recruitment of motor units may be reduced or absent shortly after injury and may take months to return to normal. Axonotmesis is associated with considerable muscle atrophy and results from a reduction in protein synthesis and myofibrillar volume as well as an elevated rate of muscle degradation.[40] Although the rate of muscle atrophy varies across species, some limb muscles may undergo as much as a 50 percent reduction in weight within 2 weeks of denervation.[41] In addition to grossly observable muscle atrophy, denervation also produces a decreased resting potential at the motor end plate and hypersensitivity of muscle membrane to acetylcholine (ACh), mainly because ACh receptors appear outside the normal end plate region.[42-44]

The prognosis for an individual with an axonotmetic nerve injury is dependent on a host of factors but is generally quite good so long as the endoneurial tubes have been preserved. When the endoneurium or perineurium is deranged by the injury, intraneural scar formation and loss of all guiding elements of the nerve trunk result in profound axonal misdirection and ultimate failure of end organ reinnervation.

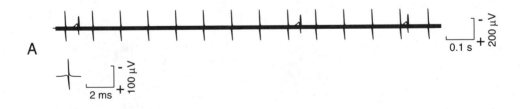

FIGURE 9–10. *(A)*, fibrillation potentials recorded at slow and fast sweep speeds. *(B)*, typical positive sharp waves. (From Goodgold, J: Electrodiagnosis of Neuromuscular Diseases, ed 3. Williams & Wilkins, Baltimore, 1983, p. 99, with permission.)

Neurotmesis denotes a nerve injury characterized by loss of axonal *and all* connective tissue continuity.[23,28] Although a severe crush mechanism can produce such a lesion, it is usually the result of rapid stretch/avulsion or complete serverance of the nerve. As with axonotmesis, Wallerian degeneration predominates during the first few weeks after injury, and clinical findings are similar to those described for the previous nerve injury category. Unlike axonotmesis, the complete disruption of axonal and connective tissue elements renders a very poor prognosis. Surgical repair is required for virtually any chance of recovery, but when accomplished, often results in a neuroma formation or aberrant reinnervation pattern. Complete severance is uncommon following most acute nerve compressions, so no further discussion of neurotmesis will be included in this review.

TOURNIQUET-INDUCED NERVE COMPRESSION

Although one might think from the preceding description that nerve injuries occur as categorical events, they rarely present as such in a clinical setting. For instance, the usual understanding is that conduction block (neurapraxia) causes muscle weaknesses or paralysis *without* significant muscle atrophy and usually with sparing of sensation.[45,46] Yet one of the interesting features of acute nerve compression palsies in humans (e.g., tourniquet palsy, thought to be a neurapraxia) is that they are usually attended by profound muscle wasting that lasts for months.[45,46] For obvious reasons, investigation of injuries of this nature is not always possible in human experiments. However, a number of animal studies provide information regarding this topic.

The pneumatic tourniquet seems to be the implement of choice for many investigators who examine the effect of pressure on peripheral nerves, because a discrete, quantifiable amount of force can be applied to the limb for a specified time using such devices. Previous animal models have used tourniquet pressures far in excess of the usual clinical range (200 to 500 mm Hg) in an effort to simulate the situation in patients characterized by a *complete* conduction block after cuff application for extremity surgery.[27,47,48] Ochoa and colleagues[27] applied a pneumatic tourniquet to baboon hind limbs with a pressure of 1000 mm Hg for 1 to 3 hours and found electron microscopic evidence of longitudinal displacement of the nodes of Ranvier by as much as 300 μm from their usual position under Schwann cell junctions. This lesion was found to be most prominent under the proximal edge of the cuff, affecting all the large myelinated fibers at this site. These investigators concluded that this anatomic lesion in animals was correlated with, and probably explained, the physiologic finding of prolonged conduction block after tourniquet application reported for some patients.[27]

Although complications following routine tourniquet application in patients are well recognized, the reported incidence of tourniquet paralysis is currently very rare.[49,50] The incidence of tourniquet *paresis* is unknown because it is not reported as such in the literature. Recent clinical studies, however, which included electromyographic (EMG) evaluation following extremity surgery performed with cuff application (200 to 450 mm Hg) have identified a 60 to 85 percent incidence of electrical abnormalities (positive sharp waves, fibrillation potentials), suggesting electrical evidence of Wallerian degeneration (axonotmesis).[51–53] The percentage of electrical abnormalities appears noteworthy because none of these individuals experienced a nerve conduction deficit (i.e., block delay), which, as previously indicated, is considered one of the hallmark signs of tourniquet-induced neurapraxia. Many of these patients with denervation also encountered severe muscle atrophy and delayed functional recovery after surgery, which seemed to be related to the denervation and consequent weakness.[51-53] In one study, patients who had tourniquet application for knee arthrotomy (meniscectomy) were tested for functional capacity 6 weeks postoperatively by expressing their single-leg vertical leap on the operated side as a percentage of that accomplished by the nonoperated side.[53] Those patients who had limb denervation following cuff pressure had a 40 percent functional capacity compared to a 70 to 80 percent capability for those patients *without* evidence of nerve injury. This method of functional testing seems somewhat unsophisticated when compared to that offered by computerized dynamometry. However, caution has recently been recommended when attempting to make clinical inferences from measurements generated by isokinetic devices.[54] Noteworthy is a recent study in which patients were examined electromyographically and isokinetically following knee arthrotomy with tourniquet application, that revealed somewhat similar results.[55] Patients with postoperative tourniquet-induced denervation had isokinetic torques for the involved limb that were roughly 20 to 40 percent of that accomplished by nonoperated thigh muscles. Conversely, those without denervation had isokinetic torque for the operated leg that ranged from 40 to 70 percent of the uninvolved limb.

The motor impairment and electrical evidence of denervation without nerve conduction block or delay experienced by these patients suggests that an *axonotmesis was present without a coincident neurapraxia*. This observation may possibly explain why some patients with symptoms of a chronic compressive neuropathy, such as carpal tunnel syndrome, occasionally have EMG evidence of thenar muscle denervation without the usual prolongation of distal motor and sensory latencies.[56] Other animal experiments have shown that acute pressure palsy often causes a "mixed" nerve lesion with conduction block (neurapraxia) in some axons and complete degeneration in others, with some small axons spared (sensation, autonomic function).[45a]

These clinical reports suggest that EMG evidence of denervation may be a more sensitive indicator of potential motor deficits following acute peripheral nerve compression than results of standard nerve conduction studies. A recent investigation indicates that integrated motor unit activity and recruitment characteristics are even *more* sensitive than standard diagnostic needle electromyography.[55] Krebs[55] reported that *all* postoperative tourniquet-aided knee arthrotomy patients had *severe* impairment in smoothed, rectified, and integrated EMG amplitude during 5- to 10-second isometric contractions.[55] However, only 53 percent of the 38 patients studied in his series had denervation potentials (positive sharp waves, fibrillations, and bizarre high-frequency discharges). He concluded that routine tourniquet use for extremity surgery causes a subtle disturbance in muscle-nerve interaction resulting in clinically significant limb function deficits in most, if not all, patients so treated. Further, EMG analysis and computerized dynamometry have provided information that standard clinical examination of such patients does not yield.[55,57]

Although this information from clinical reports contributed significantly to our understanding of the features of acute nerve compression and its functional consequences, several questions were left unanswered. Specifically, the results of clinical investigations did not clearly identify whether magnitude of cuff pressure or duration of application was primarily responsible for the observed nerve injury. In addition, debate continues about the relative contribution of nerve ischemia and direct mechanical pressure in producing this nerve deficit.[14,45a] It is nearly impossible to separate mechanical and ischemic etiologic factors because all compression forces necessarily include an ischemic component by virtue of nerve microvessel obliteration.

To address questions raised by the apparent tourniquet-induced nerve injury identified in clinical reports of postoperative patients but not answered by previous animal experiments, another model was developed in our laboratory.[13,58,59] Using *clinically relevant* tourniquet pressures (200 to 400 mm Hg) and times (1 to 3 hours), large numbers of animals (rats) were studied at various periods of time after pneumatic cuff application. Parallel motor function and physiologic and structural methods of analysis (light and electron microscopy) were used after animals had been subjected to tourniquet compression. We found that animals exhibited ambulation deficits and other motor deficits for 1 to 5 weeks after cuff application. Coincident EMG evidence of denervation (positive sharp waves, fibrillations, bizarre high-frequency discharges) was also noted, but not attended by nerve conduction delay.[59] Electron microscopic examination of these nerves revealed the expected evidence of Wallerian degeneration including disrupted myelin, degenerate axons, and numerous vacuoles. In addition, in these same nerves we identified a significant increase in mast cells and fibroblasts, as well as disrupted endothelial cells of endoneurial vessels[13] (Figs. 9–8, 9–11, 9–12). Because mast cells are believed to be involved in edema formation and vascular permeability, their presence in elevated numbers in nerves subjected to tourniquet compression suggested a mechanism of injury alluded to, but not specifically reported in, the literature. Cuff compression appears to cause mechanical damage to the endoneurial and perineurial vessel wall, resulting in elevated vascular permeability. Mast cells degranulate, which may recruit additional mast cells to the area. This attraction of mast cells may result in maintenance of the increased vascular permeability. Prolonged nerve ischemia probably results from persistent elevation of intrafascicular pressure, which causes significant metabolite deprivation in turn, leading to nerve fiber degeneration. Thus nerve injury produced by the pneumatic tourniquet inflated to pressures within the clinical range may result from mechanical forces eliciting intraneural edema, microvessel obliteration, and consequent prolonged ischemia. Neurapraxia (conduction block) does not appear to be a routine feature of such a nerve injury unless tourniquet pressures far in excess of the normal clinical limit are used.[13] Spared nerve fibers apparently continue to conduct electrical signals normally, although other axons undergo changes consistent with Wallerian degeneration.

RECOVERY FROM ACUTE NERVE COMPRESSION

Fortunately, peripheral nerve tissue has been endowed with the ability to recover from most episodes of compression, although not always spontaneously. A frequent clinical observation after surgical division of the transverse carpal ligament is the almost immediate amelioration of sensory symptoms (pain, numbness, tingling) in patients. When compared with the tissue pressure required to produce an *acute* conduction block, the pressure that results in a condition such as carpal syndrome (a more chronic entrapment neuropathy) is quite low.

An unfortunate aspect of acute, severe nerve compression lesions is the *delay* in restoration of function following injury. When myelin disruption (neurapraxia) accounts for a nerve conduction block (limb paralysis), resumption of electrical impulses through the lesion depends on the time course for the most slowly recovering paranodal block.[45,45a,46] Clinical and experimental reports have indicated that this return may

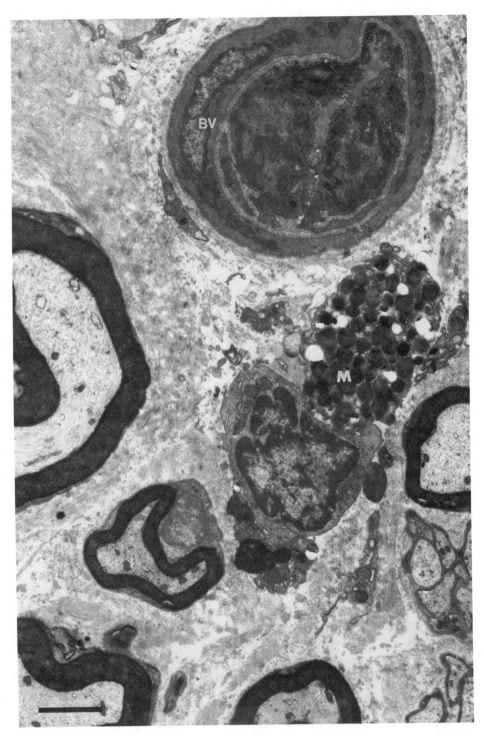

FIGURE 9–11. Sciatic nerve from an animal 1 week after tourniquet treatment of 300 mm Hg for 1 hour showing mast cell (M), blood vessel (Bv), endothelial cell (E), and basement membrane *(arrow)*.

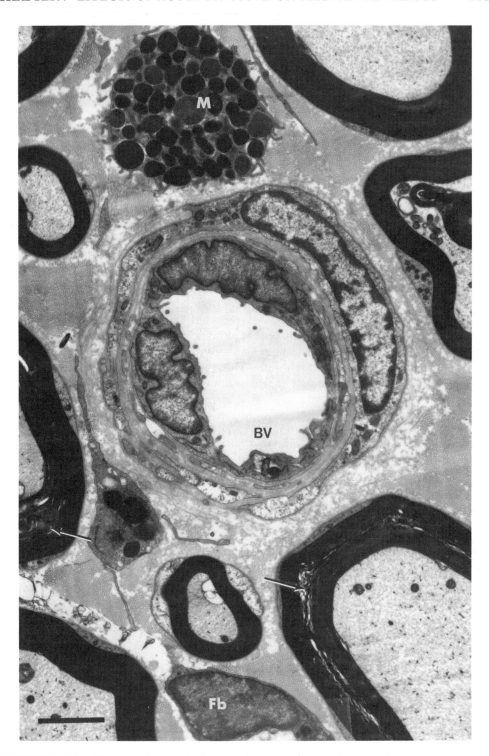

FIGURE 9–12. Electron micrograph from sciatic nerve 6 weeks after tourniquet compression of 400 mm Hg for 2 hours. M = mast cell; Bv = blood vessel; Fb = fibroblast; mild myelin disruption *(arrow)*.

take several months and is related to the length of the initial area of damage and number of affected nodes of Ranvier.[45a,46] For instance, Rudge and associates[45a] demonstrated that the demyelination resulting from a weighted (1.6 to 2.1 kg/cm^2) 1.6-mm nylon cord compressing the nerve recovered more quickly than that produced by a 5.5-cm pneumatic tourniquet (1000 mm Hg) when pressures for the two methods were normalized.[45a]

Recovery following the less severe nerve compression associated with routine tourniquet application (200 to 400 mm Hg) is quite lengthy.[53] Although not attended by complete conduction block (paralysis), EMG abnormalities (denervation potentials) persist for 3 to 6 months postcompression.[53] Whether functional deficits specifically related to the limb denervation following tourniquet-aided limb arthrotomy persist beyond the 6-month period are not well known. However, a 1-year follow-up study of patients who underwent anterior cruciate ligament reconstruction revealed deficits of 10 to 15 percent in quadriceps femoris muscle volume (as shown by computerized tomography [CT]) and isokinetic torque production.[60] Because the standard of care for extremity surgery is a tourniquet-induced "bloodless field," it is assumed (but not known!) that these persistent deficits may be related to the long-standing effects of peripheral nerve compression. A 5- to 10-year follow-up study of similar patients has identified deficits nearly identical to those reported for the 1-year follow-up group.[61] From these studies one may postulate that although the majority of limb muscle and joint function returns to presurgery levels within the first year, possibly some level of functional deficit persists indefinitely. This residual function deficit may be due, in part, to the effect of tourniquet compression on muscle-nerve structure and function.

Experimental and clinical research indicates that *severe* acute nerve compression (e.g., "Saturday night palsy"; rare tourniquet *paralysis*) causes a combinatin of neurapraxia and axonotmesis, recovery from which takes several months. More commonly, however, less intense nerve pressure, such as that produced by routine tourniquet application, causes a non-neurapraxic, axonotmesis that also prolongs recovery time and muscle-joint rehabilitation for several months. The impact of such nerve involvement on the course of rehabilitation is the next topic for discussion.

CLINICAL DEVELOPMENT AND CLINICAL DECISION MAKING

Developing a rehabilitation protocol for a patient with a suspected compressive nerve lesion requires careful documentation of a thorough history, physical examination, and, in most cases, electrophysiologic testing procedures. The results of such evaluation can then be analyzed and interpreted so that a rehabilitation plan can be implemented to meet the short- and long-term goals set for the patient. Underlying this need for careful evaluation and documentation of findings is the fact that the rehabilitation plan formulated for patients with denervation should be different from that for patients without muscle-nerve abnormalities.

Clinical evaluation of patients with complete or nearly complete conduction block (e.g., "Saturday night palsy"; tourniquet *paralysis*) will usually reveal evidence of limb atrophy below the level of the lesion, depending on the length of time postinsult. This limb atrophy is also true for patients who may have sustained a less severe limb (nerve) compression (e.g., tourniquet paresis). As noted previously, this observation suggests that such patients may have sustained a nerve injury including both neu-rapraxic and axonotmetic components. The usual method for documenting atrophy is by circumferential girth measurements, which do not provide information about the various tissue components of the limb. Because our interest in measuring girth is to obtain a rough estimate of the amount of muscle atrophy, one should combine such *quantitative* (girth) measurements with some attempt to identify the ability of the limb muscles to contract. Palpation of the limb for muscle turgidity at rest and during an isometric contraction is an unsophisticated means of accomplishing this task, because no means of grading the turgidity are available. Cross-sectional com-puterized CT and ultrasonography of the limb offer a more precise (and objective) method of determining tissue composition.[60,62,63] An example of using CT follows.

One to 2 months after medial collateral ligament injury and repair (mean tour-niquet time = 60 minutes), CT scan revealed a 30 percent *reduction* in quadriceps femoris muscle volume and a concomitant 21 percent *increase* in thigh fat volume for 84 athletes.[63a] CT of thigh muscles *1 year* after anterior cruciate ligament reconstruction demonstrated a continued 10 to 15 percent deficit in *quadriceps femoris muscle* size compared with the nonoperated leg in another series of 13 athletes.[60] This finding is particularly noteworthy because circumferential girth measurements failed to identify any significant size differential when operated and unoperated thighs were measured in the 13 athletes. Limb assessment by CT scan or ultrasonography is known to be prohibitively expensive as a routine measure.

Clinical examination of patients for sensory disturbances is also indicated when attempting to discover whether a patient has incurred an acute nerve compression. In many cases, sensory modalities of crude and light touch and pinprick are spared, not because large diameter myelinated fibers are unaffected but rather because of minimal effect of acute nerve compression and ischemia on small myelinated and nonmyelinated afferents. However, careful mapping of response to vibration and two-point discrimination stimuli often reveals subtle evidence of diminished sensory competency in either a dermatomal pattern suggestive of SNRC, or one of autonomous peripheral nerve distribution.

Muscle weakness often accompanies muscle atrophy and may conform to a myotomal or specific peripheral nerve pattern. It is hoped that clinicians will readily recognize cases of complete conduction block resulting in transient limb paralysis. With less severe nerve compression, however, *partial* denervation may occur; such a condition is not always identified with ease during clinical muscle testing. One clue that suggests a partial denervation strength deficit may be present when *passive* range of motion (PROM) is found to be considerably greater than *active* range of motion (AROM). One recognizes, however, that *small* differences between these two are normally present for most joints. Of course other factors, such as connective tissue restriction and muscle length–tension insufficiency, may also be responsible for this finding. Precisely at this point, the EMG examination is useful for determining whether partial muscle denervation is the primary cause for a significant PROM-AROM dif-ferential. When capsular restriction is noted (PROM equals AROM) coincident dener-vation should not be eliminated from consideration.

Another evidence of strength deficit that may result from partial denervation is rapid muscle fatigability. A patient with such a lesion may still be able to recruit enough motor units to generate a single maximal voluntary contraction graded as "normal."[57,64] However, quick repeated voluntary contractions will often give rise to a decremental response. The patient's history may also indicate that functional activities, undertaken for extended duration, elicit a response characterized by reduced resistance to fatigue.[57] Computerized dynamometer testing may be especially helpful at this point because torque generated by limb muscles for numerous contractions can be depicted reliably.[54,55,57] When a clinician notices a *rapid* decremental response in torque development (fatigue) or large variability in torque with repeated tests, the patient may have sustained an acute nerve compression, which has given rise to a pattern of partial denervation resulting in muscle strength or endurance deficit.

Careful clinical examination procedures such as those described above are indispensable for accumulating information about patients who may be suffering from post–nerve compression denervation. Even more precise data, however, can be obtained directly from the neuromuscular system by electrophysiologic tests. Failure or delayed conduction of a nerve stimulus across a suspected site of compression to a distal innervated muscle is evidence of a partial or complete neurapraxic lesion. Also, because the area under a surface electrode–recorded compound muscle action potential (M response) is believed to be an accurate representation of the number of viable (excitable) muscle fibers, and because muscle fibers are organized into excitable motor units that include both axons and all the muscle fibers supplied by them, considerable information is provided about the integrity of the neuromuscular unit by a rather simple procedure.[59,65] The M response can be compared to a range of values for normal subjects as well as to similar responses in the patient's *contralateral* limb. Our experience thus far with subclinical tourniquet-induced partial denervation indicates that nerve conduction velocities are almost always normal, but the amplitude and area under the curve of the M response is often reduced. This finding is consistent with a partial lesion (not all axons are involved).

Needle EMG examination of limb muscles for patients who have incurred an acute nerve compression provides evidence of muscle membrane instability (fibrillations, positive sharp waves, bizarre high-frequency discharges) if axonotmesis is present. There is some potential for confusion at this point because muscle inactivity from nerve conduction block (neurapraxia) has been associated with fibrillation potentials in two animal models.[66,67] Whether limb inactivity results in such electrical abnormalities in human subjects is unknown.

Further information about the health of muscle can be obtained by electrophysiologic evaluation of volitional activity. The configuration of individual motor units as predominantly polyphasic suggests that an attempt to compensate for partial denervation is being made by axonal sprouting. During maximal volitional effort, failure to fill the EMG screen with motor units (incomplete interference pattern) may suggest a muscle and nerve dysfunction because of denervation. One compensatory mechanism often noted during this portion of the examination is the tendency to recruit the remaining viable motor units at a significantly higher frequency—the so-called "rapid firing rate."

More sophisticated EMG technology has permitted greater refinement in identifying subtle electrophysiologic deficits, which in some cases are probably caused by acute nerve compression (tourniquet application). Specifically, volitional EMG signals can be evaluated by integration of the area under the curve or by rectifying muscle signal amplitudes during isometric contractions. As noted previously, Krebs[55] recently found a 53 percent incidence of EMG limb denervation potentials but a 100 percent incidence of deficit in smoothed, rectified EMG amplitudes in patients who had sustained a tourniquet-induced acute nerve compression.

Limb paralysis from complete nerve conduction block after tourniquet application is fortunately a rarity.[50] Electrophysiologic testing is warranted in such cases to determine if any excitable tissue has been spared to allow documenting the severity of the lesion. Prognostic information can then be formulated from subsequent serial electrophysiologic evaluations. With subtle partial denervation after tourniquet limb compression, clinical examination yields useful information about the patient's functional status. Supplemental data about muscle strength, endurance, and underlying causes of apparent deficits may be provided by computerized dynamometry and EMG testing procedures. This information is used to appropriately modify the treatment approach for such patients and constitutes the topic of the final section of this chapter.

TREATMENT REGIMENS AND TREATMENT IMPLICATION

Patients exhibiting evidence of severe limb paralysis from acute conduction block are not often sent to physical therapists for rehabilitation. Resolution of such a lesion must await recovery of the paranodal myelin and often takes several months.[44,45a] Splinting for joint protection and maintenance of joint PROM are appropriate until such time as nerve recovery nears completion. Electrical stimulation of limb muscles during this temporary period of paralysis is a matter of some controversy.[68] Once nerve recovery is complete, however, muscle strengthening exercises and neuromuscular electrical stimulation (NMES) of 50 to 90 pps frequency are useful procedures for rehabilitation. The effect of such NMES for patients with denervation or ongoing reinnervation is not known. Counseling patients about the lengthy course of recovery from a neurapraxic nerve lesion is certainly appropriate.[68]

Because patients with *complete limb paralysis* are not routinely referred to physical therapists for rehabilitation, this discussion focuses on those individuals with less severe nerve compression. Specifically, patients who have had knee arthrotomy with tourniquet application and who demonstrate a pattern of partial limb denervation will be discussed.

Patients with partial denervation have been noted to demonstrate significant muscle strength deficits. Because a principal feature of rehabilitation is therapeutic exercise and a primary goal of treatment is the most effective use of available motor units, partial denervation will likely affect the patient's ability to recruit these motor units during such activities.[69] In addition to moving joints through space, muscle has the responsibility of dampening the effect of joint reaction forces during daily activities and bouts of exercise. When fewer motor units are available because of denervation, this dampening function of muscle is diminished. Consequently, joint reaction forces during exercise, which are easily dampened by muscle under ordinary circumstances, become excessive. Deterioration in performance, caused by reduced resistance to muscle fatigue, is well documented by isokinetic dynamometry.[57] If joint reaction forces exceed a certain level, synovial tissue may respond by forming joint effusion, and articular cartilage may react by commencing degradation. Connective tissue may also bear unaccustomed stress at this point, accelerating fibrillation of collagen fibrils. Consequently, excessive exercise may be harmful because it exaggerates existing muscle weakness and may lead to "overuse" joint problems (inflammation, pain, tissue damage).[70]

Exercise protocols should be altered when postoperative partial denervation is identified by clinical and electrophysiologic testing. Specifically, because tension development and resistance to fatigue are likely to be reduced, the duration and intensity of any bout of therapeutic exercise should be limited so that no substantial deterioration in performance occurs (i.e., no greater than 20 to 30 percent decrease in isokinetic torque development over the course of a single bout of exercise).[57] Patients should exercise to this point, but not beyond. Exertion to the point of initial performance deterioration requires that exercise be undertaken in a methodical, somewhat cautious manner. As with any patient following injury, the length of exercise and intensity (amount of weight lifted, degree of tension setting on a bicycle ergometer) should begin at low levels and be increased in small increments as the patient's condition permits.

During the early phase of rehabilitation (weeks 1 to 3) the patient is encouraged to engage in brief (5 to 10 minutes), moderately intense exercise (5 to 10 repetitions of 30 to 50 percent of maximum voluntary contraction) several times (3 to 7 times) per day. As strength increases and greater resistance to fatigue is demonstrated, longer duration and more intense activities are added to the regimen. If adverse joint reaction (i.e., effusion, elevated tissue temperature, pain) or further strength decrement occurs after a bout of therapeutic exercise and is of more than a transient nature, then consideration should be given to altering the rehabilitation plan. When patients demonstrate this response to exercise, we often encourage them to use regular ice massage and a therapeutic pool, and to limit active knee exercises to unweighted static contraction. Anti-inflammatory medication, administered by the patient's physician, may also be instituted if the unwanted clinical response to exercise is identified. When joint effusion and tenderness have subsided, the more intense exercise protocol can again be resumed in a stepwise progressive fashion.

This approach to rehabilitation requires regular, careful clinical evaluation of patients before and after rehabilitation sessions. Monitoring may be enhanced by computerized dynamometry because such equipment has the capacity to reliably express torque values in such a way that decrement in torque during repeated muscle contractions serves to denote the onset of muscle fatigue. Again, it is recognized that the functional deficit correlated with an identified isokinetic measurement deficit is not known.[54]

High-amplitude NMES has been shown to have an effect on muscle tissue for healthy subjects,[71] injured patients,[71a,72] and experimental animals.[73] Completely denervated tissue does not seem to respond well to short-term NMES.[68,73a] Because the majority of patients who have had tourniquet application during knee surgery *do* exhibit parital limb denervation, the question arises as to what possible effect even intense NMES could have on such individuals. The point to recall is that if these patients exhibit *partial* denervation, they must also have partial innervation of their limb muscles. The beneficial effect of such muscle stimulation is probably directed at the remaining innervated tissue, not at that which is denervated. Consequently, muscle size and strength of the existing innervated muscle may be augmented by application of high-amplitude NMES. This augmentation of size and strength of remaining innervated muscle may be particularly important during the early rehabilitation phase, insofar as the functional impact of partial denervation resulting in decreased numbers of firing motor units is most prominent at that time.[74] Because limb stabilization has been shown to be important during NMES, no excessive joint motion is permitted,[72] minimizing potential deleterious effects of joint reaction forces during movement.

Finally, consideration must be given to improving joint proprioception and kinesthesia following joint arthrotomy attended by tourniquet application. Even though clinical assessment indicates that sensory modalities are relatively spared in the presence of tourniquet-induced partial (motor) denervation, subtle disturbances of muscle and joint position sense and length-tension relations are likely to be present. Although not examined in the recent clinical studies of tourniquet injury, joint injury is known to result in diminished proprioception and kinesthetic acuity.[75,76] Because knee arthrotomy is usually preceded, particularly among athletes, by joint injury, from that cause alone proprioception/kinesthesia might be disturbed. With the additional complication of limb (nerve) compression by the pneumatic tourniquet during surgery, further loss of joint position sense may result. For post–ankle sprain patients, training for improved proprioception and kinesthesia resulted in a marked decrease in episodes of instability and recurrent sprains.[75] From this information, inclusion of some form of proprioception/kinesthetic evaluation followed by training as patients make the transition from "in-clinic" to more functional (sports-related) activities is prudent.

In summary, patients who have sustained a nerve compression injury demonstrate clinical and electrophysiologic testing abnormalities. Careful monitoring of performance allows modification of the therapeutic protocol to permit avoidance of unwanted joint inflammation and deterioration in strength and endurance. Long-term follow-up studies currently indicate that some strength and muscle volume deficits persist for years after the surgery. One possible cause may be irreversible loss of axons and motor unit recruitment because of tourniquet-induced or trauma-related nerve injury. The challenge to clinicians directing rehabilitation for these patients is to be aware of such possible complications and make appropriate treatment modifications based on the most objective measures available.

SUMMARY

A review of the general anatomic and physiologic features of peripheral nerves revealed them to be exceedingly organized and complex structures that are very sensitive to acute nerve compression. When an injury from such compression does occur, it is usually described as representing, in ascending order of severity, a *neurapraxia*, *axonotmesis*, or *neurotmesis*. The clinical and electrophysiologic characteristics of these injury categories, as well as recovery from them, were discussed.

Pneumatic tourniquet-induced nerve injury, as a model of neurapraxia or axonotmesis, has proved to be useful for examining nerve injuries in general. The recent literature that has detailed the effects of tourniquet application on limb muscles, nerves, and function in animal and clinical studies was explored. It now appears that some measure of nerve deficit results from most tourniquet applications, and that recovery from these effects is temporally lengthy (of more than 1 year's duration) and may not always be complete.

These effects, as an example of nerve compression injuries, serve to highlight the need for close scrutiny of patients who may be exhibiting subtle signs of such lesions. Although instrumented means of measuring muscle and nerve function (EMG/NCV, isokinetic dynamometry) certainly have their limits, they serve as fairly reliable tools to document recovery from such injury or the deleterious effects of overzealous exercise therapy. Consequently, clinicians are encouraged to carefully assess patients whom they suspect may have sustained one or another form of compressive nerve injury. In addition, physical therapists must exercise flexibility as they modify therapeutic activities for patients in whom nerve-muscle lesions have been identified.

REFERENCES

1. Clark, RG: Manter and Gatz's Essentials of Clinical Neuroanatomy and Neurophysiology, ed 5. FA Davis, Philadelphia, 1975, p 1.
2. Asbury, AK: Peripheral nerves. In Haymaker, W and Adams, RD (eds): Histology and Histopathology of the Nervous System. Charles C Thomas, Springfield, IL, 1982, pp 1573–1574.
3. Wuerker, RB: Neurofilaments and glial filaments. Tissue Cell 2:1, 1970.
4. Singer, M and Salpeter, MM: The transport of ^{3}H-1-histidine through the Schwann and myelin sheath into the axon, including a re-evaluation of myelin function. J Morphol 120:281–315, 1966.
5. Revel, JP and Hamilton, DW: The double nature of the intermediate dense line in peripheral nerve myelin. Anat Rec 163:7–15, 1969.
6. Willimas, PL and Landon, DN: Paranodal apparatus of peripheral myelinated nerve fibers of mammals. Nature 198:670–673, 1963.
7. Ritchie, JM and Rogart, RB: Density of sodium channels in mammalian myelinated nerve fibers and nature of the axonal membrane under the myelin sheath. Proc Natl Acad Sci USA 74:211–215, 1977.
8. Murphy, RW: Nerve roots and spinal nerves in degenerative disk disease. Clin Orthop 129:46–60, 1977.
8a. Rydevik, B, Lundborg, G, and Nordborg, C: Intraneural tissue reactions induced by internal neurolysis. Scand J Plast Reconstr Surg Hand Surg 10:3–8, 1976.
8b. Lundborg, G and Rydevik, B: Effects of stretching the tibial nerve of the rabbit: A preliminary study of the intraneural circulation and barrier function of the perineurium. J Bone Surg [Br] 55:390–401, 1973.
9. Olsson, Y and Kristensson, K: The perineurium as a diffusion barrier to protein tracers following trauma to nerves. Acta Neuropathol (Berl) 23, 105–111, 1973.
10. Lundborg, G and Hansson, HA: Regeneration of peripheral nerve through a performed tissue space. Preliminary observations on the reorganization of regenerating nerve fibres and perineurium. Brain Res 179, 573–576, 1979.
11. Bunge, MB, Williams, AK, Wood, PM, et al.: Comparison of nerve cell and nerve cell plus Schwann cell cultures, with particular emphasis on basal lamina and collagen formation. J Cell Biol 84:184–202, 1980.
12. Makitie, J and Teravainen, H: Peripheral nerve injury and recovery after temporary ischemia. Acta Neuropathol (Berl) 37:55–63, 1977.
13. Nitz, AJ, Dobner, JJ, and Matulionis, DH: Structural assessment of rat sciatic nerve following tourniquet compression and vascular manipulation. Anat Rec 225:67–76, 1989.
14. Lundborg, G: Structure and function of the intraneural microvessels as related to trauma, edema formation and nerve function. J Bone Joint Surg [Am] 57, 938–948, 1975.
15. Korthals, JK and Wisniewski, HM: Peripheral nerve ischemia, Part I. Experimental model. J Neurol Sci, 24:65–76, 1975.
16. Reese, TS and Olsson, Y: Fine structural localization of a blood-nerve barrier in the mouse. J Neuropathol Exp Neurol, 29:123, 1970.
17. Feinstein, B, Lindegard, B, Nyman, E, et al.: Morphologic studies of motor units in normal human muscles. Acta Anat (Basel) 23:127–142, 1955.
18. Brandstater, ME and Lambert, EH: A histological study of the spatial arrangement of muscle fibers in single motor units within rat tibialis anterior muscle. Bulletin of the American Association of EMG and Electrodiagnosis 15-16:82, 1969.
19. Woolf, AL: Chronic degeneration of the lower motor neuron studied with vital staining and histochemical techniques in muscle biopsies (abstr). Proceedings of the Second International Congress of Neuropathologists, London, 1955, p 451.
20. Barchi, RL: Excitation and conduction in nerve. In Sumner, AJ (ed). The Physiology of Peripheral Nerve Diseases. WB Saunders, Philadelphia, 1980, p 1.
21. Skou, SJ: Enzymatic basis for active transport of Na^+ and K^+ across cell membranes. Physiol Rev 45:596–617, 1965.
22. Lundborg, G: Nerve regeneration and repair: A review. Acta Orthop Scand 58:145–169, 1987.
23. Seddon, HJ: Three types of nerve injury. Brain 66:237–288, 1943.
24. Seddon, HJ: Surgical Disorders of the Peripheral Nerves. Williams & Wilkins, Baltimore, 1972, p 267.
25. Lewis, T, Pickering, GW, and Rotschild, P: Centripetal paralysis arising out of arrested bloodflow to the limb, including notes on a form of tingling. Heart 16:1–32, 1931.
26. Denny-Brown, D, and Brenner, C: Lesion in peripheral nerve resulting from compression by spring clip. Archives of Neurology and Psychiatry 52:1–19, 1944.

27. Ochoa, J, Fowler, TJ, and Gilliatt, RW: Anatomical changes in peripheral nerves compressed by a pneumatic tourniquet. J Anat 113:433–455, 1972.
28. Sunderland, S: A classification of peripheral nerve injuries producing loss of function. Brain 74:491–516, 1951.
29. Sunderland, S: Nerves and Nerve Injuries, ed 2. Churchill Livingstone, Edinburgh, 1978.
30. Schlaepfer, WW and Hasler, MB: Characterization of the calcium-induced disruption of neurofilaments in rat peripheral nerve. Brain Res 168:299–300, 1979.
31. Aguayo, AJ, Epps, J, Charron, LC, et al.: Multi-potentiality of Schwann cells in cross anastomosed and grafted myelinated and unmyelinated nerves. Brain Res 104:1–20, 1976.
32. Sunderland, S and Bradley, KC: Endoneurial tube shrinkage in the distal segment of a severed nerve. J Comp Neurol 93:411–418, 1959.
33. Brattgard, SO, Edstrom, JE and Hyden, H: Chemical changes in regenerating neurons. J Neurochem 1:316–325, 1957.
34. McLean, WG, McKay, AL, and Sjostrand, J: Electrophoretic analysis of axonally transported proteins in rabbit vagus nerve. J Neurobiol. 14:227–236, 1983.
35. Gundersen, RW and Barrett, JN: Neuronal chemotaxis: Chick dorsal root axons turn toward high concentrations of nerve growth factor. Science 106:1079–1080, 1979.
36. Gundersen, RW and Barrett, JN: Characterization of the turning response of dorsal root neurites towards Nerve Growth Factor. J Cell Biol 87:546–554, 1980.
37. Gundersen, RW: Sensory neurite growth cone guidance by substrate absorbed Nerve Growth Factor. J Neurosci Res 13:199–212, 1985.
38. Politis, MJ: Specificity in mammalian peripheral nerve regeneration at the level of the nerve trunk. Brain Res 328:271–276, 1985.
39. Skene, JOP and Shooter, EM: Denervated sheath cells secrete a new protein after nerve injury. Proc Natl Acad Sci U S A 80:4169–4173, 1983.
40. Engel, AG: Morphological effects of denervation of muscle. A quantitative ultrastructural study. Ann NY Acad Sci 228:68–88, 1974.
41. Solandt, DV and Magladery, JW: The relation of atrophy to fibrillation in denervated muscle. Brain 63:255–263, 1940.
42. Stanley, FF and Drachman, DB: Denervation and the time course of testing membrane potential changes in skeletal muscle in vivo. Exp Neurol 69:253–259, 1989.
43. Thesleff, S and Sellin, LC: Denervation supersensitivity. Trends Neurosci 4: 122–126, 1980.
44. Miledi, R and Slater, CR: On the degeneration of rat neuromuscular junctions after nerve section. J Physiol (Lond) 207:507–528, 1970.
45. Rudge, P: Tourniquet paralysis with prolonged conduction block: An electrophysiological study. J Bone Joint Surg [Br] 56:716–720, 1974.
45a.Rudge, P, Ochoa, J, and Gilliatt, RW: Acute peripheral nerve compression in the baboon. J Neurol Sci 23:403–420, 1974.
46. Trojaborg, W: Prolonged conduction block with axonal degeneration: an electrophysiological study. J Neurol Neurosurg Psychiatry, 4:50–57, 1977.
47. Lundborg, G: Ischemia nerve injury. Scand J Plast Reconstr Surg Hand Surg (Suppl) 6:1–113, 1970.
48. Rorabeck, CH and Kennedy, JC: Tourniquet-induced nerve ischemia complicating knee ligament surgery. Am J Sports Med 8:98–102, 1980.
49. Flatt, AE: Tourniquet time in hand surgery. Arch Surg 104:190–192, 1972.
50. Middleton, RWD and Varian, JP: Tourniquet paralysis. Aust NZ J Surg 44:124–128, 1974.
51. Weingarden, SI, Louis, DC, and Waylonis, GW: Electromyographic changes in postmeniscectomy patients. Role of the pneumatic tourniquet. JAMA 241:1248–1250, 1979.
52. Saunders, KC, Louis, DL, Weingarden, SI, et al.: Effect of tourniquet time on post-operative quadriceps function. Clin Orthop 143:194–199, 1979.
53. Dobner, JJ and Nitz, AJ: Post-meniscectomy tourniquet palsy and functional sequelae. Am J Sports Med 10:211–214, 1982.
54. Rothstein, JM, Lamb, RL, and Mayhew, TP: Clinical used of isokinetic measurements. Phys Ther 67:1840–1844, 1987.
55. Krebs, DE: Isokinetic, electrophysiologic, and clinical function relationships following tourniquet-aided knee arthrotomy. Phys Ther 69:803–815, 1989.
56. Szabo, RM and Chidgey, LK: Stress carpal tunnel pressures in patients with carpal tunnel syndrome and normal patients. J Hand Surg [Am] 14:624–627, 1989.
57. Bohannon, RW and Gajdosik, RL: Spinal nerve root compression—some clinical implications. Phys Ther 67:376–382, 1987.
58. Nitz, AJ and Matulionis, DH: Ultrastructural changes in peripheral nerve following pneumatic tourniquet compression. J Neurosurg 57:660–666, 1982.
59. Nitz, AJ, Dobner, JJ, and Matulionis, DH: Pneumatic tourniquet application and nerve integrity: Motor function and electrophysiology. Exp Neurol 94:264–279, 1986.
60. Lo Presti, C Kirkendall, DT, Street, GM, et al.: Quadriceps insufficiency following repair of the anterior cruciate ligament. Journal of Orthopedic and Sports Physical Therapy 9:245–249, 1988.

61. Arviddson, IE, Ericksson, E, Haggmark, T, et al.: Isokinetic thigh muscle strength after ligament reconstruction in the knee joint: Results from a 5–10 year follow-up after reconstruction the anterior cruciate ligament in the knee joint. Int J Sports Med 2:7–11, 1981.
62. Haggmark, T, Jansson, E, and Svane, B: Cross-sectional area of the thigh muscle in man measured by computed tomography. Scand J Clin Lab Invest 38:355–360, 1978.
63. Young, A, Hughes, I, Russell, P, et al.: Measurement of quadriceps muscle wasting by ultrasonography. Rheumatology and Rehabilitation 19:141–148, 1980.
63a. Halkjaer-Kristensen, J and Ingemann-Hansen, T: Wasting of the human quadriceps muscle after knee ligament injuries. Scand J Rehabil Med Suppl 13:5–11, 1985.
64. Wiles, CM and Kami, Y: The measurement of muscle strength in patients with peripheral neuromuscular disorders. J Neurol Neurosurg Psychiatry 46:1006–1013, 1983.
65. Fowler, TJ, Danta, G, and Gilliatt, RW: Recovery of nerve conduction after a pneumatic tourniquet: Observations on the hind-limb of the baboon. J Neurol Neurosurg Psychiatry 35:638–647, 1972.
66. Gilliatt, RW, Westgaard, RH, and Willimas, IR: Extrajunctional acetylcholine sensitivity of inactive muscle fibres in the baboon during prolonged nerve pressure block. J Physiol (Lond) 280:499–514, 1978.
67. Bray, JJ, Hubbard, JI, and Mills, RG: The trophic influence of tetrodotoxin-inactive nerves on normal and reinnervated rat skeletal muscles. J Physiol (Lond) 297:479–491, 1979.
68. Spielholz, N: Electrical stimulation of denervated muscle. In Currier, DP and Nelson, RM (eds): Clinical Electrotherapy, Appleton & Lange, Norwalk, Connecticut, 1987, pp 97–114.
69. Lorentzon, R, Elmquist, LG, Sjostrom, M, et al.: Thigh musculature in relation to chronic anterior cruciate ligament tear: Muscle size, morphology, and mechanical output before reconstruction. Am J Sports Med 17:423–429, 1989.
70. Lundervold, A and Seyffarth, H: Electromyographic investigations of poliomyelitic paresis during the training up of the affected muscles and some remarks regarding the treatment of paretic muscles. Acta Psychiatrica et Neurologica Scandinavica 17:69–87, 1942.
71. Currier, DP and Mann, R: Muscular strength development by electrical stimulation in healthy individuals. Phys Ther 63:915–921, 1983.
71a. Wigerstad-Lossing, I, Grimbly, G, Jonsson, T, et al.: Effects of electrical stimulation combined with voluntary contractions after knee ligament surgery. Med Sci Sports Exerc 20:93–98, 1988.
72. Nitz, AJ and Dobner, JJ: High intensity electrical stimulation effect on thigh musculature during immobilization for knee sprain. Phys Ther 67:2119–222, 1987.
73. Greathouse, DG, Nitz, AJ, Matulionis, DH, et al: Effects of short-term electrical stimulation on the ultrastructure of rat skeletal muscles. Phys Ther 66:946–954, 1986.
73a. Greathouse, DG, Currier, DP, Nitz, AJ, et al.: Effects of moderate frequency electrical stimulation on partially denervated and denervated rat skeletal muscle. Anat Rec 218:52A–53A, 1987.
74. Delitto, A and Snyder-Mackler, L: Two theories of muscle strength augmentation using percutaneous electrical stimulation. Phys Ther 70:158–164, 1990.
75. Freeman, MAR, Dean, MRE, and Hanham, IEF: The etiology and prevention of functional instability of the foot. J Bone Joint Surg [Br] 47:678–685, 1965.
76. Smith, RL and Brunolli, J: Shoulder kinesthesia after anterior glenohumeral joint dislocation. Phys Ther 69:106–112, 1989.

CHAPTER 10

Modulation of Tendon Growth and Regeneration by Electrical Fields and Currents

Chukuka S. Enwemeka, Ph.D., P.T., FACSM
Neil I. Spielholz, Ph.D., P.T.

Since Du Bois-Reymond[1] discovered a large potential difference along the surface of a damaged nerve trunk, endogenous bioelectric currents and the prospects of augmenting such currents through exogenous sources have been the focus of several electrophysiologic studies. Although the earliest bioelectric investigations were primarily concerned with injury potentials generated across the membranes of damaged nerves and muscles, it was soon realized that such potentials are not unique to excitable membranes but could be measured in a variety of tissues, and even whole organisms, as demonstrated in the turtle,[2] fish eggs,[2] and in the hydroid, *Obelia*.[3] These measurements suggested that currents may be associated with healing and that tissue repair may perhaps be facilitated by modifying the electrical potential across the site of injury. Subsequently, it was shown that adult frogs, who after metamorphosis are unable to regenerate amputated limbs, can regrow them either by electrical stimulation of the brachial plexus,[4] by direct stimulation of the stump,[5,6] or by adding adrenal gland tissue to the stump.[7] Borgens and associates[8–13] have advanced this line of research. Their experiments not only confirmed that adding minute cathodal currents to a stump facilitates limb regeneration, but that the effect is not due to the by-products of electrode-tissue interaction.[8–14] Recent reports now indicate that electrical stimulation also facilitates the healing process of chronic bone lesions,[15] articular cartilage,[16] and skin wounds and ulcers.[17–22]

In summary, various tissues develop endogenous bioelectric currents, and the flow of such currents may be altered by injury. Furthermore, altered endogenous currents can themselves be modulated to facilitate healing, as when exogenous current sources are used to supplant or supplement residual endogenous currents to promote limb regeneration after amputation.[8-14,23] Because bone, muscle, nerves, ligaments, tendon, fascia, and skin are limb components, it is logical to hypothesize that electrical fields and currents of appropriate amplitude may promote the healing process of any of these tissues.

If electrical stimulation can indeed promote tendon healing, why has this modality not been used to minimize the complications associated with the 6 to 8 weeks that tendons are immobilized to ensure adequate healing after surgery? The answer to this question is partly that until recently, very little was known about tendons. The classical notion that tendons are inert "connectors," much like strings and cables, flourished for so long that minimal attention was paid to tendon research. Even today, perusal of the *Index Medicus* reveals that references to muscles and bones by far outnumber those to tendons. An aftermath of this prolonged neglect is that many clinicians have minimal understanding of tendon biology, let alone the possible effects of clinical interventions on this dense connective tissue. This state of affairs mandates a brief review of tendon biology in this chapter before we discuss the possible effects of electrical fields and currents on tendons.

THE TENDON

Embryogenesis

The initial embryogenic events leading to the development of tendons are similar to those of muscles. Cells destined to form either muscle or tendon both arise from embryonic mesoderm. Whereas the tendons of muscles derived from embryonic myotomes are likewise derived from those myotomes, the tendons of muscles derived from branchial arch mesoderm, the progenitor of most of the muscles of the head and neck, also form from this latter mesoderm. In either case, pluripotential mesenchymal cells differentiate ultimately into fibroblasts, which are responsible for producing the extracellular matrix characteristic of tendons and other dense connective tissues.

Ultrastructure, Biochemistry, and Biomechanics: A Brief Review

Tendons consist of fibroblasts and the large extracellular matrix they synthesize. The latter includes the fibrous proteins collagen and elastin, which are embedded in the so-called "ground material" made up of proteoglycans, glycoproteins, and mucopolysaccharides. The proportions of the above structural components vary slightly from tendon to tendon and with age. For example, developing tendons contain more fibroblasts than the tendons of older animals, and so do tendons undergoing repair after an injury.

With the exception of migratory and resident cells of blood vessels, fibroblasts are usually the sole cellular components of adult tendons.[24-29] In their quiescent state, fibroblasts consist of a prominent nucleus surrounded by a thin layer of cytoplasm, a few thin strands of which may project into the matrix. Under the electron microscope, the cytoplasmic organelles of quiescent fibroblasts are undifferentiated, and coarse clumps of heterochromatin frequently line the inner surface of the nuclear membrane (Figs. 10–1 and 10–2). These characteristics are rarely seen in developing or healing tendons. In either of these situations, fibroblast nuclei are rich in euchromatin and are surrounded by a relatively large volume of cytoplasm containing abundant ribosomes, numerous vesicles, well-developed rough endoplasmic reticulum (rER), Golgi complexes, and mitochondria (Figs. 10–3 and 10–4). Although these differences in the morphologic appearance of this plenipotential cell and its subcellular structures reflect its metabolic state, the terms *tenocytes, fibrocytes,* or *mature fibroblasts* have been used to describe the collagen-producing cells of the adult or mature tendon. On the other hand, in regenerating or developing tendons, these collagen-producing cells have been referred to as *fibroblasts.*[24-30]

Collagen, the major component of the extracellular matrix, accounts for as much as 86 percent of the dry weight of the entire tendon.[30] Although many phenotypes of this protein are recognized, type I predominates in tendons.[31-33] This fibrous protein is usually organized in fascicles consisting of bundles of fibers, which in turn are made up of fibrils. Whereas the entire tendon is frequently enclosed in a sheath of paratenon, each fascicle is surrounded by epitenon and the primary bundles by endotenon (Fig. 10–5). The crimped appearance of fascicles and primary bundles when viewed longitudinally is attributed to the axial alignment of fibrils within these units. The structural arrangement of the fibrils in each bundle of collagen has been described in a variety of ways. However, the frequently cited work of Kastelic, Galeski, and

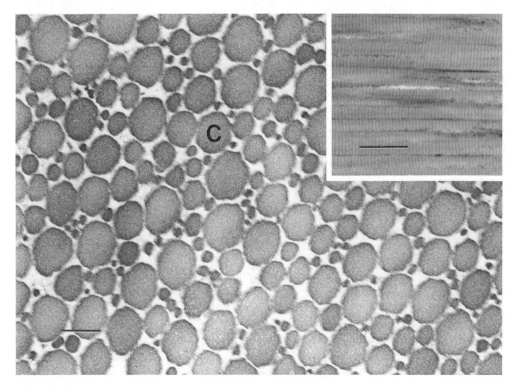

FIGURE 10–1. Electron micrograph of a cross section of a normal intact rabbit Achilles tendon showing a fibroblast (F) between adjacent bundles of fibrils (C). Note the thin layer of cytoplasm around a relatively large prominent nuclei and the coarse clumps of heterochromatin on the inner surface of the nuclear membrane. Arrows indicate the presence of a sheath around each bundle of fibrils (magnification ×14,000; bar 14.0 mm = 1 μm).

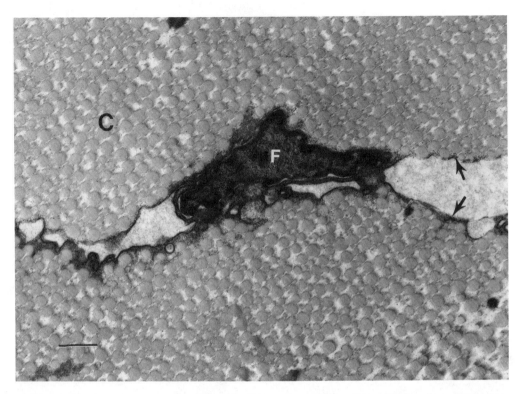

FIGURE 10–2. Electron micrograph of a cross section of the collagen fibrils of a normal intact rat Achilles tendon. Insert shows a longitudinal section of the fibrils. Note the characteristic alternate light and dark bands of the fibrils *(arrows)*. C = collagen fibril; (magnification ×17,700; bar 17.7 mm = 1 μm).

Baer[34] indicates that the fibrils of each primary bundle are made up of subfibrils, which in turn consist of microfibrils (see Fig. 1–3). Tropocollagen molecules, the fundamental molecular structure of collagen, are the primary constituents of microfibrils. Each tropocollagen molecule is a triple-stranded right-handed superhelix of three polypeptide chains.[35–38] It is the quarter stagger arrangement of tropocollagen molecules that yields the banded appearance of fibrils. Compared to collagen, tendons contain a relatively small amount of proteoglycans; less than 1 percent dry weight.

The functional requirements placed on various connective tissues are reflected in their structural organization, composition, and biomechanics. This point is well illustrated in the remarkably different macroscopic appearance of such dense connective tissues as tendons, ligaments, skin, and fascia, which consist of different proportions of the same structural materials. When the spatial arrangement of the collagen fibrils of tendons, ligaments, and skin is compared, an interesting trend becomes obvious. There is a progressive orderly longitudinal alignment of collagen fibrils as one moves from the ultrastructure of skin (which transmits only minimal tensional loads), through ligaments, to those of tendons that transmit the tremendous forces generated by their muscles. These differences are apparently related to function; and as recent studies have shown, patella tendons surgically transplanted to function as anterior cruciate ligaments progressively lose the characteristics of tendons as they assume the role and structural appearance of ligaments.[39] Thus there is a relation

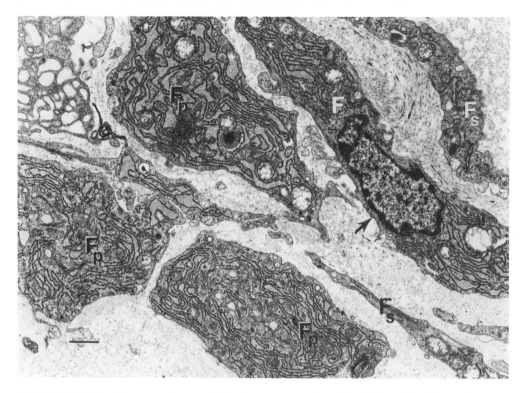

FIGURE 10–3. Electron micrograph showing a cross section of proliferated fibroblasts of a regenerating rabbit Achilles tendon 15 days after tenotomy and repair. Note the extensive network of rough endoplasmic reticulum (rER) and several electron-lucent vesicles in each fibroblast as well as the relatively large mass of cytoplasm around the nucleus. Compare this with the fibroblast in Figure 10–1. F = fibroblast; F_p = portion of a fibroblast; F_s = strands of fibroblast; (magnification × 10,700; bar 10.7 mm = 1 μm).

between the structural arrangement of collagen fibrils and the strength of dense connective tissues. In fact, evidence exists that tendon strength is mostly dependent on the quantity, sizes, and spatial orientation of its fibrils.[40–45] Thus the tension-transmitting property of mature tendon is reflected in tightly packed, longitudinally aligned, thick collagen fibrils; hence fibrils are considered the physiologic units of tendons. Because there is this relation between function and fibril architecture, it would be interesting to determine whether electrical stimulation has any effect on the ultrastructure and morphology of the collagen matrix of tendons.

TENDON HEALING

Although there is appreciable uniformity of opinion concerning events that culminate in healing, methods of subdividing these events have varied nearly as much as there are descriptions of the process.[24–29,46–52] For this reason, and in particular because of the paucity of studies on healing human tendons, the brief description provided here is based mostly on a recent study of the process in a series of tenotomized Achilles tendons of rabbits.[29] Nonetheless, inferences will be drawn from other closely related work when necessary. Based on cellular, vascular, and matrical

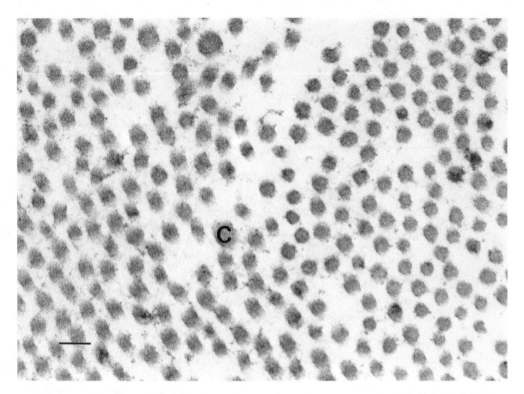

FIGURE 10–4. Electron micrograph of a cross section of the collagen fibrils of a regenerating rabbit Achilles tendon 15 days after experimental tenotomy and repair. Note the relatively small sizes of the collagen fibrils (C) (magnification ×5600; bar 11.2 mm = 1 μm).

changes, the series of events leading to healing may be divided into three aspects: (1) inflammatory response and neoangiogenesis, (2) fibroplasia and fibrillogenesis, and (3) matrix remodeling.

Inflammation and Neoangiogenesis

Following tenotomy or rupture, cellular and dissolved elements of the blood form a hematoma to which cells migrating into the wound adhere. Polymorphonuclear leukocytes (neutrophils) from intact but "leaky" capillaries are often the first cells to migrate to the site of injury, ingesting debris produced by the wounding and pathogens contaminating the wound. This migrating and ingesting proceeds for hours after the trauma. Such migration is apparently facilitated by chemicals released from platelets deposited at the site of injury as a result of bleeding.[53–55] One or 2 days later, monocytes arrive[56]; soon they are joined by macrophages and lymphocytes as phagocytosis continues (Fig. 10–6). It has been reported that at least some macrophages are transformed monocytes rather than migratory macrophages.[57] Regardless of their source, macrophages play a prominent role in wound healing. They not only phagocytize debris and debride the wound, they promote migration of fibroblasts to the site of injury and stimulate their proliferation as well.[58–60] Indeed, should the macrophage population of a wound be reduced experimentally by combined administra-

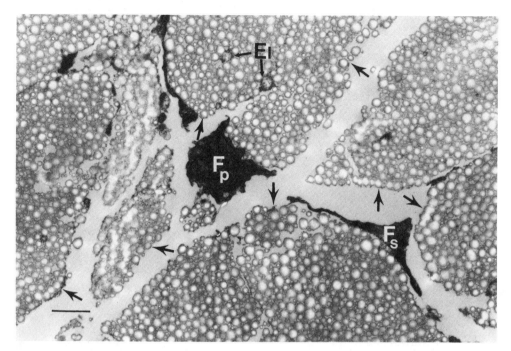

FIGURE 10–5. Electron micrograph of adjoining bundles *(arrows)* of collagen fibrils (C), and portions of fibroblasts (F_p) seen in a cross section of a normal intact tendon. El = elastin bundles; F_s = fibroblast strands; (magnification $\times 14,600$; bar 14.6 mm = 1 μm).

tion of of antimacrophage serum and cortisone, the arrival of fibroblasts is delayed, and their proliferation rate is depressed for several days.[61] How macrophages promote fibroplasia remains speculative even though the topic has been the focus of numerous investigations[58,62–70] and reviews.[71–73] However, accumulating evidence indicates that these cells produce several distinct growth factors, some of which are closely related to other well-characterized growth factors and chemotactic agents including fibroblast growth factor (FGF),[74] leukotriene B_4,[65,70] and platelet-derived growth factor (PDGF).[71–73] Thus, although fibroblasts are dominant and produce the collagen of tendons, their metabolic process may be remarkably impaired in the absence of macrophages and such cells as neutrophils, platelets, monocytes, and lymphocytes that initiate the sequence of events that precede their migration. The indispensable roles of these cells in the healing tendon demand that the effects of electric fields and currents on their function be ascertained. Unfortunately, however, this area of electrical stimulation remains ill-explored to date.

From the foregoing, it is clear that the process of inflammation involves numerous participants, each requiring an abundant supply of oxygen and nutrient materials. Oxygen is a well-known critical requirement for many metabolic processes; it is particularly so for collagen synthesis. Collagen biosynthesis is hampered when Po_2 is lower than 20 mm Hg.[75] Thus, if the mechanism for delivering oxygen and other metabolic requirements is not developed, the entire healing process may be impaired. It is understandable, therefore, why the development of new blood vessels (i.e., neoangiogenesis) precedes collagen synthesis. Ipso facto, before fibroblasts begin to synthesize collagen and other components of the matrix, vascular buds develop from capillaries in the vicinity of rupture.[76] As these buds project into the wound, they

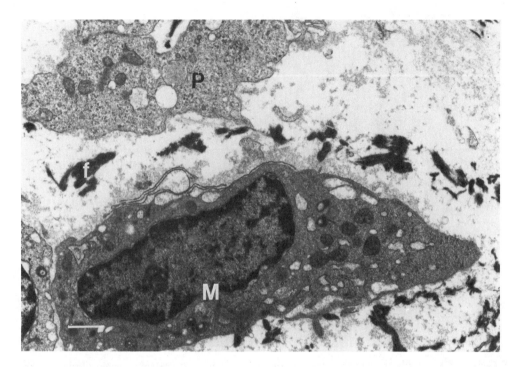

FIGURE 10–6. Electron micrograph showing a cross section of a regenerating rabbit Achilles tendon 7 days after tenotomy and repair. M = macrophage; P = platelet; f = patches of fibrin; (magnification ×10,700; bar 10.7 mm = 1 μm).

make numerous anastomoses, thus developing a rich vasculature.[76] Through this network of newly formed blood vessels, oxygen and other nutrients required for healing are carried to the healing tendon, and carbon dioxide and other metabolic waste products are removed. Angiogenesis is believed to be promoted by several components of wound fluids, including several prostaglandins, macrophageal growth factors, polymorphonuclear leukocytes, T lymphocytes, PDGF, FGF, and epidermal growth factor (EGF).[77–81] There is evidence, however, that endothelial cells, whose sprouting is necessary for angiogenesis, also promote their own growth by producing FGF.[82]

In summary, neutrophils, platelets, monocytes, macrophages, and lymphocytes play key roles during the inflammatory phase of tendon healing. Prior to collagen synthesis, new blood vessels are formed; this neovasculature provides oxygen and nutrients and removes carbon dioxide and other metabolic waste products. Not only do macrophages debride the wound via phagocytosis, they facilitate angiogenesis, as well as the migration of fibroblasts to the site of injury, and their proliferation.

Fibroplasia and Fibrillogenesis

The arrival of fibroblasts marks the beginning of collagen synthesis and the subsidence of inflammation, which is usually massive and prolonged in tendons.[29] The study by Enwemeka[29] and those of others[24–28] have shown that although fibroblasts may be seen at 5 days, fibroplasia and fibrillogenesis are not usually evident until about the seventh day after tenotomy or rupture. As fibroblasts proliferate, they develop large masses of cytoplasm each with elaborate networks of rough endoplasmic reticulum (rER), several electron lucent vesicles, some dark granules, numerous ribosomes, and a few ill-defined Golgi complexes (see Fig. 10–3). These cytoplasmic changes and the development of large nuclei filled with euchromatin indicate that these cells are actively involved in protein synthesis. In general, cells produce two types of proteins: secretory proteins and those required for cellular processes, mostly enzymes. The abundance of cytoplasmic vesicles suggests that secretory proteins are being synthesized. It is therefore not surprising that simultaneously, large quantities of collagen fibrils appear in the extracellular compartment. By the seventh day of healing, an appreciable quantity of fibrils may be seen lying in disarray in the extracellular compartment. Occasionally, pockets of well-organized, longitudinally arranged fibrils are present, and so are large quantities of proteoglycan ground material. As fibroblasts become the preponderant cell in the healing tendon, the collagen fibrils become increasingly abundant in the extracellular pool. Even though type I collagen predominates in normal intact tendons, type III collagen is first produced by healing tendons.[83] This collagen is progressively replaced by type I collagen as healing proceeds. The fate of the type III collagen fibrils remains unclear. Once produced, type I fibrils become progressively larger in size and number. How fibrils increase in size remains speculative even though a great amount of effort has been devoted to this issue (see Parry and Craig[45] for a recent review). As fibrillogenesis progresses, the fibrils become increasingly aligned in the longitudinal axis of the tendon at the same time that they are being progressively grouped into bundles. Such bundles of fibrils may be seen under the electron microscope by the 21st day of healing. Because mechanical stress ranks high among factors known to enhance fibril alignment,[84–87] it is conceivable that electrical stimulation of the homonymous muscle could produce the type of contraction that may mechanically stress the tendon and hence facilitate fibril alignment.

Matrix Remodeling

Just as there is overlap between the phases of inflammation/angiogenesis, and fibroplasia, so the processes of fibroplasia and fibrillogenesis dovetail with matrix remodeling. Remodeling entails systematic organization of the large quantities of collagen fibrils in the extracellular pool into the compact "parallel" array that is characteristic of tendons. Recent studies indicate that this process begins at about the second week of healing and continues for a considerable period of time.[29] Postacchini and associates[27,88] have demonstrated that although the healing tendon becomes progressively compact as it acquires the morphologic characteristics of normal adult tendon, collagen remodeling continues over a period of 30 weeks after partial tenotomy and repair of the calcaneal tendon of rabbits. The fibroblasts are still numerous, less uniformly distributed, and have greater amount of protein-synthesizing organelles and contractile proteins after 30 weeks of healing than before healing.[27] These observations are not unique to the partially tenotomized calcaneal tendon of rabbits. They have been observed in other experimental models, including the completely tenotomized and repaired calcaneal tendons of rats[24] and rabbits,[25] extensor tendons of rabbits,[26] tendon grafts in dogs,[46] and ruptured Achilles tendons of humans.[51]

As healing progresses, the tendon's tensile strength increases,[84,85,89–91] as has been shown in other connective tissues as well.[92] Thus there is a relation between fibril remodeling and the tensile strength acquired by the tendon.[85,93] Measurement of tensile strength and other biomechanical characteristics of the tendon is therefore valuable for assessing the modulating effects of electrical fields and electrical stimulation on the healing process of tendons.

MODULATION OF THE NORMAL REPAIR PROCESS BY ELECTRICAL FIELDS AND CURRENTS

Because electrical stimulation facilitates regeneration of amputated limbs in frogs, regrowth of tendons and other tissues in the extremities of frogs may be influenced separately by such currents. However, the complex nature of total limb regeneration and the differences between species clearly limit direct application of this simple logic to mean that tendon healing is similarly promoted by electrical stimulation. In the frog amputated limb, for example, stimulation-induced regeneration of one tissue may secondarily trigger faster regeneration in other tissues. In other words, electrical stimulation may not necessarily promote regrowth of each and every tissue directly. Hence electrical stimulation studies pertaining just to tendon injury, not to whole limb amputation, are important to elucidate the direct effect of stimulation on healing tendons.

Our review of the literature indicates that until 1982, no study had systematically investigated the use of electrical currents to stimulate tendon healing. Thus, the work of Owoeye[94] (and Owoeye and others[95]) is perhaps the first in which electrical current was applied directly on the tendon with the hope of promoting healing. This team at New York University examined the effects of direct electrical stimulation and electrode polarity on the healing of the Achilles tendons in rats. Under anesthesia, the right Achilles tendons of 60 Sprague-Dawley rats were severed, sutured, and immobilized in plaster casts. Twenty animals were then assigned randomly to one of three groups. Group one rats received anodal stimulation, group two received cathodal stimulation, and group three received no stimulation. Treatments were performed 15 minutes daily beginning from the first day after surgery using a portable high-voltage pulsed stimulator (HVPS, Electro-Med Health Industries, Miami, FL). Although a HVPS delivering the typical twin-peaked, short-duration pulses was employed, high voltage was not delivered to the tissues. Instead, treatment parameters were arbitrarily set at 75 μA at a frequency of 10 pps, monitored constantly with a current probe. After 14 days, load-to-breaking measurements were performed, and the values obtained from the three groups were compared. Analysis of variance revealed a significant difference in the breaking strength of the three groups of tendons. Post hoc analysis showed that tendons treated with anodal current were stronger than those that had healed without any stimulation and that these, in turn, were stronger than those treated with the cathode.[94,95]

This work has continued, with a number of methodologic changes. First, one of the limitations of the original study was that tendons were tested with a relatively simple strain gauge. It was restricted in the maximum force it could measure, and it could not standardize the strain rate, that is, how quickly the forces were applied to the tendons. Both these problems were overcome by obtaining access to an Instron Tester. A second change in methodology was instituted to reduce interanimal variability. The original "load-to-breaking" studies compared the strengths of treated tendons (either anode or cathode) to those obtained from nontreated control animals. In other words, tendons from three groups of animals were employed. Review of the results showed, however, that within the control group (i.e., those animals whose tendons were permitted to heal with no other treatment except cast immobilization), healing was quite variable. In subsequent experiments, therefore, to obtain more direct information concerning how electrical stimulation influences healing within individuals (as opposed to between groups), the Achilles tendons of each animal were bilaterally and identically tenotomized, sutured, had electrodes implanted, and were casted. One side or the other was then randomly chosen for treatment with the nontreated side serving as the animal's control. The assumption inherent in this design is that if it were not for some special intervention, both tendons would heal basically at the same rate.

The general trend previously reported was confirmed with the above two modifications: anodal stimulation tends to facilitate tendon healing, whereas cathodal current appears to retard it. (Note that these results are opposite to that of bone healing, where osteogenesis is facilitated by the cathode). After 14 days of healing, the average difference between tendons treated with anodal current (10 to 13 treatments, 15 minutes each, 10 pps, 200 μA) and contralateral tendons that healed without stimulation was 362.8 $\pm$ 146.59 g (range 136.0 to 680.4 g). Conversely, tendons treated with cathodal currents averaged 657.1 $\pm$ 354.85 g weaker than their contralateral controls (range 132.0 to 1610.3 g). The large range and standard error in this group was mostly the result of one cathode-treated tendon not healing at all; that is, it withstood essentially no load before breaking, so that the difference between this tendon and its contralateral control was the value of the contralateral control (Fig. 10–7).

During the course of another experiment, one animal died shortly after receiving its sixth anodal treatment. Both Achilles tendons were immediately harvested and frozen in saline until they could be tested along with other tendons. (Freezing of biologic material such as bones, tendons, or ligaments prior to mechanical testing is a routine and accepted procedure.[96–98]) During the same experiment, a second animal managed to remove the cast and electrodes from its treated leg, also shortly after receiving its sixth anodal treatment. This second rat was recasted, but because the electrodes could not be reimplanted, no more treatments were given until the animal was sacrificed on the 14th day. In both of these animals, the differences between the treated and control legs were nearly identical. Not surprisingly, the tendons of the animal that had healed for 14 days had higher absolute values than those of the animal that had healed for only 6 days, but the differences between the two sides were the same. Because both animals had six treatments, this finding suggests that the augmented healing afforded by anodal current was the same in both animals, and that even though treatment had to stop in the animal that healed for 14 days (i.e., 8 days more), the gain in strength achieved during the first 6 days of treatment was maintained after treatment stopped. Admittedly, this occurrence may have been simply a chance or coincidental happening in these two animals, but it is nevertheless intriguing and suggests yet another future experiment.

Although our findings concerning the effect of polarity on healing tendons were consistently the same in our series of experiments, others have reported contradictory results.[99] For example, Stanish and co-workers[99] found increased breaking strength in partially tenotomized patella tendons of dogs following cathodal stimulation. In spite of several experimental limitations of their study, their results cannot be brushed

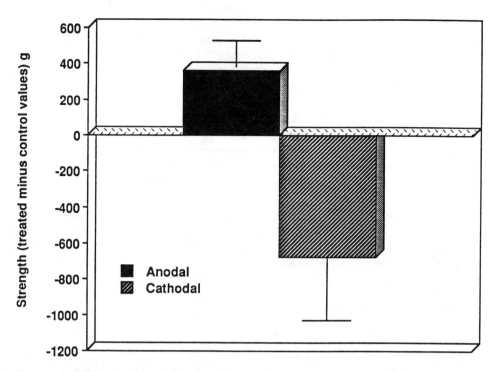

FIGURE 10–7. Comparison of load-to-breaking data of direct anodal and cathodal stimulation of regenerating rat Achilles tendons. Healing was for 14 days. Treatments were delivered with the EGS unit for 15 minutes daily at 10 pps and 200 μA. Tendons stimulated with anodal current had a mean strength of 362.8 g ± 146.59 g higher than control values, whereas those tendons stimulated with cathodal current were 675 ± 354.85 weaker than controls.

aside because cathodal stimulation is well known to promote healing in bones.[100–103] In their work,[99] the medial half of the right patella tendons of nine healthy semiconditioned dogs were severed 1 cm below the inferior patella pole. Thereafter, the wounds were closed and the dogs randomly assigned to three groups. The experimental limbs of group 1 dogs were immediately immobilized in plaster as controls, while the legs of group 2 dogs were bound in compression dressing for approximately 48 hours, after which they were permitted full cage activity. Group 3 dogs were treated in the same manner as the group 2 dogs except that the cathode of a constant current (20 μA) electrical stimulator was wrapped around the tendon, while the stimulator itself and the anode were implanted subcutaneously. Eight weeks after surgery, the tendons were excised as bone-tendon-bone units and tested with an Instron device. Although the small sample size did not permit statistical comparison of the tendons, the mean percent of normal strength obtained was higher in the group 3 tendons that were electrically stimulated. Because animals in the electrical stimulation group were not immobilized in plaster as controls, and also because stimulation and weight bearing may interact to promote healing in an unpredictable manner, it is difficult to attribute the higher mean strength obtained in this experiment to cathodal stimulation alone, especially as previous studies have shown that early weight bearing per se promotes tendon healing in both experimental rats[104] and rabbits.[84,85] Because none of the tendons were treated with anodal current, no comparison can be made between the polarities of current stimulation.

Recently, Nessler and Mass[105] also demonstrated that in vitro stimulation of whole tendons equally facilitates tendon healing. In their experiment, they tenotomized and repaired the flexor digitorum profundus tendon of rabbits, then excised and cultured the entire tendon in an acellular medium for 7, 14, 21, or 42 days. Tendons that were stimulated with a 7-μA current were then compared with controls. They showed by light microscopy and by biochemical analysis of the amount of [^{14}C]proline and [^{14}C]hydroxyproline incorporated by the repaired tendons, that electrical stimulation augmented collagen synthesis and fibroblast proliferation. However, they did not examine the effects of polarity.

In some of our other experiments, we compared the waveform produced by the HVPS to the so-called "Tsunami wave" generated by the Myo-matic (Monad Corporation, Pomona, CA). Two different studies were done. As shown in Figure 10–8, in 10 rats whose Achilles tendons were bilaterally tenotomized, repaired and casted, the side treated with the Tsunami wave healed stronger than the control side in 7 of the animals (70 percent), and averaged 179.9 g stronger than the control side, but this difference was not statistically significant ($P>.05$).

In the second experiment (Fig. 10–9), a comparison was made in six animals in which one side was treated with the Tsunami wave and the other side with an EGS unit (Electro-Med Health Industries, Miami, FL). Stimulus parameters for the two waveforms were held the same (10 pps, 40 μA, 15 minutes) except that the EGS unit puts out a very short-duration (50-microsecond) twin-peaked monophasic current (HVPS), whereas the Tsunami wave is of longer duration and of alternating polarity.

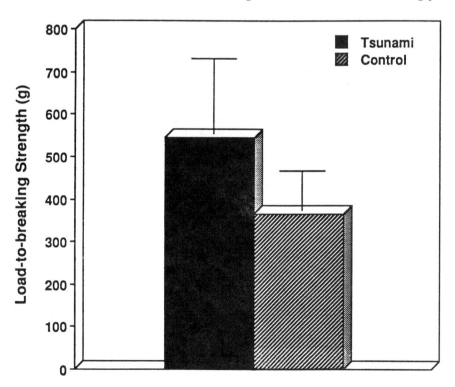

FIGURE 10–8. Comparison of load-to-breaking data of tendons stimulated with the Tsunami waves produced by the Myomatic and controls. There was no statistically significant difference between the mean strength of the two groups of tendon.

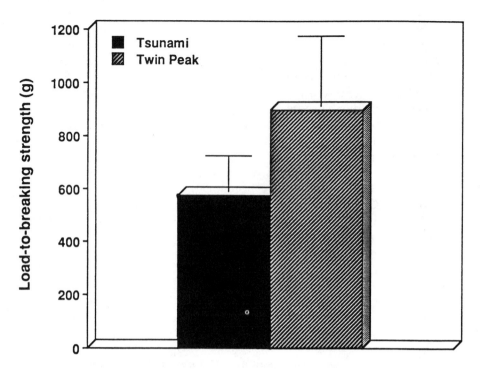

FIGURE 10–9. Comparison of Tsunami stimulation and stimulation with the twin-peak current produced by the EGS unit.

As seen in Figure 10–9, tendons treated with the EGS unit were stronger than those treated with the Tsunami wave in four of the six animals (66.7 percent) and averaged 322.8 g stronger, but this difference was not statistically significant.

To summarize, our series of experiments have confirmed the previous finding that the waveform generated by the EGS unit accelerates tendon healing when the anode is used to "treat" the tendon, and retards healing when the cathode is used. A test of the possible beneficial effects of the Tsunami wave showed that after 7 days of healing (five treatments), treated tendons were, on the average, about 180 g stronger than the nontreated tendons, but that this difference was not statistically significant. A comparison of anodal stimulation and Tsunami stimulation showed that after eight treatments (9 days of healing), anodal stimulation averaged 322.8 g stronger than tendons treated with Tsunami wave, but again this difference did not reach statistical significance.

On first thought, these three points seem to be contradictory. If anodal stimulation produces significantly stronger tendons than does control healing, whereas Tsunami wave stimulation does not, then it would seem by Euclidean reasoning that anodal stimulation should also be significantly better than Tsunami wave stimulation. However, the lack of a significant difference between the two forms of stimulation is probably because the Tsunami wave did result in stronger tendons than did control healing and therefore averaged somewhere between control healing strength and that produced by anodal stimulation. A fundamental question raised by these experiments is whether our biomechanical tests actually measured true healing. After all, we have noted that tendon healing entails fibroblast proliferation, fibrillogenesis, and subsequent remodeling of the collagen matrix, among other things. Although there is a relation between the mechanical strength of the tendon and the duration of healing, if the two ends of the experimentally servered tendon united by some other mechanism besides true healing, our biomechanical measurements would have failed to reflect true healing. Anodal stimulation may produce protein coagulation and tissue hardening,[106] which our biomechanical test cannot differentiate from true healing. To demonstrate that true healing has occurred requires a histologic study of the site in question. However, our series of experiments are not the first to demonstrate augmented healing following anodal stimulation. Other studies have shown similar results with another type of soft tissue injury, namely skin wounds and ulcers.[17–19,22,107]

POSSIBLE MECHANISMS OF ELECTRIC FIELD AND CURRENT–INDUCED ACCELERATION OF HEALING

Given the role of monocytes, macrophages, fibroblasts, and the multitude of cells that mediate healing, and given the need for optimal ionic strength, temperature, and pH, as well as the long period of remodeling required to reconstitute the collagen matrix of tendons, one may ask the question, How do electric fields and currents modulate the healing process of tendons? To address this question, we must begin by reviewing those studies that have examined the effects of electric fields and currents on the various cells and subsystems involved in tendon healing.

Drawing from the experience of several investigators who demonstrated that electric fields and currents are capable of facilitating fracture healing, Murray and Farndale[108] examined the effects of a low-frequency pulsed magnetic field on primary cultures of chicken tendon fibroblasts (the cells that are primarily responsible for collagen synthesis in tendons). The cells were isolated from 17-day embryonic chicken tendons, cultured and incubated with tritiated hydroxyproline ([^{3}H]proline). The magnetic field was then applied via a Bio-Osteogen system with a pulse duration of 230 microseconds repeated 21 times per burst. Treatment was applied from day 1, 12 hours per day at a cycle of 6 hours on and 6 hours off. Based on [^{3}H]proline analysis, a significant increase in total protein synthesis was observed in cultures exposed to the pulsed magnetic field for the last 24 hours and those treated for a total of 6 days. Compared with controls, it was specifically demonstrated that collagen production exceeded total protein synthesis in 6-day treated cultures but not in cultures treated for a shorter period of time. Although the level of cyclic adenosine monophosphate (cAMP) diminished after 6-day pulsed magnetic field treatment, the proliferation of the fibroblasts was not altered by the electric field.[108] Thus the increased collagen synthesis was induced not by fibroblast proliferation, but by modulation of cAMP metabolism.

Because local heating may account for the effects of pulsed magnetic field,[109,110] follow-up experiments were conducted to distinguish field effects from temperature effects and in particular to examine the role of cAMP in greater detail than before. Primary and passaged cultures of fibroblasts raised from bone marrow stroma of young rabbits were treated with pulsed electromagnetic field from the initiation of culture until 1 week.[111] As in the previous experiment, exposure to the field augmented collagen synthesis but did not affect cell proliferation as judged by phase contrast microscopy, tritiated thymidine incorporation into DNA, and total DNA assay.[111] A correlation between collagen breakdown and cAMP levels was demonstrated by adding dibutyryl cAMP or prostaglandin E_2 to the culture medium concurrently with [^{3}H]proline. Because the magnetic field produced less than 0.1°C rise in temperature, the observed increase in collagen production was again ascribed to the modulating effect of the field on cAMP. This conclusion is supported by other studies, which showed that the adenylate cyclase complex is temporarily inactivated or attenuated by prolonged exposure to pulsed magnetic and electric fields.[112,113] However, exactly how a decrease in cAMP levels influences collagen synthesis remains speculative, even though Brighton and associates[114,115] recently showed that desensitization of bone cells to parathyroid hormone is one mechanism of field-induced osteogenesis.

Other studies have shown that different stimulation parameters may produce different results.[116–118] In their study of cultures of human fibroblasts, Bourguignon and Bourguignon[116] examined the effects of high-voltage pulsed stimulation on protein and DNA synthesis. Using an EGS model 100-2 (Electro-Med Health Industries, Miami, FL), they exposed the cells to monophasic twin-peaked pulses of 100-microsecond duration at voltages ranging from 0 to 300 V. Stimulation was applied at room temperature at rates of 60 to 120 pps for 20 minutes. At the maximum settings of 300 V and 120 pps, the maximum time-averaged current delivered was determined to be approximately 50 μA. Protein and DNA synthesis were determined by measuring the amount of incorporation of [^{3}H]proline and [^{3}H]thymidine, respectively. Results showed that electrical stimulation induced a significant increase in the rates of both protein and DNA synthesis. Maximum stimulation of both protein and DNA synthesis was achieved at 50 and 75 V, respectively, with a rate of 100 pps and in the cells located near the cathode. At all pulse rates and locations within the chamber, amplitudes greater than 250 V inhibited both protein and DNA synthesis.

The effect of electrical current on protein synthesis has also been examined in cultures of neonatal bovine fibroblasts obtained from 2-week-old calves.[117] Current densities ranging from 0.1 μA cm^{-2} to 1.0 μA cm^{-2} were applied at frequencies of 0.1 to 1000 pps. As in the previous study, electrical stimulation was shown to modulate the incorporation of [^{3}H]proline into secreted protein. However, currents as low as 1 μA cm^{-2} triggered a 30 percent reduction in the normalized ^{3}H counts, indicating a decrease in protein synthesis. Further analysis revealed that this inhibitive effect was more pronounced when the cells were stimulated at a frequency of 10 pps and a current density of 0.5 μA cm^{-2}. Chemical by-products of electrolysis and changes in media temperature were further shown not to mediate the observed decline in protein synthesis.[117] As close as the experiments of Bourguignon and Bourguignon[116] and McLeod and colleagues[117] may seem, differences in experimental protocol do not permit a fair comparison of their results. Other investigators have, however, demonstrated elevated DNA and proteoglycan synthesis by [^{3}H]thymidine and [^{35}S]sodium sulfate uptake, respectively, in cultures of growth cartilage cells exposed to a DC current of 1.0 μA.[118] Whereas a 10-fold increase in amperage devitalized the cells, a 10-fold decrease below 1.0 μA did not produce any effect on the cells.[118] Studies on guinea pig dermal wounds covered with collagen mesh and then exposed to direct currents ranging from 0 to 100 μA also indicate that electrical stimulation promotes fibroplasia and collagen fibril alignment when currents of 20 to 100 μA are used.[119] Bourguignon and co-workers[120] have recently identified two initial cellular events that occur following exposure to high-voltage pulsed stimulation. Using their previous experimental paradigm,[116] they demonstrated increased ^{45}Ca^{2+} uptake by cultured human fibroblasts within the first minute of stimulation, and increased insulin binding a minute later. The stimulation-induced increase in insulin binding was inhibited by bepridel, a specific CA^{2+} channel blocker, thus suggesting that the influx of CA^{2+} is required for the exposure of additional insulin receptors on the cell surface. Thus these investigators concluded that one mechanism by which stimulation modulates fibroblast function is to trigger the opening of voltage-sensitive calcium channels in the fibroblast plasma membrane. The augmented intracellular Ca^{2+} thus produced then induces the exposure of additional insulin receptors on the cell surface. If insulin is available to bind to the additional receptors, increased protein and DNA synthesis may be achieved by the fibroblasts.

From the foregoing, the conclusion may be made that modulation of cAMP metabolism, increased DNA and collagen syntheses, and increased intracellular Ca^{2+} and subsequent elevation of insulin binding are possible mechanisms by which electrical fields and currents modulate tendon healing. Our experience with tendons that were immobilized without prior tenotomy suggests, however, other mechanisms of action. We have ultrastructural evidence showing that profound inactivity, such as is produced by immobilization in a cast or by denervation, results in two major changes: (1) "atrophy" of collagen fibrils can be demonstrated after just 2 weeks, and (2) changes occur in the appearance of the tendon fibroblasts. Three weeks of cast immobilization results in considerable "atrophy" of collagen fibrils compared with the tendon from the nonimmobilized side. An even more remarkable change occurs after 5 weeks of immobilization. The collagen fibrils in the 5-week-immobilized tendons are not only minuscule compared with the controls, but they also demonstrate marked matrix disorganization. Whereas collagen fibrils in normal tendon lie mostly parallel to one another, 5 weeks of immobilization in the shortened position results in a chaotic picture in many regions of the tendon (Figs. 10–10 and 10–11).

These two findings—atrophy of collagen fibrils followed by loss of orientation—are intriguing in view of the classical belief that tendon collagen is relatively inert. Indeed, our findings that atrophy can be detected after only 2 to 3 weeks of enforced inactivity suggests that collagen turnover is much more rapid than heretofore believed. Furthermore, the fact that fibril disarray is also marked after 5 weeks in the shortened position suggests that use and stretching of the tendon are both necessary physiologic stimuli for normal tendon architecture. Another interesting ultrastructural finding in the 5-week-immobilized specimens is seen when Figure 10–12 is compared with Figure 10–1. Figure 10–12 is representative of the "fibroblast" of immobilized tendon, whereas Figure 10–1 shows a fibroblast in a normal intact tendon. The most marked difference between the two cells is in the appearance of their nuclei. Cells from immobilized specimens seem to have much more dense heterochromatin than do normal cells. Does this mean that prolonged immobilization causes fibroblasts to change their normal morphology, or do these cells instead represent a different cell line altogether, perhaps one that has "invaded" the tendon as a result of the prolonged immobilization?

A major goal of our series of experiments is to understand how electrical currents of very low amplitude aid the healing process of tendons. Our hypothesis is that the effect is mediated via a low-amplitude, low-frequency electromagnetic field to which fibroblasts are sensitive. Furthermore, our model states that fibroblasts, even in mature tendons, retain an active role in maintaining the structure and do this by sensing how much the tendon is being used. We propose that the signal that couples tendon activity to the resident fibroblasts is also electromagnetic and is based on the piezoelectric properties of collagen. Use of the tendon stresses and strains collagen fibers, which then generate low-amplitude electromagnetic fields around themselves. The

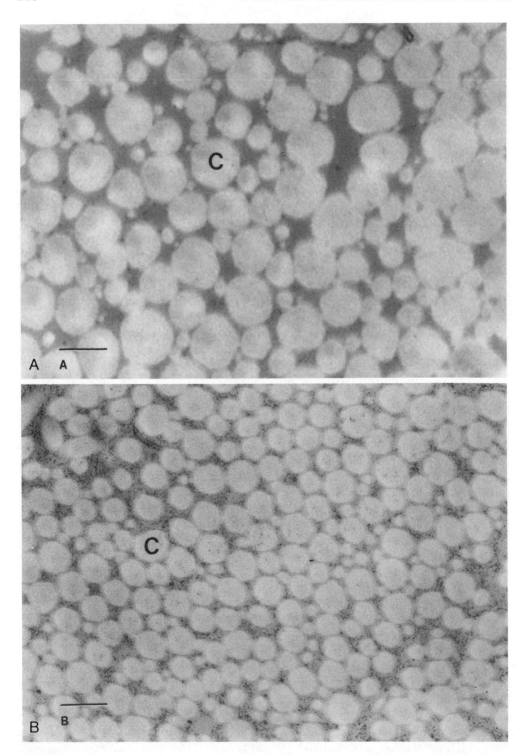

FIGURE 10–10. Electron micrograph showing two cross-sectional views of the rat Achilles tendon. *A* shows the collagen fibrils of nonimmobilized control tendon. *B* shows the collagen fibrils of a 5-week immobilized tendon. Note the remarkable difference in sizes of the fibrils even though the photographs were magnified equally. C = collagen fibrils. (magnification ×69,000; bar 17 mm = 1 μm).

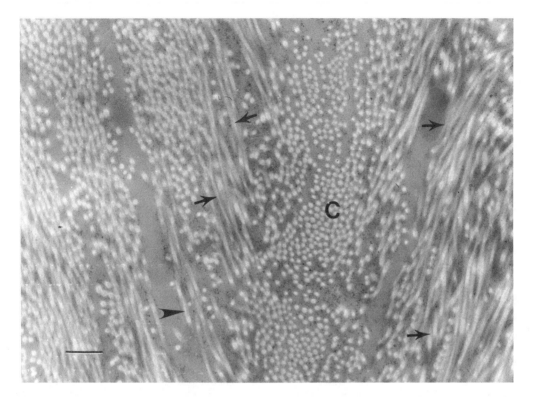

FIGURE 10–11.   Electron micrograph showing a cross section of a rat Achilles tendon that was immobilized in plaster for 5 weeks. Although this is a cross-sectional view, fibrils are seen running in different directions, indicating extensive disorganization of the orderly arrangement that is unique to tendons *(arrows)*. C = collagen fibrils; (magnification ×26,900; bar 13.4 mm = 1 μm).

presence of these fields is somehow sensed by the fibroblasts and stimulates them to repair or make more collagen. Conversely, inactivity results in a lack of these proposed electromagnetic fields. This inactivity "tells" fibroblasts that not much is going on and therefore that maintaining collagen and other ground substances is not too important. It is therefore clear that our work with the inactivity, activity, and electrical stimulation of healing tendons is really interrelated, although this may not seem to be so on superficial examination.

SUMMARY

Various tissues develop endogenous bioelectric currents, and the flow of such currents may be altered by injury. Altered endogenous currents can themselves be modulated to facilitate the healing process of injured tissues. On the basis of cellular, vascular, and matrical changes, the series of events leading to tendon healing may be divided into three aspects: (1) inflammatory response and neoangiogenesis, (2) fibroplasia and fibrillogenesis, and (3) matrix remodeling. Neutrophils, platelets, monocytes, macrophages, and lymphocytes play key roles during the inflammatory phase of tendon healing. Prior to collagen synthesis, new blood vessels are formed; this neovasculature provides oxygen and nutrients and removes carbon dioxide and other metabolic waste products. Not only do macrophages debride the wound via phag-

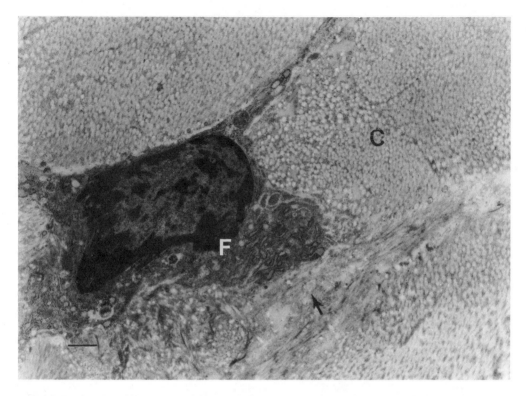

FIGURE 10–12. Electron micrograph of the collagen fibrils of a rat Achilles tendon that was immobilized in plaster for 5 weeks (another area of the tendon of Figure 10–10 *B*). Note the dense clumps of heterochromatin lining the inner surface of this fibroblast (F). Also, note that the cytoplasmic organelles within the vicinity of extensively disorganized matrix are relatively differentiated, suggesting a close relation between matrical changes and fibroblast morphology. C = collagen fibrils; (magnification ×10,700; bar 10.7 mm = 1 μm).

ocytosis, they facilitate angiogenesis, migration of fibroblasts to the site of injury, and their proliferation. Fibroplasia and fibrillogenesis occur simultaneously; and these events continue even as the newly produced matrix is being remodeled. Studies have shown that anodal stimulation augments the healing strength of experimentally tenotomized and repaired rat Achilles tendons. Electrical stimulation of tenotomized rabbit profundus tendons in vitro has been shown to enhance fibroblast proliferation and collagen synthesis, thus suggesting that the increased healing strength of stimulated tendons may be the result of the production of more collagen in these tendons. There is equal evidence that modulation of cAMP metabolism, increased DNA and collagen syntheses, and increased intracellular Ca^{2+} with subsequent elevation of insulin binding are possible mechanisms by which electrical fields and currents modulate tendon healing. However, based on our series of experiments involving electrical stimulation of tenotomized and repaired tendons, and our experience with tendons that were immobilized without prior tenotomy, we believe that there may be other mechanisms of action. We propose that the signal that couples tendon activity to the resident fibroblasts is electromagnetic and is based on the piezoelectric properties of collagen. Use of the tendon stresses and strains collagen fibers, which then generate low-amplitude electromagnetic fields around themselves. The presence of these fields is somehow sensed by the fibroblasts, which are then stimulated to repair or make more collagen. Conversely, inactivity results in a lack of these proposed electromagnetic fields. This "tells" fibroblasts that not much is going on and therefore that maintaining collagen and other ground substances is not too important.

REFERENCES

1. DuBois-Reymond, E: Cited in Borgens, RB, Jaffe, LF, and Cohen, MJ: Large and persistent electrical currents enter the transected lamprey spinal cord. Proc Natl Acad Sci U S A 77:1209–1213, 1980.
2. Hyde, IH: Differences in electrical potential in developing eggs. Am J Physiol 12:241–275, 1905.
3. Lund, EJ: Experimental control of organic polarity by the electric current. J Exp Zool 41:155–190, 1925.
4. Brodemer, CW: Evocation of regrowth phenomena in anuran limbs by electrical stimulation of the nerve supply. Anat Rec 148:441–457, 1964.
5. Smith, SD: Induction of partial limb regeneration in *Rana pipiens* by galvanic stimulation. Anat Rec 158:89–98, 1967.
6. Smith, SD: Effects of electrical fields upon regeneration in the metazoa. Am Zool 10:133–140, 1970.
7. Schotte, OE and Wilber, JF: Effects of adrenal transplants upon forelimb regeneration in normal and in hypophysectomized adult frogs. Journal of Embryology and Experimental Morphology 6:247–261, 1958.
8. Borgens, RB, Vanable, JW, and Jaffe, LF: Bioelectricity and regeneration: 1. Initiation of frog limb regeneration by minute currents. J Exp Zool 200:403–416, 1977.
9. Borgens, RB, Vanable, JW, and Jaffe, LF: Small artificial currents enhance *Xenopus* limb regeneration. J Exp Zool 207:217–225, 1979.
10. Borgens, RB, Vanable, JW, and Jaffe, LF: Bioelectricity and regeneration. Bioscience 29:468–474, 1979.
11. Borgens, RB, Vanable, JW, and Jaffe, LF: Reduction of sodium dependent stump currents disturbs urodele limb regeneration. J Exp Zool 209:377–386, 1979.
12. Borgens, RB, Vanable, JW, and Jaffe, LF: Role of subdermal current shunts in the failure of frogs to regenerate. J Exp Zool 209:49–55, 1979.
13. Borgens, RB, Jaffe, LF, and Cohen, MJ: Large and persistent electrical currents enter the transected lamprey spinal cord. Proc Natl Acad Sci U S A 77:1209–1213, 1980.
14. Borgens, RB: What is the role of naturally produced electric current in vertebrate regeneration and healing? Int Rev Cytol 76:245–298, 1982.
15. Friedenberg, ZB and Brighton, CT: Electrical fracture healing. Ann NY Acad Sci 238:564–574, 1974.
16. Baker, B and Becker, RO: A study of electrochemical enhancement of articular cartilage repair. Clin Orthop 102:251–267, 1974.
17. Assimacopoulos, D: Low intensity negative electric current in the treatment of ulcers of the leg due to chronic venous insufficiency. Preliminary report of three cases. Am J Surg 115:683–687, 1968.
18. Wolcott, LE and Wheeler, PC: Accelerated healing of skin ulcers by electrotherapy: Preliminary clinical results. South Med J 62:795–801, 1969.
19. Wheeler, PC, Wolcott, LE, Morris, JL, et al: Neural considerations in the healing of ulcerated tissue by clinical electrotherapeutic application of weak direct currents: Findings and theory. In Reynolds, DV and Sjoberg AE (eds.): Neuroelectric Research. Charles C Thomas, Springfield, IL, 1971, pp 83–99.
20. Rowley, BA: Electrical current effects in *E coli* growth rates. Proc Soc Exp Biol Med 139:929, 1972.
21. Barranco, SD, Spadaro, JA, Berger, TJ, et al: In vitro effect of weak direct current on Staphylococcus aureus. Clin Orthop 100:250–255, 1974.
22. Carey, LC and Lepley, D: Effect of continuous direct electric current on healing wounds. Surgical Forum 13:33–35, 1982.
23. Becker, RO: Stimulation of partial limb regeneration in rats. Nature 235:109–111, 1972.
24. Salamon, A and Hamori, J: Present state of tendon regeneration: Light and electron microscopic studies of the regenerating tendon of the rat. Acta Morphol Hung 14:7–24, 1966.
25. Conway, AM: Regeneration of resected calcaneal tendons of the rabbit. Anat Rec 158:43–49, 1967.
26. Rokkanon, P and Vainio, K: Healing of extensor tendons in the rabbit. Scand J Plast Reconstr Surg Hand Surg 5:100–102, 1971.
27. Postacchini, F and De Martino, C: Regeneration of rabbit calcaneal tendon: Maturation of collagen and elastic fibers following partial tenotomy. Connect Tissue Res 8:41–47, 1980.
28. Ippolito, E, Natali, PG, Postacchini, F, et al: Morphological, immunological, and biochemical study of rabbit Achilles tendon at various ages. J Bone Joint Surg [Am] 62:583–598, 1980.
29. Enwemeka, CS: Inflammation, cellularity, and fibrillogenesis in regenerating tendon: Implications for tendon rehabilitation. Phys Ther 69:816–825, 1989.
30. Williams, IF: Cellular and biochemical composition of healing tendons. In Jenkins, DHR (ed): Ligament Injuries and Their Treatment. Aspen, Rockville, MD, 1985, pp 43–57.
31. Bornstein, P and Traub, W: The chemistry and biology of collagen. In Neurath, H and Hill, RL (eds): The Proteins, Vol 4. Academic Press, New York, 1979.

32. Bornstein, P and Sage, H: Structurally distinct collagen types. Annual Review of Biochemistry 49:957, 1980.
33. Brodsky, B and Eikenberry, EF: Characterization of fibrous forms of collagen. Methods in Enzymology 82:127, 1982.
34. Hall, MC: The locomotor system: Functional Histology. Charles C Thomas, Springfield, IL, 1965.
35. Kastelic, J, Galeski, A, and Baer, E: The multicomposite structure of tendon. Connect Tissue Res 6:11–23, 1978.
36. Fessler, JH and Fessler, LI: Biosynthesis of procollagen. Annu Rev Biochem 47:129–162, 1978.
37. Olsen, BR: Collagen Biosynthesis. In Hay, ED (ed): Cell Biology of Extracellular Matrix. Plenum Press, New York, 1981, pp 139–177.
38. Nimni, ME and Harkness, RD: Molecular structure and functions of collagen. In Nimni, ME (ed): Collagen, Vol I, Biochemistry. CRC Press, Boca Raton, FL, 1988, pp 1–77.
39. Amiel, D, Kleiner, JB, Roux, RD, et al: The phenomenon of "ligamentalization": Anterior cruciate ligament reconstruction with autogenous patellar tendon. J Orthop Res 4:162–172, 1986.
40. Vogel, HG: Correlation between tensile strength and collagen content in rat skin. Effect of age and cortisol treatment. Connect Tissue Res 2:177, 1974.
41. Vogel, HG: Influence of maturation and age on mechanical and biochemical parameters of connective tissue of various organs in the rat. Connect Tissue Res 6:161, 1978.
42. Parry, DAD, Barnes, GRG, and Craig, AS: A comparison of the size distribution of collagen fibrils in connective tissues as a function of age and a possible relation between fibril size distribution and mechanical properties. Proc R Soc Lond [Biol] 203:305–321, 1978.
43. Parry, DAD and Craig, AS: Quantitative electron microscopic observations of the collagen fibrils in rat-tail tendon. Biopolymers 16:1015–1031, 1977.
44. Flint, MH, Craig, AS, Reilly, HC, et al: Collagen fibril diameters and glycosaminoglycan content of skins: Indices of tissue maturation and function. Connect Tissue Res 13:69–81, 1984.
45. Parry, DAD and Craig, AS: Collagen fibrils during development and maturatin and their contribution to the mechanical attributes of connective tissue. In Nimni ME, (ed): Collagen, Vol 2, Biochemistry and Biomechanics. CRC Press, Boca Raton, FL, 1988, pp 1–23.
46. Garlock, JH: The repair process of wounds of tendons and in tendon grafts. Ann Surg 85:95–103, 1927.
47. Mason, ML and Shearon, CG: The process of tendon repair. Arch Surg 25:615–692, 1932.
48. Stearns, ML: Studies on the development of connective tissue on transparent chambers in the rabbit's ear. I. Am J Anat 66:133–176, 1940.
49. Stearns, ML: Studies on the development of connective tissue on transparent chambers in the rabbit's ear. II. Am J Anat 67:55–97, 1940.
50. Buck, RC: Regeneration of tendon. J Pathol 66:1–18, 1953.
51. Arner, O, Lindholm, A, and Orell, SR: Histologic changes in subcutaneous rupture of the Achilles tendon. Acta Chir Scand 116:484–490, 1958/1959.
52. Flynn, JE and Graham, JH: Healing of tendon wounds. Am J Surg 109:315–324, 1965.
53. Deuel, TF, Senior, RM, Chang, D, et al: Platelet factor 4 is chemotactic for neutrophils and monocytes. Proc Natl Acad Sci U S A 78:4584–4587, 1981.
54. Deuel, TF, Senior, RM, Huang, JS, et al: Chemotaxis of monocytes and neutrophils to platelet-derived growth factor. J Clin Invest 69:1046–1049, 1982.
55. Pierce, GF, Mustoe, TA, Senior, RM, et al: In vivo incisional wound healing augmented by platelet-derived growth factor and recombinant c-cis gene homodimeric proteins. J Exp Med 67:974–987, 1988.
56. Fishel, RS, Barbul, A, Beschorner, WE, et al: Lymphocyte participation in wound healing. Morphologic assessment using monoclonal antibodies. Ann Surg 206:25–29, 1987.
57. Ross, R and Benditt, EP: Wound healing and collagen formation. I. Sequential changes in components of guinea pig skin wounds observed in the electron microscope. Journal of Biophysics Biochemistry and Cytology 11:677–700, 1961.
58. Leibovich, SJ and Ross, R: A macrophage-dependent factor that stimulates the proliferation of fibroblasts in vitro. Am J Pathol 81:501–513, 1976.
59. Laub, R and Vaes, G: Macrophages stimulate the activation of plasminogen by fibroblasts. FEBS Lett 145:362–368, 1982.
60. Laub, R, Huybrechts-Gadin, G, Peeters-Joris, C, et al: Degradation of collagen and proteoglycan by macrophages and fibroblasts: Individual potentialities of each cell type and cooperative effects through the activation of fibroblasts by macrophages. Biochim Biophys Acta 721:425–433, 1982.
61. Leibovich, SJ and Ross, R: The role of macrophages in wound repair: A study with hydrocortisone and antimacrophage serum. Am J Pathol 78:71–100, 1975.
62. DeLustro, F, Sherer, GK, and LeRoy, EC: Human monocyte stimulation of fibroblast growth by soluble mediator(s). J Leukoc Biol 28:519–532, 1980.
63. Bitterman, PB, Rennard, SI, Hunninghake, BW, et al: Human alveolar macrophage growth factor for fibroblasts: Regulation and partial characterization. J Clin Invest 70:806–822, 1982.
64. Martin, BM, Gimbrone, MA, Jr, Unanue, ER, et al: Stimulation of nonlymphoid mesenchymal cell proliferation by a macrophage-derived growth factor. J Immunol 126:1510–1515, 1981.

65. Martin, TR, Altman, LC, Albert, RK, et al: Leukotriene B$_4$ production by the human alveolar macrophage: A potential mechanism for amplifying inflammation in the lung. Am Rev Respir Dis 129:106–111, 1984.
66. Glenn, KC and Ross, R: Human monocyte-derived growth factors for mesenchymal cells: Activation of secretion by endotoxin and Con A. Cell 25:603–615, 1981.
67. Diegleman, RF, Cohen, IK, and Kaplan, AM: Effect of macrophages on fibroblast DNA synthesis and proliferation. Proc Soc Exp Biol Med 169:445–451, 1982.
68. Dohlman, JG, Payan, DG, and Goetzl, EJ: Generation of a unique fibroblast-activating factor by human monocytes. Immunology 52:577–584, 1984.
69. Baird, A, Mormede, P, and Bohlen, P: Immunoreactive fibroblast growth factor in cells of peritoneal exudate suggests its identity with macrophage-derived growth factor. Biochem Biophys Res Commun 126:358–364, 1985.
70. Leslie, CC, Musson, RA, and Henson, PM: Production of growth factor activity for fibroblasts by human monocyte-derived macrophages. J Leukoc Biol 36:143–159, 1984.
71. Shimokado, K, Raines, EW, Madtes, DK, et al: A significant part of macrophage-derived growth factor consists of at least two forms of PDGF. Cell 43:277–286, 1985.
72. Martinet, Y, Bitterman, PB, Mornex, J-F, et al: Activated human monocytes express the c-cis proto-oncogene and release a mediator showing PDGF-like activity. Nature 319:158–160, 1986.
73. Turck, CW, Dohlman, JG, and Goetz, EJ: Immunological mediators of wound healing and fibrosis. J Cell Physiol Suppl 5:89–93, 1987.
74. Gospadarowicz, D, Mescher, AL, and Birdwell, CR: Control of cellular proliferation by the fibroblast and epidermal growth factors. National Cancer Institute Moograph No. 48 1978, pp 109–130.
75. Niinikoski, J: The effect of blood and oxygen supply on the biochemistry of repair. In Hunt, TK (ed): Wound Healing and Wound Infection: Theory and Surgical Practice. Appleton-Century-Crofts, New York, 1980, pp 56–70.
76. Schoefl, GI and Majno, G: Regeneration of blood vessels in wound healing. In Montagna, W and Billingham, RE (eds): Advances in Biology of Skin, Vol 5, Wound Healing. Pergamon Press, London, 1964, pp 173–193.
77. Garner, A: Ocular angiogenesis. Int Rev Exp Pathol 28:249–306, 1986.
78. Folkman, J and Klagsbrun, M: Angiogenic factors. Science 235:442–447, 1987.
79. Clark, RA, Stone, RD, Leung, DYK, et al: Role of macrophages in wound healing. Surgical Forum 27:16–18, 1976.
80. Polverini, PJ, Cotran, RS, Gimbrone, MA, Jr, et al: Activated macrophages induce vascular proliferation. Nature 269:804–806, 1977.
81. Polverini, PJ and Leibovich, SJ: Induction of neovascularization in vivo and endothelial proliferation in vitro by tumor-associated macrophages. Lab Invest 51:635–642, 1984.
82. Schweigerer, L, Neufeld, G, Friedman, J, et al: Capillary endothelial cells express basic fibroblast growth factor, a mitogen that promotes their growth. Nature 325:257–259, 1987.
83. Nimni, ME: The molecular organization of collagen and its role in determining the biophysical properties of the connective tissues. Biorheology 17:51–82, 1980.
84. Enwemeka, CS and Konyecsni, WM: Biomechanical changes induced by early weight-bearing in healing rabbit Achilles tendons (abstr). Phys Ther 68:843, 1988.
85. Enwemeka, CS: The effects of early function on tendon healing (abstr). Med Sci Sports Exerc (Suppl) 20:33, 1988.
86. Slack, C, Flint, MH, and Thompson, BM: The effect of tensional load on isolated embryonic chick tendons in organ culture. Connect Tissue Res 12:229–247, 1984.
87. McGaw, WT: The effect of tension on collagen remodelling by fibroblasts: A stereological ultrastructural study. Connect Tissue Res 14:229–235, 1986.
88. Postacchini, F, Accini, L, Natali, PG, et al: Regeneration of rabbit calcaneal tendon: A morphological and immunochemical study. Cell Tissue Res 195:81–97, 1978.
89. Woo, SL-Y, Gelberman, RH, Cobb, NT, et al: The importance of controlled passive mobilization on flexor tendon healing. Acta Orthop Scand 52:615–622, 1981.
90. Gelberman, RH, Amiel, D, Gonsalves, M, et al: The influence of protected passive mobilization on the healing of flexor tendons. A biomechanical and microangiographic study. Hand 13:120–128, 1981.
91. Gelberman, RH, Van de Berg, JS, Lundberg, GN, et al: Flexor tendon healing and restoration of the gliding surface. J Bone Joint Surg [Am] 65:70–80, 1983.
92. Vailas, AC, Tipton, CM, Matthes, RD, et al: Physical activity and its influence on the repair process of medial collateral ligaments. Connect Tissue Res 9:25–31, 1981.
93. Enwemeka, CS: The effects of early function on collagen fibril populations in regenerating tendons (abstr). FASEB J 2:1587, 1988.
94. Owoeye, IO: The Therapeutic Effect of Galvanic Current Following Rupture of the Achilles Tendon in Rats. New York University, New York, 1982. Doctoral dissertation.
95. Owoeye, I, Spielholz, NI, Fetto, J, et al: Low intensity pulsed galvanic current and the healing of rat Achilles tenotomized tendons: Preliminary report using load-to-breaking measurements. Arch Phys Med Rehabil 68:415–418, 1987.

96. Mathews, LS and Ellis, D: Viscoelastic properties of cat tendon: Effects of time after death and preservation by freezing. J Biomech 1:65–71, 1968.
97. Woo, SL-Y, Orlando, CA, Camp, JF, et al: Effects of postmortem storage by freezing on ligament tensile behavior. J Biomech 19:399–404, 1986.
98. Frank, C, Edwards, P, McDonald, D, et al: Viability of ligaments after freezing: An experimental study in a rabbit model. J Orthop Res 6:95–102, 1988.
99. Stanish, WD, Rbinovich, M, Kozey, J, et al: The use of electricity in ligament and tendon repair. The Physician and Sportsmedicine 13:109–116, 1985.
100. Kleczynski, S: Electrical stimulation to promote the union of fractures. Int Orthop 12:83–87, 1988.
101. Bassett, CAL, Pawluk, RJ and Becker, RO: Effects of electric currents on bone in vitro. Nature 204:652–654, 1964.
102. Becker, RO: The significance of electrically stimulated osteogenesis: More questions than answers. Clin Orthop 141:266–274, 1979.
103. Black, J: Electrical stimulation of hard and soft tissues in animal models. Clinics in Plastic Surgery 12:243–257, 1985.
104. Enwemeka, CS, Spielholz, NI, and Nelson, AJ: The effect of early functional activities on experimentally tenotomized Achilles tendons in rats. Am J Phys Med Rehabil 67:264–269, 1988.
105. Nessler, JP and Mass, DP: Direct-current electrical stimulation of tendon healing in vitro. Clin Orthop 217:303–312, 1987.
106. Osborne, SL and Holmquest, HJ: Technic of Electrotherapy and Its Physical and Physiological Basis. Charles C Thomas, Springfield, IL, 1944, pp 3–38.
107. Carley, PJ and Winapel, SF: Electrotherapy for acceleration of wound healing: Low intensity direct current. Arch Phys Med Rehabil 66:443–446, 1985.
108. Murray, JC and Farndale, RW: Modulation of collagen production in cultured fibroblasts by a low-frequency, pulsed magnetic field. Biochim Biophys Acta 838:98–105, 1985.
109. Gerber, J, Cordey, J, and Perren, SM: Influence of magnetic fields on growth and regeneration in organ culture. In Burny, F, Herbst, E, and Hinsenkamp, M (eds): Electrical stimulation of bone growth and repair. Springer Verlag, New York, 1988, pp 35–40.
110. Lunt, MJ and Barker, AT: Pulsed magnetic field therapy for tibial non-union and for rotator cuff tendinitis. Lancet 38:1295, 1984.
111. Farndale, RW and Murray, JC: Pulsed electromagnetic fields promote collagen production in bone marrow fibroblasts via athermal mechanisms. Calcif Tissue Int 37:178–182, 1985.
112. Korenstein, R, Somjen, D, Fischler, H, et al: Capacitive pulsed electric stimulation of bone cells: Induction of cyclic-AMP changes and DNA synthesis. Biochim Biophys Acta 803:302–307, 1984.
113. Farndale, RW and Murray, JC: The action of pulsed magnetic fields on cyclic AMP levels in cultured fibroblasts. Biochim Biophys Acta 881:46–53, 1986.
114. Brighton, CT and McCluskey, WP: Response of cultured bone cells to a capacitively coupled electric field: Inhibition of cAMP response to parathyroid hormone. J Orthop Res 6:567–571, 1988.
115. Brighton, CT and Townsend, PF: Increased cAMP production after short-term capacitively coupled stimulation on bovine growth plate chondrocytes. J Orthop Res 6:552–558, 1988.
116. Bourguignon, GJ and Bourguignon, YW: Electric stimulation of protein and DNA synthesis in human fibroblasts. FASEB J 1:398–402, 1987.
117. McLeod, KJ, Lee, RC, and Ehrlich, HP: Frequency dependence of electric field modulation of fibroblast protein synthesis. Science 236:1465–1469, 1987.
118. Okihana, H and Shimomura, Y: Effect of direct current on cultured growth cartilage cells in vitro. J Orthop Res 6:690–694, 1988.
119. Dunn, MG, Doillon, CJ, Berg, RA, et al: Wound healing using a collagen matrix: Effect of DC electrical stimulation. J Biomed Mater Res 22:191–206, 1988.
120. Bourguignon, GJ, Wenche, JY, Bourguignon, LYW: Electric stimulation of human fibroblasts causes an increase in Ca^{2+} influx and the exposure of additional insulin receptors. J Cell Physiol 140:379–385, 1989.

CHAPTER 11

Electrical Stimulation of Articular Cartilage

A. Joseph Threlkeld, Ph.D., P.T.

Articular cartilage is a specialized connective tissue that serves as the bearing surface for synovial joints. Its unique structure provides a remarkably resilient surface capable of withstanding loading impacts several times greater than body weight and of resisting the shearing stresses of thousands of repetitive movements. In the adult human, articular cartilage averages a mere 2 to 4 mm in thickness. This thin layer of material is a key link in the production of normal, pain-free movement at synovial joints. Conversely, when articular cartilage becomes degenerate, movement often becomes pathologic, laborious, and painful. Despite the heavy toll that articular dysfunction extracts from the individual and from society, effective intervention and treatment techniques for articular degeneration remain elusive. Pharmacologic intervention targets the inflammation associated with articular degeneration rather than the cartilage itself. Surgical techniques are directed toward removing physical obstructions to movement, improving bone/joint alignment, inducing the growth of fibrous tissue to cover a degenerate surface, or inserting artificial replacement surfaces. The primary thrusts of rehabilitation have been to relieve pain, to decrease joint stress, and to educate the patient to reduce or avoid use of a dysfunctional joint. All of these strategies fail to address the most obvious and direct solution: promoting intrinsic articular cartilage repair. A growing body of theoretical and experimental evidence indicates that electrical stimulation may provide a means to reach this elusive goal. The purposes of this chapter are to (1) present the research literature concerning the degeneration, remodeling and repair of articular cartilage; (2) discuss the influence of electrical signals on skeletal tissues; and (3) present the results of an experiment exploring the effects of extrinsic electrical signals on articular cartilage remodeling.

PATHOLOGY OF ARTICULAR CARTILAGE

Degeneration, as evidenced by deterioration of the articular surface, is not a recent evolutionary trend and is found in all species possessing synovial joints. Degen-

255

erate joint surfaces have been described in the fossils of prehistoric man as well as in those of long extinct species.[1,2] The pathologic changes wrought by the various joint diseases have been documented by clinicians and researchers alike. Many elaborate therapeutic regimens have been used to ameliorate the disabling symptoms accompanying the various forms of joint disease. Despite these efforts, few real gains have been made in the prevention of joint degeneration or the repair of damaged articular cartilage.

The degeneration of the articular surface begins with mild fraying of the tangential collagen fibers (fibrillation), followed by cavitation (blistering) between the tangential collagen bundles. Blistering is succeeded by vertical splits (clefting) that penetrate the superficial layer and then the deep layers (Fig. 11–1). The clefted cartilage is gradually worn away, leading to a complete denuding of affected regions of the articular surface.[1] This progression of degenerative changes produces marked alterations in the porosity of, and thus the fluid flow through, the cartilage. As degeneration progresses, immunocompetent cells and large-molecular-weight substances (e.g., immunoglob-

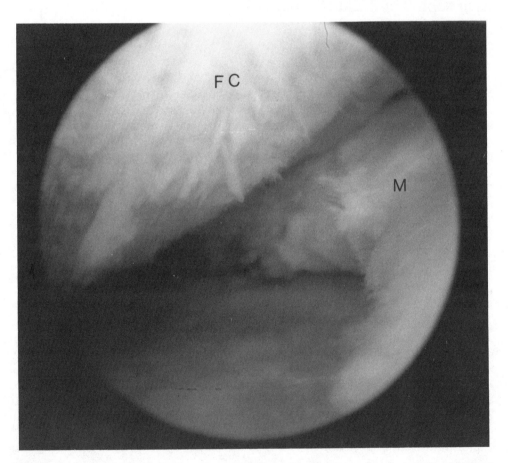

FIGURE 11–1. Degenerate articular cartilage. This photograph was taken during an arthroscopic examination of a human knee. The articular cartilage of the femoral condyle (FC) shows the ragged appearance characteristic of deep clefting. The meniscus (M) also shows degenerative change. The original magnification factor due to the arthroscope was 5 to 10 ×, depending on the object's distance from the arthroscopic lens.

ulins) may obtain access to normally protected deeper cartilage layers while biomechanical stiffness is simultaneously reduced.[3,4]

Although we do not know the initiating factor(s) in idiopathic degenerative joint
disease, articular degeneration may be induced experimentally by joint instability,
blunt trauma, overloading, and immobilization. These experimental models were
succinctly reviewed by Hulth.[5]

REMODELING AND REPAIR OF ARTICULAR CARTILAGE

All living tissues are capable of a certain amount of remodeling; replacement of
deteriorating or degenerate cellular and matrix components is essential to tissue maintenance. The normal remodeling of adult articular cartilage can be considered to
represent a minor but successful repair effort. It is suspected, but not proved, that
the failure of articular remodeling and repair in response to joint stress leads to
osteoarthritis. A few studies have followed changes within joints that were loaded
within the physiologic range but with altered force vectors. Palmoski and co-workers[6]
amputated one hind paw of a group of dogs and reported that after 6 weeks, the
femoral condylar cartilage on the amputated side demonstrated decreased thickness,
reduction in safranin-O staining, decreased glycosaminoglycan content, increased
water content, defective glycosaminoglycan structure, and reduction of net glycosaminoglycan synthesis. These alterations of articular cartilage are similar to the changes
associated with early degenerative joint disease. Unilateral hindpaw amputation has
also been shown to produce bilateral remodeling of the articular surface of the femoral
head of rats.[7] Studies of this nature to examine human joints are of course impossible,
but some case studies of human amputees are available. A clinical study of 42 below-
knee amputees by Burke and colleagues[8] reported that the amputated limb showed
an 88 percent incidence of osteoporosis, but the intact limb presented a 17 percent
incidence of degenerative joint disease in the knee. A survey by Benichou and Wirotius[9]
that examined the hips of 53 above-knee amputees reported that approximately one
half of the patients had a 50 percent reduction of hip cartilage height on the amputated
side, and that all patients had osteoporosis on the amputated side. There was no hip
osteoarthritis on the amputated side in any of the patients in the study by Benichou
and Wirotius.

Reparative phenomena in overtly damaged articular cartilage have been studied
as well. Articular cartilage that has been superficially lacerated or abraded (leaving
the underlying calcified cartilage intact) has minimal intrinsic reparative capacity.
There is a brief burst of mitotic activity in the immediate vicinity of the laceration
associated with some increase in matrix synthesis. This activity often ceases within
2 to 4 weeks after laceration, leaving the repair process incomplete.[10] If the cartilage
is lacerated through its complete thickness to the level of the underlying subchondral
bone, bleeding into the wound ensues, succeeded by an ingrowth of blood vessels.
The invading perivascular cells differentiate and manufacture a fibrous scar, filling
the defect.[11,12] Occasionally this scar matures into hyaline or hyalinelike cartilage.
Operative joint resurfacing procedures are founded on this phenomenon. The transformation from a fibrous to a hyalinelike state is strongly potentiated by continuous
passive motion of the joint during the healing phase.[13]

One could conclude from these studies that there is a relation between weight
bearing and the normal metabolism/remodeling of articular cartilage. Joint surfaces

are subject to variations in stress and loading throughout their history, variations which require remodeling and some amount of repair. At what point does the adaptive response of normal articular cartilage become ineffective and cartilage failure begin? Why is the chondrocyte's repair attempt so cursory and rapidly attentuated? There is copious documentation of the morphologic and biochemical details of degenerating cartilage, but far less is known about the adaptive responses of normal cartilage. Adaptation is essentially a successful repair effort. What signals within the articular environment incite the chondrocytes to mount a successful biologic response, and what is the nature of that response? Can these signals be approximated, produced, or augmented by external stimuli? Can the elicited responses of the chondrocytes be controlled or modified to more adequately repair joint destruction? Only when these questions have been addressed will a scientific foundation be available for effective treatment of degenerative articular diseases.

BIOLOGIC SIGNALING IN SKELETAL TISSUE

Because articular cartilage is an integral part of the appendicular skeleton, it is valuable to briefly examine the known control mechanisms for bone and see if these control mechanisms might apply to cartilage as well. Bone growth and remodeling are subject to an assortment of well-characterized endocrine and metabolic influences prior to skeletal maturity. Once maturity is reached, however, normal remodeling responses are primarily elicited by the stresses applied to bone. According to Wolff's law, bones remodel to resist an applied stress.[14] Remodeling has been linked to a series of electrical events which are generated electromechanically via the piezoelectric character of bone. As a bone is stressed, regions subjected to compression become more electronegative while areas subjected to tension become more electropositive. The osteocytes respond by manufacturing additional bone on the electronegative surface and removing it on the electropositive surface.[15–18] These mechanically generated electrical signals are monitored and averaged to influence osteocyte metabolism. Alterations of stress applied to bone appears to be interpreted locally and the resultant bone remodeling controlled and directed in the region of the stress. A bioelectric signal is generated via a piezoelectric effect and transduced by the osteocytes, which remodel the bone to resist the stress.

This principle of bone remodeling is being exploited by the use of implantable electrodes to heal nonuniting fractures. A negative electrode is placed in or near the fracture site, with the positive electrode at some distance. Fractures may also be provoked to heal through the application of externally placed inductive coils producing a pulsed electromagnetic field (PEMF)[19–22] or by capacitively coupled electrical fields.[23]

If an analogous system were present in articular cartilage, it would require that (1) an endogenous electrical signal be generated in response to deformation, and (2) the chondrocytes be able to recognize and respond to the signal. As in the case of bone, it would be useful clinically if this response could be elicited or augmented by exogenous electrical signals. First, the evidence that an electrical signal does exist in cartilage will be presented, then the studies that document the response of articular cartilage to exogenous signals will be reviewed. Finally, the results of an experiment exploring the effects of electrical signals on the remodeling process of articular cartilage will be presented.

ELECTRICAL SIGNALS INTRINSIC TO ARTICULAR CARTILAGE

The theory has been proposed that articular cartilage is remodeled in response to intrinsic electrical signals.[24] The very morphology of articular cartilage produces an electrochemical environment with a charge state that fluctuates with the movement of water in and out of the poroelastic cartilage pad. Experimental evidence of piezoelectric phenomena in articular cartilage was produced by Bassett and Pawluk,[25] who compressed plugs of bovine cartilage while monitoring the potential difference between the articular and subchondral surfaces. The onset of compression was accompanied by an immediate sharp increase in potential difference (1 to 4 mV), which exponentially decayed to a plateau value of approximately 40 percent of the peak value. This plateau value was maintained until the compression was removed. Extraction of the cartilage sample with 0.05 M NaOH, 0.05 M HCl, or soaking in 3 percent NaCl prior to testing eliminated the plateau of long-term polarization but the initial spike was unaffected. They concluded that the initial spike was a piezoelectric response due to "mechanically induced, intra- or intermolecular charge separation or dipole reorientation," whereas the plateau portion was a result of streaming potentials induced by a hydraulic flow out of the matrix.[25] These results were confirmed and expanded by Lotke and colleagues,[26] who measured the potential change within the matrix just below the articular surface of human articular cartilage plugs taken from the lateral femoral condyle. They demonstrated that the amplitude of the potential difference increased with increasing strain.[26] Similar results were obtained by others.[27-29] Much of the work on connective tissue piezoelectricity up to the early 1980s has been summarized by Grodzinsky.[30] Noteworthy is the fact that piezoelectric effect is reversible in articular cartilage. Application of an electric current to articular cartilage produces a measurable mechanical stress within the cartilage.[28]

Thus there is evidence that electrical signals are generated within articular cartilage when it is deformed by an applied load, and that the signal increases in amplitude with increasing load.

INFLUENCE OF ELECTRICAL SIGNALS ON ARTICULAR CARTILAGE

Does the maintenance and remodeling of normal articular cartilage rely on the transduction of intrinsic electrical signals? No definitive, direct, in vivo evidence exists to answer this question. However, there is a growing body of evidence indicating that externally applied electrical signals can affect articular cartilage remodeling and repair.

Direct current stimulation was used by Baker and associates[31] to aid healing of surgically created full thickness cartilage defects in the femoral condyles of rabbits. Bimetallic devices were implanted in the subchondral region of the defects in experimental animals, whereas control animals had defects but no implants. Histologic analysis showed that 62 percent of the electrically stimulated 4-mm defects were filled or nearly filled with hyaline cartilage, whereas controls demonstrated only a 14 percent rate of closure with hyaline cartilage. This latter group of animals did show defect reduction or closure via the production of fibrous tissue.[31] Sah and Grodzinsky[32] exposed plugs (explants) of immature calf articular cartilage in culture media to various magnitudes and frequencies of sinusoidal electrical current. They reported an 11 percent increase in sulfate incorporation (increased glycosaminoglycan manufacture) in response to a 10-Hz, 300-μA/cm² current.[32] The glycosaminoglycan constituent of articular cartilage matrix is responsible for the resistance of cartilage to compressive stress, and its loss is one of the principal manifestations of cartilage degeneration. The enhancement of glycosaminoglycan production by an externally applied treatment could be of benefit in the treatment of arthritis.

Smith and Nagel[33] reported an experiment designed to investigate the effects of PEMF on the closure of the cartilaginous epiphysis, the growth of long bones, and the biochemical constituents of the tibiofemoral joint articular cartilage. Immature rabbits were harnessed with a set of vertical induction coils suspended in such a fashion that the animal could walk about the cage. The stimulating device was an Electro-Biology clinical model (Electro-Biology Inc., 300 Fairfield Rd., Fairfield, NJ 07006) delivering a repetitive pulse at 72 pps.[33] This particular frequency with its associated waveform has been found to be effective in treating avascular necrosis of the hip.[21] Comparing stimulated animals to nonstimulated controls, no significant differences were found in the time of epiphysial plate closure, in bone growth, or in blood flow as measured by dispersion of radioactive technetium-99m injected prior to death. However, a 22 percent increase in glycosaminoglycan content of the condylar cartilage of the femur was reported in the stimulated group exposed to continuous (24-hour) PEMF stimulation. This glycosaminoglycan increase was not found in the tibial plateau cartilage of the continuous stimulation group, nor in any articular cartilage of a second stimulated group exposed to intermittent stimulation (12 hours on/ 12 hours off). The glycosaminoglycan content was measured by biochemically assaying dissected and minced articular cartilage. Unfortunately, there was no histology of the articular cartilage performed; therefore, the biochemical responses could not be localized to specific anatomic zones of the tibiofemoral joints.

AN EXPERIMENT: EFFECTS OF PEMF ON ARTICULAR REMODELING

To examine the effects of PEMF on articular remodeling, 29 adult Sprague-Dawley rats (90 days old, 306 to 380 g) were randomly assigned to one of three groups. A group of eight rats remained as normal controls (Norm). Twelve rats underwent unilateral hindpaw amputation and were placed in standard rat housing for 8 weeks (AmpCont group). A final group of nine rats underwent unilateral hindpaw amputation but were exposed to PEMF for 8 weeks (AmpStim group). The housing for the AmpStim rats consisted of individual lucite cages (24 × 24 × 16.5 cm) surrounded by four horizontally mounted Helmholtz coils. The coils were mounted such that the bottom coil was at the horizontal level of the cage floor and the top coil at the top of the cage with the remaining two coils spaced evenly between (5.5 cm on center). Adjacent coils were of opposite polarity, producing a Helmholtz-aiding configuration. The vertical magnetic field resulting from this coil architecture was very consistent and nearly homogeneous within the living space of the cages. The peak strength of the magnetic field was 20 gauss (G) with an average field strength of 2 to 3 G.[34] The voltage induced in the tissue of the stimulated rats has been calculated to range from 1.5 to 15 mV/cm and approximately 1 μA/cm².[35] The coils were turned on 12 hours during the "daylight" cycle of the animal quarters and turned off during the 12 hours of darkness. Thus the stimulation period coincided with the relatively quiescent activity period of the nocturnal rodent. Details concerning the PEMF stimulation parameters are given in Figure 11–2. More detail about the materials and methods used in this experiment have been previously described with respect to the Norm and AmpCont groups by Threlkeld and Smith.[7] Statistical analysis of the data was carried out with an unbalanced split plot analysis of variance with a general line models procedure. The significance level was set at $P \leq .05$. Significant effects were further analyzed with individual contrasts. Subpopulations of each of these groups were used in the various

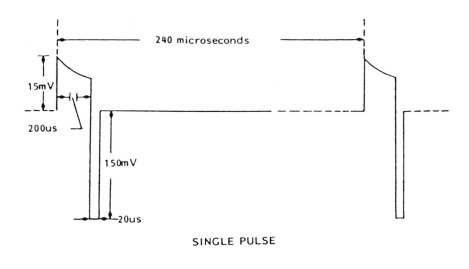

SINGLE PULSE

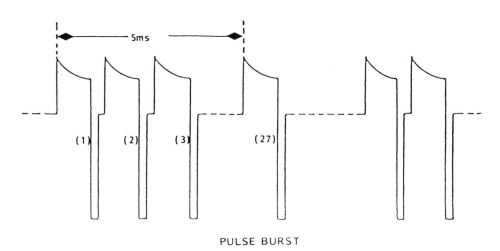

PULSE BURST

FIGURE 11–2. PEMF time and voltage parameters. Schematic diagram of the waveform parameters used in this experiment. The drawings are not to scale. The upper diagram *(single pulse)* shows the time and voltage characteristics of an individual pulse. The lower diagram *(pulse burst)* shows how the individual pulses were grouped into a train of 27 pulses, or "pulse burst," within a 5-millisecond period. The burst of pulses is repeated at 15 Hz.

analyses. The exact number of femora used for each analysis is indicated in Figures 11–3 through 11–5.

This experimental model produced mechanical environments that promoted differential remodeling responses of each hip without superimposing the effects of trauma or inflammation on the joint under examination.[7] In the AmpCont and AmpStim animals, the intact hind limb was often adducted with respect to its usual position, so as to support the weight of the hindquarters during gait. This relative adduction of the femur moved the femoral head within the acetabulum such that the central foveal region of the femoral head relocated from its mediodorsal position to a position closer to the vertical, where it would participate more directly in the transmission of body weight. By this same logic, the lateral edge of the femoral head was moved outward, away from the acetabular shelf, and was exposed to less weight-bearing force than usual. Conversely, the limb with the hindpaw amputated was often carried in an abducted position such that the lateral edge region of the femoral head was moved further beneath the acetabulum. With normal coxofemoral joint alignment, the lateral edge of the femoral head infrequently abuts the zenith of the acetabulum and is not considered a region of primary load transmission. Thus, a position of relative coxofemoral abduction would tend to place the lateral edge of the femoral head into a region of the acetabulum where weight-bearing forces were higher than those usually experienced by the lateral region of the femoral head. It is postulated

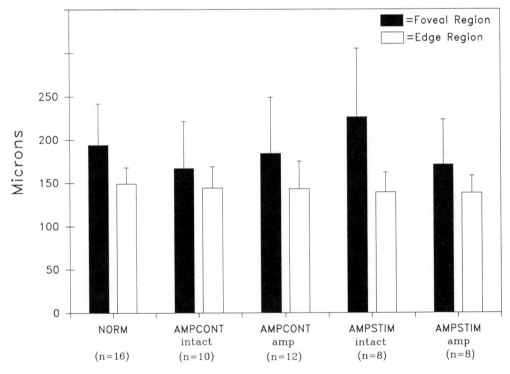

FIGURE 11–3. Articular cartilage thickness. The mean (± SD) of the articular cartilage thickness of the femoral head in the foveal region *(black bar)* and in the edge region *(white bar)* in the normal (Norm) animals, animals with a unilateral hindpaw amputation (AmpCont), and animals with a unilateral hindpaw amputation that were exposed to pulsed electromagnetic fields (AmpStim). The numbers of femora (n) used to calculate the means are indicated.

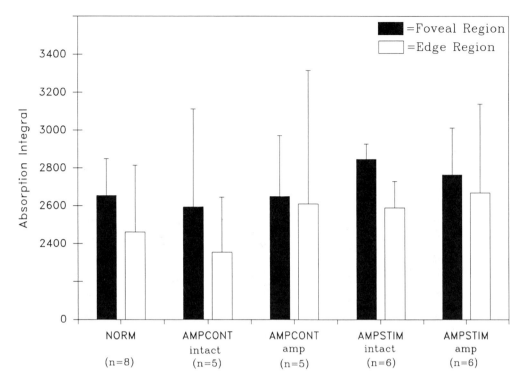

FIGURE 11–4. Proteoglycan density. The mean (± SD) of the articular cartilage proteoglycan density of the femoral head as measured through absorption densitometry of safranin-O staining. Results are shown for the foveal region *(black bar)* and the edge region *(white bar)* in the normal (Norm) animals, animals with a unilateral hindpaw amputation (AmpCont), and animals with a unilateral hindpaw amputation that were exposed to pulsed electromagnetic fields (AmpStim). The numbers of femora (n) used to calculate the means are indicated.

that (1) a remodeling response of the articular cartilage would be seen in the AmpCont animals when compared with the Norm animals, (2) the remodeling response would be regional and would vary with the weight-bearing status of the limb involved, and (3) the remodeling response would be altered in the AmpStim animals exposed to PEMF.

The cranial weight-bearing region of the femoral head articular cartilage was evaluated for morphologic and biochemical changes that would indicate articular remodeling. The weight-bearing region was divided into two subregions: the central weight-bearing region nearest the fovea capitis femoris (foveal region) and the peripheral weight-bearing region nearest the lateral edge of the femoral head (edge region) (Fig. 11–6). Articular thickness, cellularity, proteoglycan (PG) density, and PG production were assessed. There were no significant changes in cartilage cellularity due to the experimental manipulations; thus only the data concerning changes in thickness and PG will be presented here. (See Figs. 11–3, 11–4, and 11–5.)

Articular Cartilage Remodeling in the Intact Limb

The articular cartilage of the Norm animals was thickest near the fovea and thinner toward the lateral edge ($P<.008$). (See Fig. 11–3.) The AmpCont animals did not lose

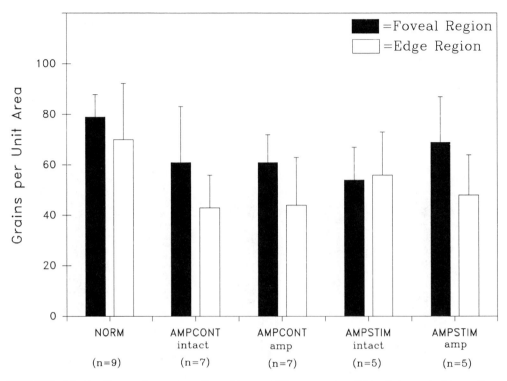

FIGURE 11–5. Proteoglycan manufacturing rate. The mean ($\pm$ SD) of the articular cartilage proteoglycan manufacturing rate of the femoral head as indicated by incorporation of $^{35}SO_4$ and measured through autoradiography and grain counting. Results are shown for the foveal region *(black bar)* and the edge region *(white bar)* in the normal (Norm) animals, animals with a unilateral hindpaw amputation (AmpCont), and animals with a unilateral hindpaw amputation that were exposed to pulsed electromagnetic fields (AmpStim). The numbers of femora (n) used to calculate the means are indicated.

cartilage thickness in the hip of the intact limb when compared with Norm animals; rather, the cartilage thickness was redistributed. There was no significant difference ($P<.07$) between the thickness of the foveal and edge regions in the AmpCont animals. The foveal cartilage of the AmpCont animals demonstrated a relative thinning with respect to the cartilage of the lateral edge region. The result was to yield a rather even cartilage thickness across the superior articular surface of the AmpCont femoral heads rather than the wedge shape demonstrated in the normal animals.

The animals of the AmpStim group showed a much different response in the intact limb. (See Fig. 11–3.) The foveal cartilage of the intact limb was distinctly thicker than the edge cartilage ($P<.0001$). The mean regional cartilage thicknesses of this group were not different from those of the Norm animals, but the normal wedge shape was maintained. The mean thickness of the foveal region of the AmpStim group was significantly thicker than the foveal region of the AmpCont animals ($P<.04$).

Absorption densitometry was used to assess PG density.[7] The Norm animals had more PG in the foveal region than in the edge region ($P<.01$), as did the AmpCont ($P<.04$) and the AmpStim animals ($P<.001$) (see Fig. 11–4). The proteoglycan density of the foveal region of the AmpStim animals was much greater than the foveal PG density of the Norm group ($P<.007$) or of the foveal PG density of the AmpCont animals ($P<.009$).

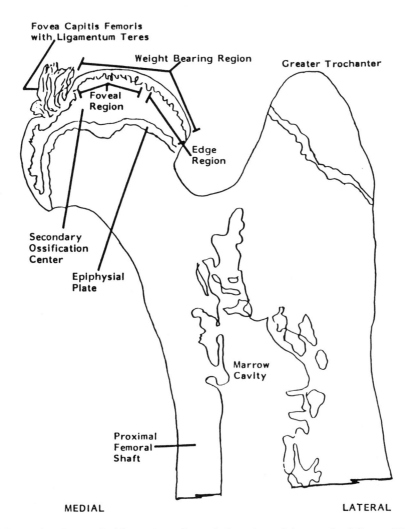

FIGURE 11-6. Camera lucida tracing of a typical section of the proximal femur. The weight-bearing region was classified into two subregions for analysis: the foveal region and the edge region.

Twenty-four hours before the animals were euthanized, subpopulations of all groups were injected with $^{35}SO_4$. Sulfate is incorporated into the cartilage proteoglycan; therefore the amount of radioactivity assimilated into the cartilage was an indicator of the relative proteoglycan manufacturing rate at the time of the injection. Quantitative autoradiography was used to assess the radioactive sulfate content.[7] The Norm animals had similar proteoglycan manufacturing rates in both the foveal and lateral edge regions. (See Fig. 11-5.) The AmpCont animals' mean PG manufacturing rate in the foveal region of the intact limb was lower than, but not statistically different from, that of the foveal region of the Norm animals. The PG manufacturing rate in the edge region of the AmpCont animals was less than that in the edge region of the Norm animals ($P<.01$). However, the AmpCont animals had a greater mean PG manufacturing rate in the foveal region when compared with that of their own lateral edge region in the intact limb ($P<.05$).

The AmpStim animals demonstrated a PG manufacturing rate in the intact limb that was not statistically different in the foveal and edge regions. (See Fig. 11–5.) The AmpStim PG manufacturing rate was not statistically different from the Norm rate in either region in the intact limb.

DISCUSSION OF THE RESULTS FROM THE INTACT LIMB

The foveal cartilage in the intact limb of the AmpCont animals was relatively thinned with respect to the edge region. The thinning could have been a response to the increased compressive and shear forces one would expect in this hip and region. There was a strong trend toward diminution of the mean PG content and mean PG manufacturing in both regions of the AmpCont animals when compared with normal levels. (See Figs. 11–4 and 11–5.) This diminution was statistically significant for the PG manufacture in the edge region of the AmpCont animals. The long-term implications of these articular remodeling responses can only be guessed from this experiment, but the decreased cartilage thickness and reduction in PG are usually associated with degenerating cartilage. Postulation could be made that a more appropriate response to increased compressive stress would be cartilage thickening and increased PG. None of the animals in the AmpCont group demonstrated frank articular degeneration in the hip of the intact limb. On the other hand, the morphologic changes associated with this remodeling response do not appear to be appropriate for resisting increased articular stress.

The articular response in the intact limb of the AmpStim animals appeared to be more suitable. The normal wedge shape was maintained, and the foveal cartilage of the AmpStim animals was significantly thicker than the foveal cartilage of the AmpCont animals. The PG concentration in the foveal region of the AmpStim animals was higher than that of the foveal regions of both the Norm and AmpCont group. The PG manufacture in the AmpStim group was similar to the normal.

Apparently the mechanical environment accompanying the increased articular stress in the intact limb did not by itself provide an intrinsic signal capable of directing articular remodeling of the femoral head in a manner that might be considered desirable (e.g., in response to increased stress, the cartilage thinned rather than thickened and contained less PG rather than more). When the intrinsic signals were combined with an extrinsically produced electrical signal, the articular remodeling response appeared congruous with the mechanical demands on the joint in that the cartilage thickened and had a higher PG concentration. (See Figs. 11–3 and 11–4.)

Articular Cartilage Remodeling in the Limb with an Amputated Hindpaw

The hip cartilage on the limb with an amputated hindpaw (amp limb) of the AmpCont animals maintained a wedge shape, with the foveal cartilage thicker than the lateral edge ($P<.02$). The amputated limb of the AmpStim animals had no significant difference in thickness between the foveal and edge regions. (See Fig. 11–3.) The foveal and lateral edge regions of the amp limb of the AmpCont animals showed no statistical difference in PG density. The PG density in the lateral edge region of the AmpCont animals was significantly greater ($P<.04$) in the amp limb than in the intact limb of the same group. (See Fig. 11–4.)

The PG densities in the foveal and lateral edge regions of the amp limb of the AmpStim group were not significantly different from one another, nor were they different from their regional counterparts in the intact AmpStim femora or the amp limb of the AmpCont femora. The mean PG density of the edge region of the amp limbs in the AmpStim femora was significantly greater than that of the foveal region of the intact limb of the AmpCont femora ($P<.04$) and approached, but did not reach, a statistically significant difference from the edge region of the Norm femora ($P<.058$). (See Fig. 11–4.)

The mean PG manufacture in the amp limb of the AmpCont animals was greater in the foveal region than the lateral edge region ($P<.05$). The PG manufacture in the edge region was less in the AmpCont animals than in the Norm animals ($P<.01$). (See Fig. 11–5.)

The mean PG manufacture in the amp limb of the AmpStim animals was not statistically different in the foveal and edge regions ($P<.07$). The edge region of the AmpStim animals had a lower PG manufacturing rate than the edge region of the normal animals ($P<.05$).

DISCUSSION OF RESULTS FROM THE LIMB WITH AN AMPUTATED HINDPAW

The articular cartilage of the AmpCont animals maintained its wedge shape in the amputated limb with the foveal cartilage thicker than the edge, like that of the normal animals. Because the amputated limb is held in a relatively abducted position, one would expect the lateral edge region to be moved medially, further beneath the acetabulum. In this way it would be positioned to mate more directly with the acetabulum (become more congruent) and could thereby incur more compressive stress than the normal. Because the animal bore weight on the stump of the amputated limb less often than through the intact limb, the net ground reaction forces would be reduced in the amputated limb. However, one could reasonably assume that the powerful musculature of the hip joint imparted significant stress to this hip whether the limb was actually bearing weight or was being held in a non–weight-bearing abducted position.[7,36] It would be necessary for the hip musculature to be very active to splint the amputated lower extremity in a compensatory position of abduction. The expected remodeling response would have been to increase the thickness of the edge region or to increase the PG density, or both, to resist the increased stress. The lateral edge thickness was not increased, but an appropriate response to increased stress was manifested in the increased PG density in the lateral edge region. (See Fig. 11–4.) The increased PG density would stiffen the cartilage of the lateral edge region. Coupled with the increased PG content, the AmpCont animals had a reduced PG manufacturing rate in the edge region compared with the normal animals. (See Fig. 11–5.) These data lend to the postulation that cartilage remodeling requiring increases in PG content is accomplished by reducing the regular removal of PGs rather than by boosting the manufacturing rate of PG. However, there are no data from time points other than at the end of the 8-week remodeling cycle to shore up this postulation.

In the amputated limb, the remodeling response of the animals that were exposed to PEMF varied from the response of the unexposed AmpCont animals primarily in the foveal cartilage thickness. There was a loss of the wedge shape of the AmpStim cartilage (thickness of the foveal and edge regions was not statistically different)

because of a diminution of thickness in the foveal region. (See Fig. 11–3.) This diminution of thickness would appear to be an appropriate biologic response to decreased
loading in the foveal region due to relative abduction of the amputated limb. The
regional PG density response was similar in the amputated limbs of the AmpCont
and AmpStim animals in that there were statistically similar PG densities in the foveal
and edge regions because of increases in the mean edge PG density. (See Fig. 11–4.)
Again, this response appears to be appropriate to increased stress on the lateral edge
of the femoral head in conjunction with the abducted hip position. When compared
with the norm group, the PG manufacturing rate was depressed in the edge region
of both the AmpStim and the AmpCont animals. One can generalize that the biologic
remodeling in the femoral head cartilage of the amputated limb was similar whether
or not the animal was exposed to PEMF.

Conclusions

The following conclusions can be drawn from this experiment. First, the articular
cartilage of the femoral head in the Sprague-Dawley rat did remodel in response to
alterations of weight bearing. The remodeling response was more energetic in the
femoral head of the intact limb. Second, the articular cartilage of the femoral heads
of Sprague-Dawley rats exposed to PEMF demonstrated a modified articular remodeling response when compared with those animals with a unilateral hindpaw amputation but not exposed to PEMF. The data obtained from this study unquestionably
support the contention that compressive force, as reflected by weight bearing, plays
a major role in the control of articular cartilage metabolism and remodeling. There
were distinct alterations in the cartilage morphology in response to both decreased
and increased weight bearing in the amputated animals. These changes were reduced
or eliminated in the amputated animals that were exposed to pulse-burst PEMF. The
mechanism by which these changes were brought about may be common to both
altered weight bearing and exposure to PEMF: The remodeling of the cartilage was
in response to electrical signals. Intrinsic electrical signals produced in the cartilage
by the action of weight bearing, as well as electrical signals extrinsically imposed on
the cartilage by PEMF, are transduced to guide articular remodeling and repair.

SUMMARY

Articular cartilage is a dynamic tissue that is capable of appropriate remodeling
and repair. There is ample evidence that mechanical phenomena powerfully affect
the remodeling and repair efforts of articular cartilege. A growing body of evidence
exists that electrical signals can influence articular cartilage metabolism and potentially
influence the long-term health of the tissue. Failures in the reparative efforts of chondrocytes might be ameliorated or reversed if the intrinsic signal(s) or repair could be
augmented or replaced by externally produced stimuli. Exogenous electrical signals
may be capable of supplying the necessary stimulus for repair, and the experiment
described in this chapter demonstrated the biologic influence of induced electrical
signals on articular remodeling. These results warrant further investigation into the
therapeutic effects of electrical stimulation on the arthritides.

ACKNOWLEDGMENT

The author thanks Joseph Dobner, M.D. of Frankfort, Kentucky for providing the arthroscopic photography.

REFERENCES

1. Jurmain, RD: The pattern of involvement of appendicular degenerative joint disease. Am J Phys Anthrop 53:143–150, 1980.
2. Gardner, DL: General pathology of the peripheral joints. In Sokoloff, L (ed): The Joints and Synovial Fluid, Vol. 1. Academic Press, New York, pp 325–425.
3. Cooke, TDV: The interaction and local disease manifestations of immune complexes in articular collagenous tissues. Studies in Joint Disease 1:158–200, 1980.
4. Elves, MW: The immunobiology of the joints. In Sokoloff, L (ed), The Joints and Synovial Fluid, Vol. 1. Academic Press, New York, 1980.
5. Hulth, A: Experimental osteoarthritis. A survey. Acta Orthop Scand 53:1–6, 1982.
6. Palmoski, MJ, Colyer, RA, and Brandt, KA: Joint motion in the absence of normal loading does not maintain normal articular cartilage. Arthritis Rheum 23(3):325–334, 1980.
7. Threlkeld, AJ and Smith, SD: Unilateral hindpaw amputation causes bilateral articular cartilage remodeling of the rat hip joint. Anat Rec 221:576–583, 1988.
8. Burke, MJ, Roman, V, and Wright, V: Bone and joint changes in lower limb amputees. Ann Rheum Dis 37:252–254, 1978.
9. Benichou, C and Wirotius, JM: Articular cartilage atrophy in lower limb amputees. Arthritis Rheum 25:80–82, 1980.
10. Ghadially, FN, Thomas, I, Oryschak, AF, et al: Long term results of superficial defects in articular cartilege. A scanning electron miscrocope study. J Pathol 121:213–217, 1977.
11. Mitchell, N and Shepard, N: The resurfacing of adult rabbit articular cartilage by multiple perforations through the subchondral bone. J Bone Joint Surg [Am] 58:230–233, 1976.
12. Mitchell, N and Shepard, N: Healing of articular cartilage in intra-articular fractures in rabbits. J Bone Joint Surg [Am] 62:628–634, 1980.
13. Salter, RB, Simmonds, DF, Malcom, BW, et al: The biological effect of continuous passive motion on the healing of full-thickness defects in articular cartilage. J Bone Joint Surg [Am] 62(8):1232–1251, 1980.
14. Wolff, J: Das Gesetz der Transformation der Knochen. A Hirschwald, Berlin, 1892.
15. Fukuda, E and Yasuda, I: On the piezoelectrical effect of bone. Journal of the Physiological Society of Japan 12:1158, 1957.
16. Bassett, CAL and Becker, RO: Generation of electric potentials by bone in response to mechanical stress. Science 137:1063, 1962.
17. Black, J and Korostoff, E: Strain-related potentials in living bone. Ann NY Acad Sci 238:95, 1974.
18. Pollack, SR, Korostoff, E, Starkebaum, W, et al: Microelectrode studies of stress generated potentials in bone. In Brighton, CT, Black, J and Pollack, SR (eds), Electrical Properties of Bone and Cartilage: Experimental Effects and Clinical Applications. Grune & Stratton, New York, pp 69–82, 1979.
19. Bassett, CAL, Pawluk, RJ, and Pilla, AA: Augmentation of bone repair by inductively coupled electromagnetic fields. Science 184:575–577, 1974.
20. Bassett, CAL, Valdes, MG, and Hernandez, E: Modification of fracture repair with selected pulsing electromagnetic fields. J Bone Joint Surg [Am] 64:888–895, 1982.
21. Bassett, CAL: The development and application of pulsed electromagentic fields (PEMF's) for ununited fractures and arthrodeses. Orthop Clin North Am 15:61–88, 1984.
22. Heckman, JD, Ingram, AJ, Lloyd, DD, et al: Non-union treatment with pulsed electromagnetic fields. Clin Orthop 161:58–66, 1981.
23. Brighton, CT, Hozack, WJ, and Brager, MD: Fracture healing in the rabbit fibula when subjected to various capacitively coupled electrical fields. J Orthop Res 3:331–340, 1985.
24. Kaye, CF, Lippiello, L, Mankin, H, et al: Evidence for a pressure sensitive stimulus receptor in articular cartilage. Transactions of the Orthopedic Research Society 5:155, 1980.
25. Bassett, CAL and Pawluk, RJ: Electrical behavior of cartilage during loading. Science 178:982–983, 1972.
26. Lotke, PA, Black, J, and Richardson, S: Electromechanical properties in human articular cartilage. J Bone Joint Surg [Am] 56:1040–1046, 1974.
27. Lee, RC, Frank, EH, Grodzinsky, AJ, et al: Oscillatory compressional behavior of articular cartilage and its associated electromechanical properties. J Biomech 103:280–292, 1981.
28. Frank, EH and Grodzinsky, AJ: Cartilage electromechanics. I. Electrokinetic transduction and the effects of electrolyte pH and ionic strength. J Biomech 20:615–627, 1987.

29. Frank, EH, Grodzinsky, AJ, Koob, TJ, et al: Streaming potentials: A sensitive index of enzymatic degradation in articular cartilage. J Orthop Res 5:497–508, 1987.
30. Grodzinsky, AJ: Electromechanical and physicochemical properties of connective tissue. Crit Rev Biomed Eng 9:133–199, 1983.
31. Baker, B, Becker, RO, and Spadaro, J: A study of electrochemical enhancement of articular cartilage repair. Clin Orthop 102:251–267, 1974.
32. Sah, RL-Y and Grodzinsky, AJ: Biosynthetic response to mechanical and electrical forces: Calf articular cartilage in organ culture. In Norton, LA and Burstone, CJ (eds), Biology of Tooth Movement. CRC Press, Boca Raton, FL, 1989, pp 335–347.
33. Smith, RL and Nagel, DA: Effects of pulsing electromagnetic fields on bone growth and articular cartilage. Clin Orthop 181:277–282, 1983.
34. Smith, SD and Feola, JM: Effects of duty-cycle distribution on pulsed magnetic field modulation of LSA tumors in mice. Journal of Bioelectricity 4:15–41, 1985.
35. Pilla, AA: Electrochemical information transfer and its possible role in the control of cell function. In Brighton, CT, Black, J, and Pollack, SR (eds), Electrical Properties of Bone and Cartilage. Grune & Statton, New York, 1979, p 455.
36. Steindler, A: Mechanics of the hip joint. In Kinesiology of the Human Body Under Normal and Pathological Conditions. Charles C Thomas, Springfield, IL, 1955, pp 285–286.

Index

A "t" following a page number indicates a table; an "f" indicates a figure.